Bioethics' Rise, Decline, and Fall

Bernard J. Ficarra

University Press of America, Inc.
Lanham • New York • Oxford

4720 Boston Way
Lanham, Maryland 20706
UPA Acquisitions Department (301) 459-3366

12 Hid's Copse Rd.
Cumnor Hill, Oxford OX2 9JJ

Printed in the United States of America
British Library Cataloging in Publication Information Available

Library of Congress Cataloging-in-Publication Data

Ficarra, Bernard J. (Bernard Joseph), 1914-
Bioethics' rise, decline, and fall / Bernard J. Ficarra.
p. cm
Includes bibliographical references (p.).
1. Medical ethics. 2. Bioethics. I. Title.

R724 .F457 2001 174'.2—dc21 2001054032 CIP

ISBN 0-7618-2167-8 (pbk. : alk. paper)

™ The paper used in this publication meets the minimum requirements of American National Standard for Information Sciences—Permanence of Paper for Printed Library Materials, ANSI Z39.48—1984

Dedicated
to the Memory of
My Father and Mother
Who Taught
Their Four Sons
the Beauty of Truth
and
the Virtue of Goodness

Contents

Introduction

> Right is right even if no one is doing it.
> Wrong is wrong even if everybody is doing it.
>
> St. Augustine [354-430]

There is an immense difference between a spoken lecture and a written text. It is a great pity that even those with scholarly credentials do not appreciate this invulnerable dissimilarity. This book is meant to be read silently in quietude at a moderate pace to suit personal stride. Thereby the words can be examined closely—even minutely. Eliminated, prior to assimilation partially or totally, are preconceived preferences, biased convictions, irreligious prejudices, and premature judgments.

The topics selected for this book have been evaluated carefully as to present need. Not on purpose some subjects may not be included. But this is not to be construed as a pre-programmed elimination. To encompass in one textbook every conceivable bioethical encounter, however desired, is a speculative accomplishment. Salient features of medico-surgical dilemmas in clinical experience have been accentuated.

These decisional conclusions were not adopted easily even as they are hopefully models of ultimate perfection. Capacity for accurate judgment is not always its own reward. Judgment is a precious, priceless, privileged attribute given sparsely in limited quantity even to exceptional people. It is sown in the field of honesty, grows in the soil of knowledge, is watered by the perspiration from hard work, is tempered in the heat of failure, is nurtured into maturity by the wisdom born through the complications of painful labor, and is mindful of sad experiences.

Designed for practicing physicians, active surgeons, ethicists, allied consultants, sociologists, philosophers, and those in academia at university and postgraduate levels, this book will provide auxiliary assistance in solving medicomoral encounters when similar or like circumstances are confronted. Without indulging in an *apologia*, bioethical digressions do invoke morality, temptation, and sin, no matter all the attempts to dissociate and disperse them from the main subject. These discussions are not a series of pastoral homilies but an intricate element as to culpability for miscalculations and bad judgments.

Ethics and morality can not be sifted in a colander into two separate entities in which watered-down morality runs out through apertures allowing ethics to remain alone by itself. Both are fungible and inseparable as mutual contributions to the composite collated bioethical unit.

Responsibility increases when talent is bestowed upon someone. Greater is the duty of a bioscientist whose primary purpose should be to employ medical knowledge to assuage the painful grief of those who seek surcease from the ravage of illness. Health ministry as a learned discipline is rooted in an honest commitment to respect, promote, and defend human dignity through its natural destiny. As such the ministration's demonstrative energy should be directed to the welfare of people. This dictum is mandated under the aegis of distributive justice as an ethical directive. Scientists distinguish themselves when by service and advocacy they help those whose civil status places them at the margin of society. These unfortunate people are in depressed situations that expose them to particular vulnerability in sociomedical insufficiences.

Benevolence Prevails

The wonderful sensation of goodness is that it generates a feeling the person doing good is marching forward in the right direction. Exhilaration and sentient ecstacy are the rewards for doing what is correct. Because doing what is just and right is goodness in action. Goodness is a euphemism for God. Hence it is that while doing evil, the doers become unscrupulous scoffers of God. As the biological clock unwinds true values in life are realized. Honor is to be desired as a worthwhile possession at all ages.

To be meaningful and valid, honor must inspire. This is necessary since honor has an internal, personal driving force with high-minded motivation. Morality is a component of honor. Both are self-imposed. Each is a coercive, sustaining power to the other. One leads the other to the ultimate conclusion that ethical conduct is the unified expression of this lofty duality.

Honor is a trait, an attribute, no person can bestow upon another. High standards in human behavior incorporates it into the formative structure of character. Upon honor rests the morality from which is derived guided ethical performances. Such upright deportment should be an innate element in the composition of every scientist worthy of the name.

Professional advancement, financial gain, and being a recipient of awards by wrongdoing is cheap nobility that is dethroned easily. Compounding the loathsome evil is when a scientist is caught *in flagrante delicto* (while performing it). Culprits seem chafed while yammering against allegations of impropriety. Whining and whimpering with peevish attitudes, the accused almost always complains of prejudicial unfairness.

Misguided, envious ambition laced with false zealousness can taint the most idealistic scientist. Naively some bioscientists fail to appreciate the loftiness of their solemn commitment to humanity. No estimation with accuracy is possible of the destructive influence from the ethical misbehavior of blathering bioscientists when what they either say or write has neither style nor heft.

When ignorance importunes scholarship evil attacks goodness, lies distort truth, commercialism invades bioscience, irregularities supplant standards, carelessness overcomes empathy, and conscience is obtunded as bioethical guidelines are abandoned easily. Slowly, silently the symbolic poetry of propriety is stripped away brusquely from the smirking mind. Whenever human dignity is either disregarded or degraded evil thrives. Even in its perpetuity evil is limited in its potency. Goodness in its own splendor has no confining boundary whose luster is never darkened.

Bioscientists with an impaired perspective are no exception to impediments. Some do relegate proper professional behavior to some distant corner of their lives. Soon they become a segregated breed from their colleagues in the moral camp. Economic distress can lead to a missed appraisal of ethical measurements. Searching for wealth may lead to ill-gotten gain which is a mirage not the anticipated financial oasis.

Exploitation of any kind may bring some degree of success. But the invisible force of retribution is never far behind. Cooperation with an inducement to financial acquisitions is easier than confrontational denial of the temptation. There is no counter-balance to strong, ethical performance. Failure to adhere to ethical values eventually has disastrous endings, consequences of which are like a predestined obituary.

Moral standards, ethical codes have been changed, modified, and bent out-of-shape by cultural determinants. From the superficiality of this wide variety of ignored misbehavior arises diversity of opinion. Under these circumstances bioethical propriety loses uniformity becoming extremely subjective and very flexible. Loss of critical evaluation occurs effortlessly as respect for the principle of subsidiarity is discounted. Then prevails the dictum that just because something can be done, it should be done. Although something is scientifically and technically feasible does not *ipso facto* make it permissible morally.

Medicine, and its descendant bioscience, was considered a noble, almost religious, pursuit. Hence the physician was looked upon as above the average citizen. As a person of wisdom, integrity, and morality in antiquity physicians were not associated with either lucre or commerce. Nonetheless medicine was evaluated as an activity for which the physician had the right to request payment. According to Galen [130?-201? floruit], the Greek anatomist, physiologist, and physician, the ideal practitioner of medicine was a philosopher. Who, like all philosophers, was temperate, disdained money, loved knowledge, and did his work relentlessly even without any recompense [Fridolf, 1976].

The Place Of Science

A rightful rôle for scientists is not new. From time immemorable science was dedicated to the benefit of humanity, the animal kingdom, vegetation, and the environment. Science is a limited tool. It does not have all the answers. Therefore its service is restricted. Hence it is not able to satisfy every need and fulfill all purposes.

The task of scientists is to fit the tools of science [knowledge, reason, methodology, and research] to the disposition and purpose of the user. A truly dedicated scientist is not an irascible curmudgeon who indulges in scientific folly. Horrors have been committed in the name of science. When not abused, science can provide much hope for the betterment of the future for those who are seeking relief from specific anxieties and infirmities. Dire distress is unable to redeem itself. It requires assistance.

"There are no crimes in science" said the fanatic, Nazi scientist Joseph Mengele. A cold bioscientist, he impressed those in authority who gave him unrestricted leeway in medical experimentation. His scientific credentials were awesome. Doctor of Medicine, Doctor of Philosophy in anthropology gave him an exclusive recognition. Unemotional, always professorially professional, and imperturbable even when he performed unspeakable experiments on innocent children. His immoral activities and criminal intentions negated his own educational background. Most people say it is the intellect which makes a great scientist. They are wrong: it is the character [Albert Einstein, 1879-1955].

Science in the service of a political, pseudo-ideological system is incarcerated. In effect it is forced to abandon the search for truth in favor of predetermined goals. Thus it ceases to be science because it is bereft of free, right reason. Automatically are suspect scientific findings/conclusions that are subservient to self-interest and/or a false ideal. Only rigorous, exclusive values protect the integrity of a scientific manifesto. Procrustean science dominated by dictatorial oppression is disbarred and immobilized from addressing any bioethical situation. Questions are forbidden. Answers are not allowed. In essence, such oversight forbids the free-will to weigh the difference between good and evil.

A learned historian in one of his books overturns the vision of science as a pristine enterprise driven by pure reason. He argued that science moves erratically and not always toward the truth. Direction is heavily influenced and moved in the way determined by the scientific communities [Kuhn, 1962]. This is termed by some pertinent authorities in their textbooks as "Kuhn's paradigm shift" [Goertz, 1997]. Sociological considerations can never affect truth as to the paucity and/or the gravity of matter which is offensive since truth is transcendental. However unpalatable this may be, it is a known fact to proven philosophers and those who are not victimized by subjectivism, irrationalism, relativism, hedonism, pragmatism, and misaligned psychology.

The biosciences have fallen wounded by the pervasive, crass immorality that is undermining to the point of collapse its exalted status. Without the unqualified adherence to the primacy of the person, human rights, dignity, and life can be destroyed. To avoid this catastrophe a firm moral dimension is to be preserved in authentic bioscientists who strengthen sublime truth. Full maturity with intellectual development is paramount in an ethically oriented, productive profession.

Objective reality justifies disassociation from arbitrary, devious, flexible, bioethical conduct. Unstable codes are counterproductive in attempting to preserve the dignity and ethical orderliness of learned bioscientists. This necessity is not an issue of religion. It is based upon right reasoning. All thinking bioscientists, however innominate, believe in and defend the validity of unbiased reason and the humaneness in humanity.

During purgatorial purification, bioscientists like all other human beings will receive their just punishments. Then they will understand fully the difference between what was expected of them because of their individual talents, what they did, and what they failed to do. Human memory may be short. But sins, transgressions, and evil are recalled with ease while in purgatory. Out of the labyrinthine circle of purgatory, the contrite penitent finds paradise.

Morality Is Nature's Gift

There is no new morality to supplant what has been established. When Moses descended from Mount Sinai with the divine tablets the ethical and moral directives were written upon it. Nothing can be added or detracted from these Ten Commandments of God. No human intelligence can invent right and wrong. The free-will to differentiate between them is a divine gift housed in the educated conscience of mankind. People of all nations and all cultures had and have an upright code of proper behavior. Disobedience was attached to punishment of various kinds depending upon the evil deed.

When a person turns his/her back on God, hero worship is dismissed. Having no one to emulate, some people look into a mirror where the person sees himself/herself. In this fable each one is a deity for any intended purpose. Being one's own inspiration engenders egotistic narcissism that is boundless. Left to their own desires such people do not separate right from wrong. Confusion enters their minds so that promiscuity becomes freedom of expression. Liberation from social bondage is an excuse for sin. Forgetting what is wrong does not endure forever.

Far too many human beings in adopting misleading new culturisms have lost their moral guidon. Immorality, whose sibling is unethical conduct, deludes even the wise to become traitors to their souls. It is delusory to think that falsity of any category will go undetected forever.

In Samson Agonistes, John Milton's epic poem, Samson says of Delilah, "She sought to make me traitor to myself." Evil does the same.

Moral imperatives are influential in the formation of ideal ethical deportment which is the defining dimension of the format for a life worth living. Uncommon courage is needed to make apt choices in order to be morally good. Even when the cloud of censure darkens the blood in the bravest heart, there is comfort in thinking of posthumous rebirth in paradise gained.

Formulation of basic ethical statutes is not left to chance, choice, serendipity, and individual whim. Fundamentally the laws of Moses are the template. Freedom of will may discard them but their intrinsic, divine merit remains intact. Every human conscience must be formed to discern the objective moral law which preserves the common good in civil society. Although the human conscience is not infallible, it can be formed in such a manner that it does identify truth. This discernment distinguishes the moral from the immoral, right from wrong, the ethical from the unethical, and the saint from the sinner. By its invocation to action the conscience becomes a teacher of immutable truth and an unyielding witness to the moral law.

Properly formed consciences are the military police that insist upon following divine directives. Consciences are not independent, exclusively personal, autonomous, and do not have the ultimate criteria to determine what constitutes good and evil [Pope John Paul II, 1998]. Because the conscience is the sanctuary of the human person where men/women are alone with God who instills within it the strength to love good and to despise with avoidance all evil. Goodness of a person resides in living according to a truthful conscience as guided by God's laws [Pope John Paul II].

Rejuvenation Of Ethics

The hard-driving advancement in scientific technology, biomedical engineering, and weapons of destruction have produced situations that are highly improbable for the average person to comprehend. Without understanding how can the morality of these productions be evaluated? In most instances an ethical guide-book is missing. Obviously the complexity of many moral questions requires a system of values and norms. Without which the subordination of humanity to convenience, self-gratification, economic stress, and political chicanery is inevitable. This occurs when the mental disposition of some scientists avoids ethical conflicts by associating them with religion which they either impugn or label as an interloper of science.

Moral consensus in a pluralistic, democratic society is difficult to achieve. Complexities inherent in the ethical problem presented brings forth additional disagreements. Even when cynicism and skepticism are forceful antagonists, proper ethical standards remain intact. Although arguable and debatable the ethical positions on reproductive technology, withholding/withdrawing treatment, organ transplantation, the culture of death, practicing intubation on the recently deceased, and for-profit medicine have not been standardized. The lack of uniformity is exemplified by some bioethicists who in their writings opt for open debate on these moral questions. One author in three closing essays in his book advocates freedom within policy constraints and a democratic process for decision-making on vague bioethical questions [Caplan, 1998]. In this way strong opinions can be asserted freely and without restraint according to the writer.

No matter how it is distorted, ethics is not removed as a subdivision of philosophy which seeks the ultimate criterion of truth. Even when moral dilemmas arise in an amoral atmosphere the problem does not evaporate. Reprised ethical misbehavior is kindred to moral turpitude. Without alertness to what is occurring a depraved indifference to righteousness can eventuate. This burnishes automatically immoral credentials. Moreover, degradation and pollution of human behavior in any aspect is accelerating the pace to the annihilation of personal morality.

Unethical acts are symbolic of the general dissolution of values that besmirch modern society. They discount those intangible qualities of integrity, honor, probity, and dedication to honest labor. Under this credo ethical relevancy succumbs to economic pressures. This yields to an unending tsuris.[1]

---

1. Yiddish word for trouble, distress, and series of misfortune with suffering.

Matrix Of Ethics

An absolute base, an immutable foundation for ethical behavior can be found only in God's laws. When God is denied, His laws are not known. Atheists, agnostics, and other non-believers are ignorant of divine guidance. To them is lost the blessing that upstanding ethical conduct is good intellectual hygiene. Such purity of mind avoids the dangerous vertiginous slide downward to perdition. Moreover it generates magnetism that inspires other persons to do the same.

Ethical conduct is not an illegitimate subject for scholarly inquiry. No rational argument is persuasive against such studies. Even for those who ignore the importance of bioethics, it is a vital nucleus in the composition of bioscientists of merit. Without a supervisional command, scientists are doomed to disgrace like any miscreant. It behooves the academically learned to recall that fragmented morality is deviation from wisdom.

Biomedical activities in the new millennium years appear to have gone awry. Efforts by upright bioethicists seem ineffectual in filling this empty lacuna. Because many bioscientists look upon ethical standards as a farrago of individual choices selected cafeterially to suit the project at hand.

A disregard of normative bioethics dismisses deterrence against unconventional, unconscionable scientific behavior. Such grotesque irregularities become instigators of poor judgment, misinterpretation, illusion, and the inability to distinguish accurately. Out of the deviation from recognized normal conduct comes crime. Auto-suggestion then becomes a persuasive medium that dismisses an improper action as a moral casualty.

Irrationality can penetrate the mind to formulate a pattern for justification of what has been done—no matter the depth of the wrong. Philosophical analysis of unethical performances indicates they are overlooked examples of the social dimension of either a perverted, corrupt society or one that determines legitimacy by intentional ignorance.

Bioscientists who wend their way through ethical perplexities with indifference can collide with dishonor. Easily they become denizens of dishonesty without any qualm. When small moral infractions do not undergo valid recension, the future becomes bleak for ethical stability. Misbehavior patterns easily perpetuate themselves into iniquities. Depletion of bioethical values may not destroy the biosciences totally. However the real threat is that it may diminish bioethics into taxonomy, as a scientific nonentity.

The peccant, persistent phage of bad memories will bring melancholy to those bioscientists who participate in ignoble practices. Dark phases in the history of medicine will mar its radiance. Dethroned bioethics should not be the brash expression of the bedlam with moral recession by the irregularly contoured morality of this century. Anonymous though they may be, there are those of high professional rank who are shields behind which others may hide to do damage. Simultaneously both create the facade of encyclopedic experts on bioethics. Becoming their own thesaurus they are looked upon as the bioethical Oracle of Delphi.

The establishment of highly publicized, much-sought-after awards for achievements in various sciences can bring about accomplishments that are ethically bankrupt. Bestowed fame is not worthwhile if it changes the high esteem of investigative researchers. Especially is this a valid conclusion when the honorific is more defined by publicity than pedigree.

Distortion, deviation from, and destruction of honesty in seeking scientific acclaim can render the reward a satirical travesty. Exaggerated value is placed on the acquisition of some professional awards. Beneath the outward veneer of the recipient may be an unsavory trait in the moral portraiture of infamy that does not glow even under the blaze of squishy publicity.

The appetite for celebrity status can exchange character for caricature. To some people, notability is more gratifying than an untarnished, highly respected reputation. Renown is no longer ligated to the traditional definition of attainments obtained by sacrifice and honorable hard work.

Pervasive insensitivity to fundamental principles has diminished to disappearance in some instances many respectful, disciplinary ways of living, acting, and researching. Adherence to religious beliefs is discounted by many faculties of higher learning. Often considered as *passé*, puerile, unrealistic, and useless, discussions on religion are forbidden.

A caveat for bioscientists is that the indoor world of laboratory studies and solitary scholarship with their intellectual insularity is conducive to ethical misguidance. At times solitude allows the conscience to be deadened to well-founded ideals.

Quietude opens the frontal lobes of the brain to subtle mental gymnastics. There with clever machination of sophism, evil can be made harmless. Lost may be the concept that dishonesty is wrong and not eradicable. No matter how one tries to run away from ethical mischief, no one is able to hide from it. Trashy behavior is an everlasting whipping thong in those burdened by a heavy heart from imprudent indiscretions.

Upright, untampered bioscientific research and ethical clinical medicosurgical practice are chosen goals to pursue. Under this admirable duad, bioscientists will rise to the height of awe inspiring truth with the freedom of an eagle flying to heaven. Seminal wisdom sustains the philosophical proposition that impeccable moral behavior is adherence to truth as both a cultural and scientific treasure. Every human being with an educated conscience is obedient to moral deportment which is founded upon intransigent truth.

Let not the words of the Rubaiyat, Stanza 93, by Omar Khayyam [1070-1123] be applicable to American bioscientists.

> Indeed the idols I have loved so long
> Have done my credit in this world much wrong:
> Have drowned my glory in a shallow cup,
> And sold my reputation for a song.

Monotonous cants and hoary pretensions of iconoclastic ultramodernists make impassioned calumniating attacks against virtue. They espouse casual, nonrepentant, no-conscience stricken revolution against morality, ethical normalcy, and uncompromising, high-standards of deportment. Today the daily mood is to live without restraint, no matter the danger of falling off that high precipice to disaster. The utmost desire is to satisfy personal ambition, appetites, feel the thrill of domination, and pleasure of avarice. No one appears embarrassed in these quests. Even if horrendous methods are used to achieve them. Ignored is the grave disturbance of the pathetic, agony of self-defeatism.

Social Liberty

Freedom of behavior is sociologically attractive; defendants of which are found in august academic positions, under whose *nihil obstat* faculty stalwarts bombard former ethical criteria as either antediluvian or anathema. Nothing of substance is offered to sustain the denunciation comparable to this high-voiced oral terrorism. Any reference to the Bible elicits scorn. Roseate retrospection to the high-minded etiquette of past decades is not even a factoid of the imagination. An awkward silence, denial, and faltered credibility are the inept reactions when inquiries are made, especially as they relate to historicity when rancor appears that was concealed in the tormented conscience.

History has clear warnings with described detailed patterns which are not recognized. Numerous incidents repeat the peril when humanity *in lieu* of assimilating the preferable morality places a *moratorium* on it. Stultifying misconduct has an inward fickle sentiment built on the abuse of truth. To overcome this negligence requires unsurpassed courage to recognize it and have sufficient intelligence to shun it. No universal remedy is available like the mercury of Paracelsus[2] to assist in this effort. Whining a passageway through myriad discussions develops a martyr complex. But it does not eliminate the immoveable debasement even in dialogue with putative, educationally oriented adults.

During the 1960s rebellions against established codes of honor sanctioned preaching of a good life bound to total freedom of thoughts, words, and actions *in camera et in pays*. Neither restraint nor inhibition was required. Traditional, patristic values were antiques. Encouragement was given only to what was compatible with the scripted scenario of the day. Those who emulated the old ways were relegated to the Mesozoic era of dinosaurs. Many tripped on this speculation.

Having fallen, the majority of adherents to this hypothesis could not rise from this infirmity because of their morbid moral and intellectual impairments. The inability to be healed from these invisible injuries was sordid television, the recording industry, the live theatre, seamy movies, and sullen journalism. With servile devotion all promoted the agenda in their fashion but unanimously flaunting immorality overtly without ambiguity. The glorifying of evil and sanctioning misdeeds was their grandiose *forté* that encouraged a dismal lifestyle.

Many times well-educated people are equated with moral worthiness. Erroneously, the proposition that intelligence quotient is in parallel relationship to ethical stamina and moral measurement is the belief of many with celebrity standing in academia. The speculation is the higher the caliber of the intellect the greater is the appreciation of ethics, morality, and goodness—but always with the person's own spin. Supposedly

---

2. Paracelsus, Theophrastus Bombastus von Hohenheim [1493-1541] was a Swiss alchemist and physician who wrote extensively on medicine. Mercury was his cure for every illness.

this fortuity lessens the complexity of life since all actions are to favor the self.

Not difficult to find are those in sophistry who separate the intellect and free-will from the social environment as molders of character. Such distinct division diminishes any scientific suggestion that sophisticated technology can discern a biological etiology for misdeeds by electro-encephalography.

The intellect as a divine attribute is unbiased. When called upon to function it assists free-will in the selection process as to choice, direction, and decision-making. Both exist in the human life-principle [the *anima*]. Wisdom is melded by them when properly used in performances according to their creation as originally ordained.

Wisdom is not value-neutral. As a teacher it instructs the acumen to arrive at accurate judgments. Mature wisdom enlightens even the uninitiated to the reality that deliberate ignorance of evil-doing does not eliminate its presence. Wisdom's poignancy disallows straddling the fulcrum between good and evil. Lacking it picro-people lose their moral gyroscopes and ethical rudders, becoming pitiable vagabonds like a derelict ship without a compass.

Contemporary philosophers attempting to operationalize the notion of culture in terms of an hierarchy of canonical structures (conceptual and artistic) must include in the evaluation ethical and religious beliefs. Thus are characterized communities on an often overlapping ethnic, religious, functional, intellectual, territorial background, and every other category to reach the global level of recognition. Eventually the entire human community is encompassed in this philosophical Utopia.[3]

Which recalls the notion of Noösphere. The neologism is derived from the Greek noun *nous* (mind) meaning literally, "the world of the mind."[4] As the thinking layer of the earth it concerns also the biosphere

---

3. Utopia is the name of an imaginary island that served as the subject and title of a book by Saint Thomas Moore in 1516. The island was described as a place of perfection in moral, social, and political life.

4. Initially employed in the 1940s, used by Julian Sorell Huxley, Pierre Teilhard de Chardin, Marshall McLuhan, and others to refer to the thinking layer of the earth. It is an extension into the realm of knowledge and thought [plus its products] on the concepts of geosphere, lithosphere, atmosphere, hydrosphere, and biosphere. Random House Dictionary defines neösphere from an ecology standpoint as the biosphere including and modified by such human

[biology + spherical earth] from which the word bioethics is derived. The ethical preservation of biological life in the world was the reason for its coming into existence.

Academic efforts at the professorial level give the term "noösphere" an empirical content. Explained in the sense of its emergence from a global consensus in regard to the structure and content of the so-called high culture represented by university curricula worldwide. The courses of studies offered are consensually accepted on the subjects of science, agreement on artistic, literary critical methods, and canons. Cultures as traditionally known and *weltanschauungen* become objects of inquiry and systematic exposition.[5] Witness the chair for Catholic Studies at Yale University as an illustrative example [Dechert, 1999].

Bioethics is part of the effort to present an all-encompassing plan for universal knowledge. A systematic approach includes a place for ethics and morality as both are philosophically and unconditionally committed to truth. This is difficult in a world increasingly demonstrating a cognizable rise in cultural and ethical relativism. Sometimes verging on a nihilism there is a fear that it could corrupt the fine arts, literature, and the biosciences into instruments of power for evil.

Caught in this web is bioethics which will be victimized by misinformation that intoxicates right reason into anesthetic inertia. Denigration of this ilk is not sloth to twisted exaggeration, sterilization of logic, discourteous intelligence, no enthusiasm for social justice, and courage goes out of style. Persuasive falsehood will be worded easily in the finery of a very fantastical banquet [Modified from Shakespeare's Much Ado About Nothing, Act II Scene 3]. Like Antaeus,[6] a false theory that

---

activities as agriculture, forestry, animal husbandry, urbanization, and industrialization. A synonym for noösphere is anthroposphere. The Oxford English Dictionary uses Pierre Teilhard de Chardin's notion of the "stage or sphere characterized by the emergence of consciousness and mind which follow the stage of the establishment of human life."

5. According to the American Heritage Dictionary the German word *weltanschauung* means a world view. It is a comprehensive philosophy of the world or of human life. Political and economic interpretations indicate global homogenation in terms of democracy and free markets as an economic goal.

6. Antaeus in Greek mythology was an invincible giant when his feet touched ground. He was defeated by Hercules who lifted him into the air and crushed him to death.

all truth is relative to the individual, to the time, and to the place in which the action takes place can become attached to the biosphere, removable only by Herculean super-intelligence assisted by divinity.

Only through a complete understanding of the obligations to self, neighbor, society, nation, and God can anyone hope to conform to morally defined human conduct. Thorough acquisition of this informative knowledge for good is the basis for understanding why bioethics is a driving force for the preservation of a moral society. Justice contributes to the format of true ethical values. Without which there is no appropriate requisite to the definition of admirable civilization.

Subversion of Society

Worldwide inhabitants are encased in an evanescent culture momentarily fortified by symptoms, signs, and signatures that glorify the opposites to morality, integrity, honor, and respect. There was a time in flowering civilization when it was not difficult to decide what to ignore, what to contradict, and what to defend. Historically, correctness was preferred with ease minus hesitancy. Every day answers were positive, decisive, accurate, and in the right direction. Daily activities reaffirmed the rigid facts of a firm social order in which the place of each person was known, fixed, and stabile. The central target envisioned was the resplendent reward for adherence to theology.

Nowadays negativism to lofty endeavors prevails as the paradigm. Die-hard, hard-eyed, hard-headed modernists, and self-termed realists, might argue that national morality no longer remains in the world. Since it is dead only minimal signs of mourning are left for what no longer exists. For those believing this lie, a return to religion may open the door for them to pass through the portals where those people of faith and virtue live.

> If we are able to enjoy properly the good things that the Lord showers upon us every day of our earthly lives, then we have begun to experience the joy, which will be completely ours in the next life [Pope John Paul II].

Modern society has a commentator personality that has forgotten the good things of yesterday. Judging tomorrow by today each day's horizon is yesterday's dawn. Heritage is easily obliterated. Lost to the cultural reconstructionists is the failure to realize nothing is more tragic to civilization than the loss of its wholesome traditions. Too great is the tendency to categorize respect with antiquity and heritage as being synonymous with reactionary.

The refusal to accept precepts evolved from experience, avoiding the wisdom of previous generations, and not heeding advice from elders encourages restlessness of spirit into indecisiveness that hinders mental, moral, and mechanical productivity. Persons unable to live serenely with themselves can never live calmly with other people. Human beings not at peace with themselves are incapable of sharing peace with neighbors, relatives, and God. Without spiritual pacificity the age in which we live becomes emotionally impetuous, morally tempestuous, and ethically frivolous.

Misperceptions of values has produced blatant displays of multiple fissiparous[7] chicanery, gullibility, greed, vanity, lying, and immorality in the past century. This is the unfolding ingratitude erupting from the consummate narcissism of the most affluent generation in world history.

Subconscious subduction by the pursuit of convenient self-gratification was the mode of the former decades which are almost the apothegm for the 20th century. Discarding what is historic authenticity each person invents his/her reality. Creating current climates of abundant liberty and plenitude of freedom to choose have discarded previous cultural limits. The result is moral illiteracy that is unable to stop mental carnage. Increased are psychiatric disorders, massive anxieties, and serious risk-taking. Added to this is the deception in attractive financial ventures, gambling, greed, misdemeanors, felonies, grand larceny, and crime. If wealth is the end-game, what is going to happen when the golden calf dies?

Added to the bedazzling dissonance in uncivil society is lack of sufficient reason. Individual success, the blooming economy, national prosperity, the envious spectacle of Wall Street add to the misconception that everything is permissible because of these favorable richnesses. The cornucopia is so intoxicating it fosters the misbelief that dishonesty, unethical business transactions, and political correctness are acceptable since they satisfy the person—not the ideal.

---

7. Fissiparous means reproduced by fission; multiple divisions.

Such misconceptions have an adverse influence on personal conduct. Malicious deportment has detrimental, destructive effects beyond its initiation. Unethical means to riches gives the owner a deceiving mask. This travesty adds to the devaluation of an already unreprimanded society. Misguiding ideologies have squandered morality, dethroned admirable leadership, and degraded idealists. Bioscience is not excused from this indictment.

Brash moral decay is visible on every day's horizon. Nothing decelerates its progress as a cataclysmic explosion is marking time for disaster to happen. Once there were great nations that stood for moral international law and procrustean ethical performance. Where are they now? None of them appear to have sensitivity either to embarrassment or debasement. Dwindling down to their populations are these same defects. In this regard the universal *lingua franca* of the nations' laity is to speak in terms of social norms formed by themselves. No counterbalance slows down runaway individualism as expediency is chosen over resolution, and the palpable triumphs over the impalpable.

Behavior that is a departure from the straight, narrow, well-plowed path of goodness is prompted by desires over and above the necessaries of life. Excessive desires ignore the virtue of temperance which disposes to the avoidance of excesses of all descriptions. Without the gyroscope of temperance within, endangerment to self and others is a constant threat. Minus self-control respect for the self is in peril, temperance diminishes, and immorality becomes an enemy.

Loss Of Love

Down through the ages of recorded time, the world authors, poets, and historians have accumulated the inspirational thoughts on the blessings of life. Animated wisdom unfolds the intrinsic value of meritorious living, the imperfections to be avoided, how to overcome disappointments, enjoy inner peace, find somatic contentment, and a tranquil mind. Apropos is the old Chinese proverb:

> You can not prevent the birds of sorrow from flying over your head.
> But you can prevent them from building nests in your hair.

Good lives are founded on love of God and His Commandments. From divine love human nature is identified with all things beautiful in the physical, spiritual, and moral orders. Love fosters goodness in every category of life.

Nothing on earth is more pleasing than pure love that is returned unselfishly. Because love is born of God, rests in Him, always is perceived in Him. Life's supreme happiness is found in the strong conviction that God loves us. This love is a gleaming taper light that guides the way with bright rays even when day into night grows darkest. Love gives courage to combat evil, strengthens the faint-hearted, and gives fortitude to those threatened by adversity. It is love that bestows the will to conquer it.

God's people go on despite calamities. Even when forced into the gray twilight between defeat and victory. When waiting patiently each particle of time is like a year until a decision is made. Patience is the nutrient that feeds virtue into maturity. As a matter of choice virtue is worked for, a plane to be achieved. Virtuous ideals are like celestial stars. No one succeeds in touching them. Like the seafarer on the massive, wide ocean who sees them as guiding lights they lead to the ultimate sidereal destiny. This applies to bioscientists.

Honesty In Bioscience

Philosophy, religion, science, and art have culled a unifying power that created an omnifarious systematization of knowledge. Each contributed to the ubiquitously integrated formal patterns that are not now universally accepted. Applied to clinical medicine, the scientization of which the last half of the twentieth century has instituted, gave a long-term flexible perspective on bioethics. The revolutionary changes generated by complex biotechnologies invaded society bringing forth hesitancy, questioning, and pauses that looked into the ethical propriety of the products engineered. Known and unknown was the discernment that the more scientific medicine became, the greater the abuses evoked. Many did not elect to follow positive bioethics in the search for the perspicacity that leads to the unravelling of the scientific unknown.

Bioscientists are mesmerized by the prefigured productions of their intellects with the freedom of action enjoyed. The alert, moral conscience with a concern for ethical responsibility as a fundamental imperative of the intelligentsia has become distorted on many occasions. Moral danger is associated with many bioscientifically engineered experiments. The presumed ethical monitor in the medical laboratory seems to be elsewhere on too many occasions. Established credos that bound science and ethics for rational performance have been modified. Both exist for the same purpose as explorers for and guardians of truth. For worthy success mutual cooperation is a necessity. Right reason, moral firmness, and earnest faith are needed to prevent their separation.

Unconscionable use of the mystique of science to promote invented ideas that are either untrue or not scientifically verifiable is the antithesis to science's legitimacy. An example in the 19th century was Karl Marx and Frederick Engel who applied the term scientific socialism to their aim at civil corrections. This gross misnomer borders on misology for *Das Kapital* as false propaganda as if it was reality. Most scientific endeavors are applied beneficially. Wrongfully adapted they can be offensive—an ethical felony.

Deviation from required bioethical probity is unacceptable and merits dissatisfaction with taunted resentment. Gentle correction is in order without any Calvinist asperity or Knoxian belligerency. The tenor of serenity is advisable even in the presence of overt abusion—the perversion of truth.

Honesty is the defining feature of the research scientist. Encased in the constricted world of pursuing knowledge in unknown, undiscovered, uninvented realms the scientist lives in solitude. Other particulate characteristics are patience and forbearance to ponder pensively how to solve the project with a continuous peaked interest to the receptive brain. Justification for recognition received is in the honest completion of a tedious undertaking that even makes the greatest stoic gasp.

An undertone of resentment with dissatisfaction has tainted the practice of health care. Exploration and analysis of this uncertainty has indicted decreasing physician autonomy, interruption of care continuity by the primary physician, the unfavorable supervised climate, and creeping commercialism as the progenitors for the disenchantment in medicine. These accusations are not to be dismissed hastily. They are not the entire core for the disillusionment. A deeper study discloses the devaluation of medicine's historic purpose. Which is the care of the sick in accordance with the highest traditional standards of ethical professionalism. Lost to many physicians is their time-honored function to give health care during life and comfort in death as the crown of respected professionalism.

Honesty in ethical codes supports them as an *ens a se* [stand by self] having been formulated philosophically from metaphysics and epistemology. Some physicians ignore or choose to be uncommitted to philosophic principles. Others are neutral and/or indifferent in their posture concerning bioethics. In ancient times philosophers were the physicians. The closeness between the two disciplines facilitated a medical code of ethical conduct that was pleasing and followed unquestionably. Hence Hippocratic teachings had few objectors. Physicians were taught they do not exist for themselves but for those who are in need of their medical skill. Hellenic and Roman medical principles were prized highly giving to physicians an honored place in society.

Modern-day bioscientists could profit by this historical example. Medical technology can neither replace nor think for the physician. Mechanical items however useful, awesome in appearance, attractive in their movements on a screen, and mesmerizing are lifeless. Impersonal computers, monitors, and laboratory machinery should not become persuasive in dissociating the physician from humaneness. Erosion of this compassion evaporates altruism which is replaced surreptitiously by legislated artificial medicosurgical care.

Faith In The Medical Profession

What a physician should be is not defined by each individual according to personal interpretation and self-creation. This attitude is not hidden in today's medical doctors. Even the simple and timeless ideals are not encouraged by newer generations of physicians. Resentment is evident. When elders try to impose past ideals attentive ears are not eagerly present. Forgotten is that professionalism is honed on the whetstone of acquired wisdom oiled by die-hard experience.

Sir William Osler taught high ideals that were acquired by familiarity with the great minds of ages long-gone. He called them the "saints of humanity" [Cushing, 1925]. Their ultimate goals were gained by bolstered ideals that gave stride toward absolute perfection. Such men/women were standard models to be emulated as the best of their kind.

Sir Robert Hutchinson wrote many wise essays, instructive medical papers, and gave fine lectures. In addition he composed an anthology of comments for and against doctors of medicine. Among these is one that simulates an excerpt from a Franciscan Litany.

> From inability to leave well alone,
> from too much zeal for what is new, and

> contempt for what is old,
> from putting knowledge before wisdom, science
> before art, cleverness before common sense;
> from treating patients as cases, and making the
> cure of the disease more grievous than its
> endurance, The Good Lord deliver us [Bean, 1972].

Receiving the Doctorate in Medicine brings an inexplicable dawn of hopes, dreams, and fulfillment to the recipient. The word doctor means teacher that equates with being learned. Medicine is defined as "The science and the art of dealing with the prevention, care or alleviation of disease" [Frommeyer, 1971-1972]. The Hippocratic oath concurs in this definition with an inclusion of ethic deportment which is part thereof.

The mandate of Hippocrates is carried down to this century. Physicians do this by teaching medical students, residents, and those who obtain medicosurgical fellowships. In non-academic settings they teach myriads of health assistants and instruct many through the medium of a thousand scientific meetings. These are the hard, cold sides of medicine as a science but not its totality.

As opposed to the better known science of medicine there is the art of medicine which not every physician possesses, practices, and understands. On the art of medicine Paracelsus in the 16th century wrote:

> Medicine is not only a science: it is also an art. It does not consist of compounding pills and plasters. It deals with the very processes of life which must be understood before they may be guided.

The art of medicine includes bioethics as the formative network that embellishes it.

In its performance bioethics represents belief in God and compassion. As its adherence reflects humility, truth, integrity, and love proving that material things are not important, people are. The responsible physician tries to do that which is proper and correct at all times. This is what a physician should be and is the prayer of all good samaritans. The adjective professional has been elongated to include athletes, actors, and singers. Why is medicine called a profession by comparison? Because it is a *bona fide* profession by definition.

"A member of a profession pursues a scholarly discipline in a way that inspires confidence and trust, and that prizes expert performance of a skill above financial gain" [Ingelfinger, 1976]. The vital element in medical professionalism is its humanitarian leadership and secure technical knowledge. Because of the latter doctors are licensed by the state. The idealism of the horse-and-buggy doctors and their counterparts at medical schools has vanished. With this disappearance has gone the respected social position once a mark of a doctor's distinction. In former days physicians were expected to be unworldly, dedicated, and idealistic with a high sense of human responsibility. This tradition was prevalent before World War II. Its luster commenced to dim in the 1960s [Page, 1977].

Professionalism is concerned with the serious behavioral aspects of medical practice in every way. Hence dignity and authority are part of it which enables physicians to manage life-or-death situations. Wearing a white coat, serious deportment, and professional manners are neither arrogance nor playing God. Majority of physicians have not forgotten they participate in a learned discipline in a special way that inspires confidence, trust, and places expert performance above financial gain. The vast majority of physicians are workers in the field, treating and comforting patients. They are honest and try to keep abreast with the rapid technical advances in medicine. More importantly they value professionalism and the earnest responsibility it entails. Professionalism is the mental force that teaches how to avoid mistakes, rather than to learn by making them. Even as it encourages a willingness in doctors to be skeptical of fads and fearless in criticism of themselves. Thus recognition is given to the necessity for preserving the stature and status of medicine and surgery.

It is equitable to state that during the past 50-60 years the medical profession has made more contributions toward lengthening the life, improving the health, and comfort of patients than in all previous decades. Yet all is not harmonious between physicians and the public they serve. Criticism of and evidence of dissatisfaction are increasingly alarming. Invidious comments, vitriolic insinuations, and dire predictions have been made from all segments of society. This includes the President, members of his cabinet, Senators, Representatives, and all classes of authors who add to the unpopularity of physicians. The number of malpractice allegations and the giant awards by juries against doctors have not diminished. Physicians know they are providing a vastly improved quality of health care to the public. Apparently the public either does not know it or ignores it. This is a grave departure from the complete empathy once enjoyed and lack of appreciation of the fine services doctors have to offer.

The American genius for organization that has been so well demonstrated in industry etc has been conspicuously absent in the field of health [Clagett, 1968]. Insurance carriers, HMOs, Medicare, Medicaid, research grants, and other enterprises have taken away what was once the individual, profoundly personal nature of medicosurgical practice. Less enthusiasm is militated against socialized medicine as expenditures for health purposes soar.

Health care is big business, among the largest in the nation. Society will no longer tolerate the present disorganized services and payments currently in existence. Since the medical profession has not been effective in solving the chaotic system, politicians and those outside the medical profession will insinuate themselves into the reorganization and management of health care.

What these external agencies do not have and will not be able to take away from physicians and their colleagues in the health care industry are two precious elements. These are judgment and virtue. Each has been and continues to be a specialty living naturally within the medical profession. Both have indigenous application and meaning in medicine. Judgment is a priceless, privileged attribute given sparsely even to scholars.

Defined variously, virtue in Aristotle's Greek philosophy is that state of a thing which constitutes its peculiar excellence that enables it to perform its function well. Particularly applied to human beings, virtue is the activity of reason and of rationally ordered habits. The word is derived from the Latin *virtus*. In Roman philosophy virtue was associated with virility and strength of character. During the Italian Renaissance the word was interpreted as shrewd prudence which was invigorated by Nicolo di Bernardo Machiavelli [1469-1527]. The quiddity of virtue rests not only in the performance of specific good actions, but also in the essence of a positive, willful determination to accomplish them to a beneficial conclusion. Virtue is inherent to medicine.

> All are but parts of one stupendous whole,
> Whose body Nature is and God the soul.
>
> Alexander Pope [1688-1744]

Nobility of character is the ambition of those who participate in the activities of bioscience. This respected desire has endured in spite of caustic invectives and fiction novelists who have portrayed doctors as Frankenstein makers, Dr. Jekyl, and Dr. Rappacini. Even Jack-the-Ripper is suspected of being a physician according to the author's innuendo. Non-medical writers at times describe doctors as disorganized, absent-minded professors. Similar negativism is attached in real life to those physicians who deviate from bioethical norms.

Great scientists of every category generally are inclined preternaturally to do useful things. Intellectual urging makes an imperative to do what is beneficial. To accomplish a worthy objective has its demands. Meaning abstinence from most social amenities, long hours of work, orientation to a specific goal, and no thought of réclame.

Scientific achievements that contribute to the advancement of health care hoists the doer upward to the sunlit uplands of inspirational scholarship. Performers of excellent deeds in the biosciences are enlisted in the closed ranks of those who persist in self-set tasks to satisfactory conclusions. Even when gloom dampens the probability for success. Undaunted physicians are encouraged knowing that their profession is immensely valuable and is beneficial to humanity.

Chapter 1

Brief History Of Bioethics

> The God of this World raged in vain:
> He bound Old Satan in his chain,
> And bursting forth his furious ire
> Became a chariot of fire
>
> [William Blake 1747-1827].

Codes of behavior for those who administered cures for illnesses were not known as physicians in antiquity. They were referred to as scholars who knew what to do under all circumstances. This included the effects of ravaging diseases that were described in terms which were unrelated to the underlying pathologic process. Hence the original reference to a physician as a man [occasionally a woman] who treats illnesses is the one who knows. This concept descends from Oriental, Egyptian, Persian, and Mesopotamian histories. The distinct presence of ethics in medicine is attributed to the Hippocratic Oath which has been the moral guideline for physicians since its publication.

However in the twentieth century the dint of revolutionary changes in scientific research, the introduction of medical commerce, and the business of health care established bioethics as a vital ingredient in the widened range of bioscientific enterprises. In the 1970s bioethics became a necessary discipline defined with care, specificity, but not always accurately in medical, legal, English, and worldwide dictionaries. Coinciding with this ethical renaissance was noted the establishment of Institutes of Bioethics on university campuses. Formal courses in bioethics were adapted to comply with the curriculum in vogue. Outstanding professors were recruited to teach this burgeoning subject.

Bioethics has become an invaluable, needed arbiter to moderate some of the most contentious and passionate debates in present-day bioscience. As a subdivision of philosophy, bioethics urges practical, moral applications of biotechnology to avoid legal embarrassment and to be aware of the detriments in molecular genetics which may produce deformities, create monsters, and result in other unseen disasters.

A dedicated mission of bioethics is to advise against excessive enthusiasm in publishing research data that has not been tested with established certification. Likewise it warns against premature conclusions made without a repeated reassessment of the results claimed. Bioethicists of acute acumen warn against unproven information on genetic engineering in agriculture, animal husbandry, ecology, bioscientific research, and medicosurgical practice. As monitors, bioethicists oversee progress in science. They call attention to the peril accompanying premature publication in non-scientific media of unsustained opinions, unsubstantiated medical material stated as facts, and incompleted research to an emotional, anxious public whom they may confuse more than enlighten.

Bioscientific technology, the lowering of the moral environment, and the secularization of general ethics has brought about a transformation of bioethics as discerned in a survey of essays and books on this delicate subject. In the early 1950s, this author's book, *Newer Ethical Problems in Medicine and Surgery*, appeared as an oddity in the bibliography of science [Ficarra, 1951]. Since that time bioethics has become a determined discipline. It grapples with the many moral dilemmas arising out of the laudable advancements in medicine, surgery, and bioengineering. Bioethics flourishes today as a necessary subject in medical schools, nursing schools, hospitals, and universities. It is taught to all students who are to be participants in medicosurgical care. As an urgent necessity it is a valuable subject in the prescribed curriculum.

From its primordial beginning bioethics was concerned with moral correctness. This was the promise. Now the popular cry is patient's autonomy which is a threat to the purpose and the promise. Disappointing as it may be, rugged individualism has become stronger than the desire to uphold the moral principles once held so dear to physicians. Invasion into medicine by philosophers, sociologists, attorneys-at-law, advocates of new cultural movements, and nonanalytic politicians have brought about conflicts that can destroy the medicosurgical profession's historic, idealized identity. With the changes came the patient's arrogation for major decision-making pertinent to his/her own medical treatment. Under the right of patient's autonomy it became the primary factor in the new "principlism".[1] This gave autonomy a higher place than respect for the person. Contemporaneously the physician was demoted as the person venerated for great knowledge and love of humanity. This beneficence in the medical profession is evaporating.

Bioethics and ethicists have been strongarmed by sociologists, philosophers, and others, into a practical discipline. It has been driven into a corner by high profile publicity on medical controversies, malpractice, and dishonesty in health care administration. Subject to all forms of criticisms the medical profession had to defend itself in courts of law bringing bioethics with it as it became more secularized than its early proponents could have anticipated.

The greatest rise in bioethics was discerned in the latter half of the twentieth century. During those years bioscientific experimentation rose dramatically. This was an intellectual stimulus prompting imaginative investigators to explore uncharted territory that brought forth the need for moral interpretations and guidance.

From the viewpoint of medical history the impact of bioethics as a discipline of its own is remarkable. Fostering serious public discussions morality in medicine became a new topic aired in printed journals and newspapers. Later the impact was so severe that television and the internet now includes ethics as part of human research either in progress or proposed.

Bioethicists have the duty to prevent abuses of human beings in any experiment that is morally repugnant. Beneath the carapace of bioscientific research can be found a cabal of researchers who disregard human rights in the eagerness to succeed. In the name of scientific research ethics is discarded as an impediment to the search for knowledge, a false premise for seekers of truth.

Hence it is that a sincere assessment of the deep meaning of bioethics in medical practice and medicosurgical research is not what it should

---

1. From *Daedalus* [Fall 1999] publication of the Hastings Centre in Garrison, N.Y. Principlism is used by Daniel Callahan founder of that bioethical centre in 1969. The leading theory in bioethics today is principlism which stresses "the principles of respect for persons [generally understood as respect for autonomy], nonmaleficence, beneficence, and justice. . . . In practice the principle of beneficence, gets the least play." From *Wilson Quarterly*, Spring 2000, 113-114.

be. Ethical precepts do not change even if the profound alterations in experimental biophysiology demands it to satisfy intellectual curiosity. Much has changed in the objectives of well-educated bioscientists. But this does not grant permission to discard basic ethical norms. Regardless of the progressive intent of scientists, they do not have the authority to legitimatize unethical procedures. They are not to be dictated to by those who shape and mold the social conventions and the political correctness of these present and emerging years.

Ethical transitions and transactions are not to be considered superficially. Authority and autonomy of institutions is not a *nihil obstat*[2] to sanction the "anything goes" philosophy of members on their faculties. This same *caveat*[3] is applicable to external commercial forces that have a profound influence on academic research programs because of financial incentives which erode easily obvious ethical rules.

Essential restraints recognize that assumptions are not in themselves the grantors of permission. The inner drive that arrives at the conclusion "I can do it," does not mean it is morally correct to do it. Even when the parameters of bioethics have not been defined at the moment, the broad guidelines have been stated with clarity. Some advocate that: "We will need more empirical research on practices associated with ethics both in patient-provider relationships and in our healthcare institutions and systems" [Brandt, 2000]. The pitfall to avoid in this dialogue expressed as a "need" is that the advances in medicine will force downgrading of bioethics to accommodate changes which may be made for immoral reasons.

Another danger is: "Whenever one chooses a course of action in a morally problematic situation, one is in effect declaring that the same choice can justifiably be made in all morally equivalent situations" [Culver, 2000]. This non-syllogism is a thinking which is the specific being greater than the general process, which contradicts the logic that the specific is the subaltern to the general classification. Retrospection and prospective reflection should warn against adoption of ethical permissions that have internal defects. Failure to do so will turn back the pages of medical history to the chapter on medical ethics which will be a blank page.

---

2. *Nihil obstat* is Latin for "Nothing obstructs it."

3. From the Latin verb *cavēre* to beware. Caveat means a warning or caution.

Bioethics Defined

By definition bioethics is an area/field of special study concerned with the comportment [ethics] and philosophical implications of certain biological and medicosurgical procedures, technologies, bioengineering, surgical procedures, and medical treatments. Among the specified subjects are organ transplantations, genetics, manipulation of cells, care of the terminally ill, and thanatology.

In general ethics as a discipline is a system of moral principles to be applied in human behavior. As rules of conduct ethics is recognized in regard to particular actions performed individually. It is a branch of philosophy[4] dealing with values as they relate to human conduct, specifically, to the rightness or wrongness of certain acts, the goodness or badness of the motives and the intended ends of such actions. Applied to bioethics it is the moral outrigger that supports and gives stability to uprightness in the medical profession.

Bioethics as a noun is not listed in the older medical dictionaries. What is defined in an updated dictionary was known as medical ethics. In a religious application it was termed pastoral medicine. Although a medical dictionary is an inventory of the language of medicine, it is not a guide to proper professional behavior. As a literary, moral monument from an instructive viewpoint, bioethics must be accepted as derived from general ethics as adapted to the biological sciences.

Therefore ethics is the study of the general nature of morals as to specific choices made by an individual in relationship with other people. Called the philosophy of morals, it is also termed moral philosophy. It is the rules and standards governing conduct. Hence ethics is a set of good principles and values. It is the moral quality in a course of action. This definition as applied to medical clinical practice, research, teaching, and legal medicine is bioethics.

To be a bioethicist is both a professional challenge and a public trust. Each person so proclaimed is dedicated to the preservation of the highest ideals, to the identification of the best qualities in the biosciences,

---

4. For the purpose of this essay, philosophy is the science that treats of the ultimate criterion of things in the light of pure reason. Hence it is the rational investigation of the truths and principles of being, knowledge, and demeanor. Three branches of this science make it an entity. These are natural philosophy, moral philosophy, and metaphysical philosophy.

and sharing them with others for the benefit of the common good. In recognizing and discharging this responsibility, bioethicists promote and promulgate the best bioscientific information with laudable moral excellence. This is their epitome.

Moral choices and actions thus made are the basis upon which virtuous bioethics finds its merit. Among the virtues relevant to medicine are those derived from theology, added to which are compassion and integrity. Bioethicists have added phronesis as a cardinal mores. They call phronesis "the capacity to discern what moral choice or course of action is most conducive to the good in a given set of circumstances. It embodies prudence, the link between the intellectual, moral, and supernatural virtues" [Pellegrino and Thomasma, 1993].

Ancient History Of Bioethics

Rules of proper conduct are not the creation of the latest civilizations. Ethics, although not specified as such, was founded in antiquity. Its strong seed was planted in fertile soil whose durable roots have grown. Socrates and his interrogations stimulated discussions on morality. Well-known for evolving rhetoric into the adversarial system now called Socratic dialectics, he was an ethicist. Some historians intimate he is the originator of Hellenic ethics. Hippocrates by his historic, promulgated oath is the father of bioethics. This eponymic oath fortifies the concept that ethics is natural to bioscience [Spratt, 1998]. Highly opined scientific debates with unsubstantiated conclusions and illogical solutions are unable to change this inchoation.

Perhaps Celsus was the most persuasive and knowledgeable physician of classical Italy as recorded in European medical history. His great intellect allowed him to include all the desirable features of the enormous treasure of philosophic speculations, theories, hypotheses, and practical experiences that had been accumulated from Egypt, Greece, and Rome. Familiar with the medical literature preserved before his career, he was an ardent reader, calm critic, and keen observer. His natural instincts encouraged him to preserve in writing the current ideas of his time.[5]

---

5. Celsus [Aulus Cornelius Celsus] lived in Rome at the beginning of the Christian era. An encylopedist he gathered everything that was known in his

A worthy disciple of Hippocratic medical ethics, and medical history, he recognized and proclaimed loudly that physicians should admit their errors. His belief was that "the simple avowal of an error committed is proper for a man of great intelligence" [Castiglioni, 1941]. This he taught because the physician may be useful to those who follow him and prevent others from being mistaken as he was mistaken. The honored status of Celsus is justified. His professional life was exemplary. He was the embodiment of the best Roman tradition in his nobility of style, elegance of form, clarity of expression, and in the practicality of his medical recommendations [Castiglioni, 1941].

Celsus can be estimated as a Hippocratist in the sense that he was imperturbable in his reasoning, accurate in his interpretative observations, and firm adherent to ethical standards. Occasionally historical notes indicate he was far in advance of his own time. Reference is made to his defense of and the moral permissiveness of autopsy study. Well documented this advocacy is found in writing. "*[R]ationalem guidem puto medicinam esse debere; mortuorum corpora incidere discentibus necessarium.*" [I am of the opinion that the art of medicine ought to be rational; to open the bodies of the dead is necessary for learners].[6]

Considered to be the earliest medical writer of note, Cornelius Celsus, like Hippocrates, recommended vinegar to clean wounds and the application of dry dressings. Cleanliness of body, mind, and spirit were taught religiously. Hence it was automatic thinking for him to address morality and ethics as the means to a clean mind and pure spirit. The Roman motto, *Mens sana in corpore sano* [Sound mind in a sound body], was his credo. By his personal conduct, teachings, and writings Celsus brought to the history of ancient medicine remarkable contributions to medical ethics.

Medical jurisprudence in earlier times was equated with medical ethics according to the definition of the illustrious law-giver, Justinian.

---

lifetime about many subjects. Not being a medical practitioner he was a *philiatros* [a friend of physicians]. A man of extensively vast culture, learned in natural sciences, medicine, and philosophy he could express his opinions with valued appreciation by his listeners and colleagues on medical subjects and ethical problems.

6. *De Medicina, Proemium*. Sect 74 is quoted by Castiglioni. The usefulness of this text is its plethora of medical references, professionalism, morality, and ethics as important canons of medicine.

To him jurisprudence was understood to include moral injunctions as well as positive ordinances. *Juris praecepta sunt haec: honestè vivere, alterum non laedere, suum cuique tribuere* [Inst. Justin, Liber I, pagina 3]. Justinian I [483-565 AD] in history is known as "the Great," a suffix attached to his name. A Roman Caesar of renown, he was Emperor of the Eastern Empire from 527 to 565.

From Roman beginnings a code of professional ethics was sanctioned because codes of behavior improve courteous communications among colleagues, learned disciplines, and with patients. Jactation [boasting] was frowned upon as being of inferior degree, not befitting physicians. The deportment of physicians down through the centuries united tenderness with steadfastness, and humility with substantially reliable authority, so as to inspire others with gratitude, respect, and confidence. Concomitantly physicians tried not to give the impression of any misapprehension that could magnify either real signs/symptoms of illness or create imaginary ones. Roman physicians believed high ethical values invigorate and enlarge understanding giving an ample and honorable atmosphere of professional etiquette even under delicate, critical circumstances.

Guy De Chauliac

Contained in Italian literature is a famous letter of Petrarch[7] written to Pope Clement VI. This writing instigated an interminable quarrel with Guy de Chauliac, physician to the Pope. The humanist poet wrote: "I know that your bedside is beleaguered by doctors and naturally this fills me with fear. Their opinions are always conflicting and he who has nothing new to say suffers the shame of limping behind others. They learn their art at our expense and even our death brings them experience: the physician alone has the right to kill with impunity. Entirely appropriate to our time is the prophesy of the ancient Cato:[8] 'When the Greeks

---

7. Francesco Petrarca [1304-1374], Italian humanist poet, designed the Petrarchan sonnet consisting of two parts: an octave and a sestet rhyme patterns.

8. Marcus Porcius Cato [95-46 BC], surname Uticensia, called the Younger, was a Roman statesman, an opponent of Cataline and Caesar. He was the great-grandson of Cato the Elder [234-149 BC] Roman consul and censor.

have flooded us with their literature and especially their physicians, they will ruin everything for us. As we fear to live without physicians, although countless nations have lived better perhaps and healthier without them. Pliny[9] says the Romans themselves lived so for more than 600 years at the time of their greatest epochs. Then find yourself a single one of their band who is worthy, not on account of the grace of his expressions, but because of his knowledge and integrity'" [Petrarch's Letters]. This was a subtle way of saying Guy de Chauliac was an incompetent physician which he was not. Contrarily, his reputation was one of outstanding scientific scholarship whose character was unblemished. Moreover it was splendored with high attributes of ethical, medical performance. In the 14th century Chauliac was recognized for his penetrating writings on ethical conduct and medical wisdom of the past.

Guy de Chauliac [circa 1300-1367] was born near Lyon. He was among the celebrated pupils and later a master at Montpellier University, whose Latin designation is *Mons Pessuhanus*. Next to the School of Salerno which was first in advocating standards for physician behavior, Montpellier was among the earliest schools in western Europe to establish rigid codes for physician behavior in the 12th century. Being a strong advocate of the Montpellier code Chauliac was the chief glory of the university. He was considered to be the most famous surgeon of the Middle Ages. His best-known publication was *Chirurgia Magna* printed in Venice during 1498. In this book he writes about the necessary qualifications for the surgeon, his moral duties to patients and ethical courtesies to colleagues. In his own manner he established a standardized professional code that can be called bioethics as it is understood today.

Because of Chauliac's exceptional reputation he was called to Rome to be physician to Pope Clement VI during the great plague. Now in Rome he was in the same category of Italian physicians who were ridiculed unceasingly and unmercifully. This was the time of Petrarch, a strong critic of physicians. Famous were the quarrels between them which resulted in the many written satires of Petrarch against physicians. The constant carping did much good as it elevated medical conduct to a progressively high level of professional performance.

---

9. Pliny, Gaius Plinius Secundus [23-79 AD] called The Elder was a Roman scholar, man of letters, orator of distinction, and author of *Historia Naturalis*.

"Thus we find well-organized medical schools at the end of the 15th century and laws governing the practice of medicine, with severe penalties for those who practiced without the necessary license. Ethical rules not observed had fines and suspensions enforced. It was forbidden to a physician to make a grave or even qualified prognoses about his patient's disease without consultation with a colleague. A fine was inflicted on any physician who spoke evil of another physician in public. The practice of medicine was entirely in the hands of the laity. It is at this time that historians find a body of professional laws so adequate and well thought out that even up to our own times it has not been necessary to make any considerable changes" [Castiglioni, 1941].

Bioethics In 15th/16th Centuries

Revival with forcefulness of medical ethics in Europe is attributed to Zerbi. Under the title of medical prudence, pastoral medicine as the forerunner of bioethics was advanced in the Middle Ages by the authors who wrote *De Cautelis Medicorum*. Translated it concentrates "on the rules of caution for physicians. The theme was continued into the Renaissance by the Paduan professor Gabriele Zerbi [ca. 1435-1505]. He was a recognized seminal author of repute who wrote on a multiple variety of medical subjects. From 1471-1504 Zerbi served as full professor of philosophy and medicine at the Universities of Padua, Bologna, and Rome. Medical historians acclaim in writing: "The Medical Ethics of Gabriele de Zerbi recognize him as a demotic, avatar pioneer of bioethics" [French, 1993].

To define *cautela* correctly and precisely requires a descriptive sentence. "*Cautela* means both caution and precaution" [Lind, 1975]. Legally it implies security against malpractice. Zerbi defines the word as "the avoidance with diligent attention to deception, fraud, delusion, infamy, ignominy, and shame which can occur to the physician in his operative activity upon the human body which his practical reason directs him to preserve for the honor and usefulness of his profession. Thus is expressed all the material, formal, efficient, and final causes of *cautela*" [Linden, 1999].

Most historians and writers interpret *De Cautelis Medicorum* as an authentic acquisition to early specimens of a treatise on medical ethics. "The *De Cautelis Medicorum* is a textbook of ethics in the sense that it consists partly of advice, devices, and strategies that the doctor can employ to enhance his reputation . . . that will encourage the patient and his family to call a doctor a second time, rather than one of the different kinds of unlicensed practitioners" [French, 1993]. Constructive criticism indicates that the concept of ethics as a tool administered by a medical group to secure financial success appears to be narrow-minded, circumspect, and self-serving. Bioethics fosters morality, and is not a means to economic gain.

However interpreted, the postulates of the *cautelae medicorum* were recommendations divided into six groups. Briefly presented succinctly they are the following.

1. Rules for the studies and perfection of the physician according to "the congenital disposition of the soul and the body" [French, 1993]. The original Latin writing is: *secundum dispositiones tam animae quam corporis a generatione contractas*.
2. The obligation of the physician to God.
3. Recommendations for acquired dispositions and general conduct, concerning the dispositions of the body and soul acquired in the course of time [French, 1993].
4. The proper professional attitude toward the patient.
5. Rules for the attitude toward the patient's family and other people involved in the treatment of the sick person.
6. Regulation of the physician's relationship with the general public [French, 1993].

This division reflects the general pattern of traditional codes of medical practice which have been set by the Hippocratic Oath and the [subsequent] treatises on medical etiquette. It is Zerbi's explicit aim to convey the views of the medical authorities with these words: "imitating . . . whatever had been written by the ancients and particularly by Hippocrates, our guide to all that is good" [Kühn, 1821]. Zerbi emphasized that true perfection in medicine can be attained only through practical experience. Galen taught that without clinical experience and empirical research there is an insufficiency of doctrinal knowledge [Kuhn, 1821].

Hippocrates, Galen, Zerbi, and Giovanni Battista da Monte of Padua contributed to the formation of physician conduct that aimed at trust of the patient in the physician. Each in his own inimitable fashion urged physicians to acquire honorable habits whose shrewdness would separate physicians from the category of those morally corrupt. With this objective paramount, these molders of physician character advised men of medicine not to blur their profession. That honor requires the avoidance of ambition, blasphemy, ambivalence in words, pride, drunkenness, and have no devotion to luxury, and always to strive for the maintenance of confident deportment [Siraisi, 1990].

Added to the recommendations made, physicians were advised to be prudent, honest, and in control of their emotions. For personal well-being physically they were to abstain from gluttony and excessive venery. The Hippocratic Oath is not demised. "It ought to be obeyed in its affirmation of confidentiality, both *intra* and *extra curam*. Zerbi's last piece of advice with regard to the physician's person is to protect his own health" [fol. b2]. Otherwise he will be ridiculed with the famous proverb '*Medice cura teipsum*' [Physician heal thyself], St. Luke's Gospel, chapter 4, line 23 [Siraisi, 1990]. These words are the seeds from whence grew the evergreen tree of professional conduct and medical appropriateness. Hence green is the color of the academic hood indicative of medicine.

Bioscience and biomedicine are the glamorous sciences of the future. Physics and chemistry have lost the limelight and their former starry stage presence to biology. Celebrity status in science by revolutionary research has fallen upon biologists who now wear the laurel wreath of fame. The crown is not free of thorns because of tampering with divine, natural orderliness. Biologists are the recipients of academic accolades and prestigious awards/prizes given easily, previously, and frequently to physicists 30-40 years ago. No longer are physics and chemistry the undisputed prestige sciences in the world of scholars. The salvation of physics and chemistry is when they supplement medical research in molecular biology, biochemistry, genetics, and other studies on living organisms. This does not intimate that the innovative capacity for all scientific research is not to be encouraged and nurtured in every conceivable way.

Medical Ethics And Jurisprudence In 18th/19th Centuries

An address to the fellows of the Royal College of Surgeons of London was made by John Armstrong in 1825. It was a rebuke with reprimand that chided the membership on its injurious conduct, lack of ethics, and defective state of that corporation. With special reference to professional rights, medical science, and public health it excoriated the medical profession.

The acerbic criticism appeared in book form. First edition of this fascinating attack on the conduct of the Royal College of Surgeons had an almost savage response because the author was a very popular and a most successful physician. Armstrong came into conflict with the college over their attempts to discourage private medical teaching by refusing to accept certificates of medicine from institutions other than those of recognized English hospitals and their medical schools. Armstrong was an excellent, highly appreciated teacher of medicine. Also he was a lecturer at a school founded in Webb Street which was considered one of the most important in London.

In his book he cites the opposition encountered by his own associate and two other capable surgeons who had run into direct conflict with the Court of Examiners of the college. The three candidates were refused fellowship in that august community of surgeons. The *corpus* of this literary work mentions many other areas of ethical concern which the author felt needed urgent attention. He appeals to the fellows of the Royal College to review their codes of practice and correct abuses [Armstrong, 1825].

Strange to relate before the advocacy of Sir John Armstrong there were persuasive publications that advanced laws by medical societies. In 1803 the Laws of the Medical Society of Edinburgh were printed. It contained a history of the organization together with a code of professional ethics which was a main-stay of medicine throughout Scotland since its incorporation [Edinburgh, 1803].[10]

---

10. The Edinburgh Medical Society was founded in 1737 at a time when Edinburgh was one of the leading medical centres in Europe. The Medical School grew in importance from 1726 when the Leiden-trained Alexander Monro, the elder, became professor of anatomy. In the following century, Edinburgh boasted a galaxy of talent including all three members of the Monro family. Black in chemistry, Cullen and Gregory in theoretical and practical medicine, and may others. Through the influence of Leiden, the school's strength lay in imparting the elements of anatomy, surgery, chemistry, medical theory and practice. Such success, inevitably led to the formation of a flourishing Medical Society, which was granted a Royal Charter in 1778.

In the English-speaking world medical ethics as a discipline is thought generically to have originated in the 18th century. Acknowledgement is given to the medical philosophy propounded by the Scotsman John Gregory [1725-1773] and his two younger colleagues in other countries. The two were the Englishman, known as the Dissenter, Thomas Percival [1740-1804] and the famous American physician Benjamin Rush [1745-1813], a signer of the colonists' Declaration of Independence. These three scholars combined the thoughts of Francis Bacon [1561-1626], the English philosopher essayist. It was he whose enlightenment ideas organized the science of morals and the morals of science. Their medical ethics was an adaptation of traditional moral ideas to the dramatically changing medical world. "In accounting for the dynamics of this process, [an author] rejects the anachronism that modern medical ethics was a new paradigm" [Haakonssen, 1997].

With the rising tide of ethical codes, there was no elimination of deceptive medical therapy. An example was an account of some experiments made with the vapor of boiling tar in the cure of pulmonary consumption [tuberculosis]. Written by the renowned physician Sir Alexander Crichton it had many believers among his patients. His colleagues did not share in this enthusiasm.

Even though he was Physician in Ordinary to their Imperial Majesties the Emperor and the Dowager-Empress of Russia his ethical manner was questioned as was his unproven claims of cure. His book was published in French and printed at St. Petersburg in 1816. One year later it appeared in England [Crichton, 1817].[11] Shortly after its appearance the word fraudulent was whispered about it. Crichton was originally inspired to try this form of treatment by John Mudge's *A Radical and Expeditious Cure for a recent Catarrhous Cough* [Mudge, 1778].[12] In

11. Crichton was appointed as physician in ordinary to Alexander I of Russia in 1804 and went on to become head of the civil medical department. He was much respected at the Russian court, and his efforts to mitigate the horrors of an epidemic which devastated the southeastern provinces in 1809 were rewarded with him being conferred the knight grand cross of the order of St. Anne and St. Vladimir, third class, and then in 1814, for his long and faithful service, that of second class.

12. First edition of this interesting work of popular medicine was a handbook to cure chest infections associated with the common cold and other respiratory complaints. This uncomfortable symptom of cold and "flu," should be

the course of his observations Mudge says he believes, that much of the benefit which consumptive persons experience from sea-voyages, is derived from the tar vapour constantly on board a ship. After carrying out initial and successful trials, he gained permission from the Empress Dowager, with whom he had a close association, to pursue further trials at the Hospital for the Poor. "This favor was directly granted; and one Ward, containing four or five beds was devoted to this purpose." Two physicians, Messr Bluhm and Roos, were charged with overseeing the trials, and their reports are included, six case histories being cited. The fumigation was achieved by placing the tar in an earthen vessel over a lamp or heated iron, to cause a slow volatilization until the air of the ward was sufficiently impregnated. Despite a few set-backs, including the realization that although the vapors provided relief, the burnt fumes of tar could be very harmful, he nevertheless felt the method worthwhile and advocated further trials. It appears, however, that Crichton's appeals met with some resistance. In a review found in the *Edinburgh Medical and Surgical Journal*, 1, January 1818, the anonymous writer states that: "We are extremely sceptical of the possibility of curing pulmonary consumption, and we are well read in the history of supposed remedies, which have from time to time gained the confidence of the public, only to fall successively into oblivion." Clearly physicians were alert to ethical transgressions. There was no hesitancy to call attention to conduct unbecoming a physician.

During the pontificate of Pope Pius XII [1939-1958] references to ethical matters were termed Pastoral Medicine. This was the Pope's field of expertise. His great pronouncement spoken before an audience of international physicians is a memorable milestone in the history of bioethics.[13]

---

treated promptly to prevent it from developing into "diseases truly formidable to tender constitutions." The remedial inhaler, as designed by Mudge, was described and illustrated, and won widespread acclaim and acceptance. Mudge studied medicine at Plymouth hospital. In 1777, his Dissertation on the Inoculated Small Pox advanced several new theories on the subject and was much respected. He became a fellow of the Royal Society in 1777 and was a friend to Sir Joshua Reynolds and Dr. Samuel Johnson, who described him as "the celebrated physician who was not more distinguished for quickness of parts and variety of knowledge, than loved and esteemed for his amiable manners."

13. Pope Pius XII, November 24, 1957 in an address to the gathering of Catholic Physician Guilds and world anesthesiologists.

> But normally one is held to use only ordinary means—according to circumstances of persons, places, times, and culture—that is to say, means that do not involve any grave burden for oneself or another. A more strict obligation would be too burdensome for most men and would render the attainment of the higher, more important good too difficult. Life, health, all temporal activities are in fact subordinated to spiritual ends. On the other hand, one is not forbidden to take more than the strictly necessary steps to preserve life and health, as long as he does not fail in some more serious duty.

Tersely the duty of the diligent physician, without any intimation of negligent supervision, is to pursue ordinary means but not extraordinary means in the treatment of patients to preserve life. Thus a moral decision based upon substantial bioethics is well-founded on this Pian dictum.

Some two decades later when environmentalists became hyperactive, the atmosphere was referred to as the biosphere. Appended to which was the ethical requisite to preserve it from contamination of water and pollution of the air. To attract attention to this hygiene the word bioethics was coined. Finding it an engaging noun, the medical profession adopted it with alacrity and celerity. Pastoral Medicine and Medical Ethics became preterits. Bioethics supplanted them becoming the biobehavioral main-stay of the life sciences. Its tenets should forestall, thwart, and ward off professional errantry. Especially nowadays with the debates raging over human experimentation, genetic engineering, organ/bone marrow transplantation, xenophysiology, new reproductive technology, abortion, euthanasia, assisted suicide, termination of life-sustaining treatment, and other issues of conscience [Jonsen, 1999].

Chapter 2

Energetic Bioethics

A philosopher is a physician of culture said Friedrich Nietzsche [1844-1900]. Little did he realize that subsequent generations would be participants in moral philosophic decision-making by physicians. Bioscientists caught in the accelerated momentum of progressive medicine are confronted with numerous moral questions which require honest answers. Erring bioscientists can mislead the laity who easily become victims of misguided ethics.

Allegations of ethical misconduct may be dismissed without adequate investigation. Supporters of proper ethical standards often find themselves expending their efforts against an eternal void. Some bioscientists resort to the fable that whatever they do is named medical progress. They fail to know that what is technically feasible is not always ethically permissible.

Natural human functions are not alterable to accomplish an unnatural result. Proper ethical conduct is an appended duty, a sacred obligation not to venture against the natural human order. What was not acceptable years ago seems to be permissible currently. Medical ethics is not exempted from this laxity. The association of philosophy with the biosciences has become a specialty termed bioethics. As an overseer, bioethics is a potent "guide in the moral dimension of clinical decision-making" [Fletcher, 1987]. Hence it is concerned with many daily medicosurgical encounters centering on the quality-of-life questions. The litany of which is elective death, proxy consent powers, resuscitation, patient's rights, artificial reproduction, the transmission of genetic/infectious diseases, what to do with comatose patients, selective termination of pregnancy, selling of ova, and many more subjects.

Associated with the need for bioethical determination is the economic evaluation of long term treatment of comatose patients and other associated problems pertinent to cost-containment. Danger lurks when a financial reduction concern becomes a greater consideration than moral correctness [Dyer, 1979]. Professionalism diminishes when the physician is enmeshed in economics.[1]

Looking through the prism of experience it is noted that medical ethics began as a slender body of advice on medical manners, deportment, etiquette, and duties toward fellow physicians. Superficial in solemnity it proposed no critical reflections on the physician-patient relationship. From this insignificant origin it has grown into a biophilosophical discipline with the name bioethics. With medicine as its core bioethics embraces all the life sciences. Modern ethical considerations are directed to the patient as the classical description of medicine defines. A physician is a failure in clinical practice if personal qualities of morality are missing. The high quality of medicine finds its foundation on the ethical character of its clinicians and all those called assistants or associates.

Redoubtable bioscientists as clinicians are foremost advocates of ethical norms in medical practice. Having acquired insight in the care of critically ill patients they implement answers to medicomoral questions. Trying as they do to explain the problems arising out of the biomedical revolution, some opposition to their conclusions is inevitable. As an impediment this antagonism is a digression occasionally from the Hippocratic mission which is the source for ethical structure of medicine and surgery.

Bioethics serves on a case-by-case basis. Not always easy to solve, many require the wisdom of Solomon and the patience of Job prior to arriving at a just conclusion. Due to massive social changes plus multiple cultures pluralistic approaches are necessary and often defeating. Separate religions do not have a common bond of tradition to allow facile communication. The difficulty is compounded when the physician is a stranger to the patient's culture and finds resistance to professional

---

1. A professional person is described historically as one who professes to perform specific acts which become a self-imposed duty. To profess is to take a vow. Physicians traditionally at the time of graduation after receiving their parchments attesting to their worthiness to receive the MD degree took the Hippocratic Oath which was tantamount to taking a vow to serve humanity ethically.

advice. The ethical imperatives used in decision-making are firm but to bring about understanding varies from culture to culture. Disparity increases the physician's ineffectiveness when some non-caucasian patients/ families do not understand good intentions which bring about doubt and suspicion. Other groups are immersed in the generality that criticizes conformity as their societal policy. Many people either individually or collectively seal themselves off from all other neighbors. These factors present dilemmas to the bioethicist [Feuerherd, 1991].

After many decades of discussion, discord, debate, and ethical upheavals, the medicosurgical community is poised to do more good than moral harm in vaunted, glowing promises. The bioscientific disciplines of pharmacy, genomes, tissue engineering, gene therapy, immunology, and other undisclosed research are included in the conglomerate of the new millennium bioworld. Obscurity no longer hides the professional conduct of scientists. Whether easily decipherable or complex, their actions theoretically are scrutinized via peer review. Ethical principles are not contraband to be hidden from those who observe as ombudsmen.

Ethical Norms Are From Teachers

Instructors in bioscience, those in medical research, and others in similar positions are educational navigators. They are looked upon as directors of studies who give true knowledge. Even when confronted with acrimonious controversy each is bound in honest conscience to uphold intellectually proven truths. Scientific feasibility tainted by falsity may gain a competitive edge. This does not excuse erosion of proper scientific transactions sustained by truthful, honest study. The Bible teaches: "Such is the irresistible quality of truth that all it asks and all it wants is the liberty of appearing" [Thomas Paine, 1737-1809].

Dividing standard bioscience that does not preserve, enhance, or strengthen bioethical guidelines is malfeance in teaching. Although of the same origin, to differentiate the end-result by selectivity is a divisive play that weakens what is taught as correct. Bioethics does not support two opposing systems. An absolute component as the essential key-point does not allow relativism to departmentalize truth to obscure it. Delineation of right from wrong is not to be blurred by any intentional haziness. To do this is to weaken the pedestal that supports strict adherence to truth with all that flows from it. Teachers of merit are the champions of truth. Because:

> They that are learned shall shine as the brightness of the firmament; and they that instruct many to justice, as stars for all eternity [Daniel XII, 3].

An example illustrative of academic discord is in reference to the appointment of a controversial professor that occurred at Princeton University. An Australian philosopher appointed to the endowed chair in bioethics caused tremendous furor. What is shocking to the academic world is the indifference to the appointment of a bioethicist who is an advocate of death. This did not stir criticism from other university professors. Contrarily, there are moral philosophers, psychologists, and academicians who agree with the new appointee. "He believes it is wrong to eat animals but not necessarily immoral to kill disabled human babies or senile adults. He opposes the use of animals in medical experiments but advocates the right of parents to kill their infants if they suffer from a debilitating condition such as hemophilia" [Chavez, 1999].

Neonaticide as a cultural betterment has many supporters on university faculties. To some the practice is a triage whereby parents might decide to eliminate sickly newborn babies in favor of healthier infants [Steven Pinker quoted by Chavez]. This false reason seeks justification in the excuse that killing a defective child induces the parents to have another child who is born without a congenital disease. "The loss of a happy life for the first infant is outweighed by the gain of a happier life for the second . . . This is total utilitarianism" [Peter Singer quoted by Chavez].

Here is an incident of an international reputation founded on killing a disabled infant is not morally equivalent to killing a person. Very often it is not wrong at all according to some professors. They do not see the evil upon which reputation was founded. Practical Ethics is the course to be taught by the Australian bioethicist. Arguments against its contents will not be heard as false. Immoral bioethics will be taught to students who in turn will spread this culture of death—a human abomination that is intrinsically immoral.

> Who learns and learns
> But does not what he knows
> Is one who plows and plows
> Yet never sows [Old Persian Proverb].

Disagreement with the appointment of the Australian bioethicist by a solitary member of the university's board of trustees was fruitless. Requests to rescind the appointment were denied. The new tenured faculty member's "views, which challenge the moral values of Judeo-Christian faiths and most secular philosophical systems, have been the subject of growing criticism and have sparked protests" [Billups, 1999].

The irony of this university appointment is that this professor for death is the chairman of the department in human values. Disabled persons were the strongest protesters with an equal vociferous group of anti-abortionists. Influential alumni and a member of the board of trustees had no effect in their protestations. Most of the university population was faint-hearted at a time when a stout-hearted spirit was needed.

Moral, militant leadership was absent to counteract the defenders of the appointee who supported him as an issue of academic freedom. But critics stated the "appointment sends a dangerous and debilitating message that anything goes, that there are no bounds when it comes to life and death" [Billups, 1999]. Teachers who advocate death of the disabled should listen to those who are handicapable when each joins the other to say, My life is worth living.

Chapter 3

Dignity Of Human Nature Preserved

The union of bioethical excellence with dedication to old-fashioned caring for the welfare of patients is mutually supportive. Standards do not vary as to age, severity of the illness/injuries, and economy. From infants unborn, the neonates, teenagers, adults, and those in the geriatric age group the moral principles of care do not change. The sacredness of human life does not vary according to the external appearance of the body that contains it. Challenges of the century with its plethora of promises, predictions, and pretenses are not to alter time-tested bioethics.

No matter the magnificent achievements prophesized with preordained admiration, the moral and ethical dimensions of health care must not be diminished. Contrariwise, the fullest attention is to be given the practice of and teaching of it in hospitals, nursing schools, and schools of medicine. The 21st century will witness major developments in undisclosed directions that will enhance present medical technology. Biological research, teaching, and medicosurgical clinical practice may be redesigned. Newer alterations may change traditional commitment to health service. With it there should not be any denigration of lofty, value-based bioethics no matter how difficult the situation and powerful the opposition.

Retention of the highest moral standards is compatible with worthwhile, advanced scientific accomplishments. The aggressive pursuit of knowledge in the overt clinical arena and in the covert recesses of the secluded laboratory respects the ethical and moral enthusiasm of successful accomplishments. Intellectual honesty includes the humane concern in bioscientific endeavors of all classifications. Scientific objectivity does not license elimination of moral values, and those core principles that are beyond ethical questioning.

Leaders in health care that include physicians, nurses, medical technicians, and hospital employees should have the character to match the trust patients place in them. They are expected to respect the whole person under their supervision as human beings with the same dignity they themselves would like to receive. The moral heritage of medical practice is its crowning glory that has given it the honor it deserves.

This is a major reason why ethical relativism is not to be allowed to cross the protective threshold of the medical sciences. If it does, illicit and disturbing behavior will flourish. Illusory manipulations from self-glorifying temptations will rise. Respect for human beings is one of the basic, inexorable demands of the moral law. "It is on this eternal law that the universal and unchangeable nature of the moral law is based, a law which shows us the boundless horizon of the good and indicates the limit not to be transgressed by those intrinsically evil acts that no circumstance or intention can make acceptable and good" [Pope John Paul II cf. *Veritatis* splendor, nn. 80-81].

Chapter 4

Truth Telling In Medicine

Patients often request from their attending physicians to know the truth about their illnesses. Especially is the request made for personal reasons, such as estate planning and making a final will and testament. Physicians usually disclose facts to the relatives but often are reticent to give bad news to the patient directly. At times the effect of learning the truth has an adverse effect on the patient. Unvarnished disclosure may affect the course of the patient's spirit to live, thereby influence the quality of dying.

From the physician's side there is always the threat of malpractice. Previously a mistake somewhere may have been made which restrains the physician from being positive in statements. Hesitancy because of the possibility of a quantified mistake masks the physician as a mistake maker. Human error does not exempt even the exalted physician and most talented surgeon. Hospital records attest to errors and mistakes regarding missed diagnoses of patients which gave an unfavorable, even a terminal, prognosis. Although such incidents are rare, they do occur.

Ambiguity is not truth. This is a manner of avoiding lying. Thus the physician succeeds in preventing a patient from having an illusion about the severity of the illness. Half-truths cause equal devastation as the whole truth. Serious illness can instill panic in those who are its victims. Sickness and mental anguish are in a state of continuous interaction that add acute stress to an existing disease.

It may be argued that once the physician is convinced that death is certain, he has an overriding obligation to impart that truth with complete candor—regardless of the effect. Yet his sense of certainty concerning the inevitability of the patient's death does not deter him from taking strenuous measures to save the patient—chemotherapy, surgery, radiation. If he thinks that everything should be done, whatever the odds to help a patient, then by the same token he should regard his communications with the patient in the same light.

Why should not a sense of professional obligation lead the physician to invoke and employ the full array of psychological tools and approaches open to him? The patient's attitude—his will to live, his confidence in the physician and in himself, and his determination to fight the disease—is an important element in therapy. It is well known that the physician's treatment is enhanced by a favorable psychological environment. Such being the case, it may be reasonable to suggest that anything that impairs the possible usefulness of treatment—including truth telling—ought to be avoided or appropriately modified [Cousins, 1980].

In the ever-expanding panoply of individual rights, the psychiatric profession now wants to add a new one: the right to lie . . . to do for lying what some wish to do for drugs: decriminalize it . . . This should lighten the burden of guilt from those who have been indicted for perjury . . . Lying is considered to be a social achievement—a social lubricant—a natural by-product of psychological growth [Thomas, 1988].

Lying in a large measure is due to the denial of a fixed set of absolutes and definition of truth. Lying is seen "as much a part of normal growth and development as telling the truth" [Goldbert, 1988]. "Also this view has led to the 'doctrine' of moral equivalence, which sees all people and nations as equal and the concept of evil [as in evil empire] as outmoded and unfit for debate" [Thomas, 1988]. Lying unravels the social fabric lacerating the seamless garment of theology. If it is human nature to lie, it is the higher goal to be ever truthful.

Bioscientists by training and pursuit of their professional goals know that they must adhere to truth for success in their quests. Those who fail to achieve these ends are those who have abandoned truth. Not to be truthful is to lie. Lying is the enemy of bioethics that weakens it to a debility that makes it a limping cripple. Weak bioethics in clinical medicine and bioscientific research leads to artful deception, lying, and falsehoods. These bring about professional divisions that divide and conquer what is good. The true value of bioethics is found in that fixed, predetermined policy which disavows lying, and preserves its cultural guardianship of worthwhile, honest bioscience. The greater the ethical heights reached by bioscientists the broader becomes their medical horizons. This gives them joyous communion with the creative medical minds that went before them whose characters were impeccably glorious and stamped with grandeur.

Ethical Responsibility Of Medical Students

A physician's bioethical norms must be formulated long before undertaking the care of patients. Schools of medicine have an academic obligation to instruct medical students in bioethical conduct indigenous to their future careers. It is assumed that they are a highly selected group whose character traits made them stand taller than the other pre-medical applicants whom they have surpassed.

These young people have crossed the threshold leading to scientific professionalism. As a chosen few they should be instilled with the burden that their future life's work places upon them. Medical school experiences include the denial of petty immature envy that brings forth fierce competition. Curtailment of excess emotionalism must be taught. Failure to do so may arouse discontentment that breeds unfettered desires which lead to relentless evil behavior.

When the toga of professionalism is worn it may rechart an entire future. It is well to remember that it is easier to be a medical student and physician on paper than to perform as such in the world as we know it. Realism demands a deep commitment not one that is deceptively thin. Lip service is not the logo of medicine. The heart of every profession must be honor. Only then can be found the true love of a learned profession that has no equivalent.

Medical discipline grants certain rights. To these rights are appended special tangible duties with attached responsibilities. Members of any esteemed, learned profession are looked upon with respect, admiration, envy. Often they are idolized. Hence it is imperative that people of medicine compose themselves with deportment that is made of stern substance. Exceptional physicians disenthrall themselves from all fictitious, illusory mirages of grandeur. Medicosurgical superiority is founded upon correct, repetitive rites of ethical intellectual rehearsals strengthened by excellence in learning. If a motto is sought consider, *Semper docere et paratus doceri*. In translation it signifies: always prepared to teach and always prepared to be taught.

The adoption of medical professionalism has attached to it certain obligations which are direct supplements to the rights it bestows. Among these are the personal, ethical, necessary responsibilities to be honorable, to adhere to propriety, probity, integrity, personal dignity, and respect for the patient in his/her physical person as well as in his/her confidentiality. The *noblesse oblige* of dignified physicians is the inspiration it engenders in all health care personnel toward increasing proper ethical conduct among them. Uplifting ethical deportment becomes contagious as it replicates itself.

Professionalism arises first and foremost from a deep-seated conviction on the part of a well-defined, selected peer group. The acknowledgment is that they owe their principal duty to the specific people they serve and in the residual extent to the general community. Arrogance and self-glory, while not being submerged entirely, must be kept far in the background, recessed from observation, and well under personal control. Pride in accomplishment is laudable. However inordinate pride can become a personal sin. It leads to a fall in spiritual stature. Theologically, pride is acknowledged to precede human disaster.

The professional person stresses constantly "the service ideal" and the sacred obligation of striving for perfection in his/her workplace. Hence there is the tedious burden of a long university curriculum, the prolonged formal training after graduation, the recurrent reinforcement of knowledge by continuous experience and continual medical education. These activities bolster the unyielding pledge to the demands of prime professional performance. Strict adherence to these distinctive impalpables is necessary to arrive at perfection thresholds. The alternative is a loss of precious benchmark attributes that are not replaceable or regained.

An academic institution of medical learning does not create scholars by parenteral infusion. Any intellectual achievement in medicine is not acquired through the fabric of university buildings. The ivy-covered walls, the massive portals, the marble corridors are not the creators of men or women of distinction. The mark of supremacy in learning is produced through the noble character of the teaching physicians/surgeons who enter the granite portals, open the massive doors, walk to the lecture halls, and the laboratories. Scholastic surroundings may induce an unmatched atmosphere of education but real contributions to medicosurgical advancements must come from within the spirit of the person dedicated to the pursuit of knowledge. Remember well that Madame Curie discovered radium while doing research in a barn.

Professional people are organized around problems that touch human core values and invade the matrix of society at its foundation as well as in its mundane changes. This is the classical perspective of medicine. Contemporaneously it makes aware to the universe the physical/mental toll that such stressful and exacting labors takes on its practitioners. From this traditional overview medical professionalism is an exemplification of rendering the personal service ideal, a counterpoint to the more worldly commonplace commercial activity of daily life. Any attendant reward is not needed to motivate individuals to take upon themselves such arduous labor as is the study and practice of medicine.

People to be professionalized are the product of a period of tedious formal training, an elevated code of ethical conduct, professional associations, and marked devotion to duty. Dignified personal conduct is part of this composite. In order to obtain such respect one must earn it. The uninterrupted contribution a physician can make that brings forth respect is visible professionalism in all that it implies. This is aroused from within by obvious personality traits many of which are attributed to the empathy inspired by medicine itself. Medical professionalism does have its own distinctive charisma that increases as the passing years fade into the annals of history.

In the face of newer studies, recent inventions, biochemical engineering, and other current technical exploits that medical scientists are developing it is urgent to arrive at a heightened conscious differentiation between good and evil in medical actions. This distinction will lead to a moral appreciation for divine creation and an absolute respect for human beings who transcend every material thing.

All medical school activities as daily performances should be above reproach. Elevated individual ethical standards are the splendors of medicine's hidden spirit. Recollect from hidden memories that reputation is what people think you are, but character is what you really are. Medical students are not to retain the childish prank of cheating. They should not be tempted to falsify either chemical analyses, laboratory reports, or medical records. Shun the temptation to harm or embarrass fellow students by rumors, improper nods, false becks, and wreathed smiles of deception. Colleagues should be friends—help them. Do not place obstacles in their pathways. Rejoice not in their sorrow. Do not laugh at their tears. Medical students must eliminate from their minds animosity and envy of each other. There but for the grace of God anyone may have been in the place of another.

Each medical student should look upon classmates as future professional colleagues, as similar laborers working in the vineyard of life. What one is as a medical student he/she will be as a doctor of medicine. A cheating medical student becomes a cheating doctor. Numerical/letter grades are printed on ephemeral papier-maché. Thus they have neither eternal mundane importance or infinite spirituality. They do not represent progressive intellectual growth, increasing knowledge, or true learning capacity. Moreover they are not indicators of moral virtue. Patients will not ask what were your marks in medical school but rather can you help them. To do this one must possess competent medical skills founded upon the highest ethical standards applied capably without prejudicial judgment. High marks may be necessary to acquire a certificate from Alpha Omega Alpha. Memberships in honor societies are laudable rewards but they are not a prerequisite to being acclaimed a Nobel laureate in medicine or acquiring distinctions of equal solemnity.

Medical students learn early that physicians are charitable to those in need. They give of their personal sustenance, not merely of their financial surplus. Physicians do not contribute to the problems of life: but try to be contributors to their solutions. They have learned to respect one another's culture differences as they work for justice via communications with physicians in other parts of the world. Honor in professional behavior at all levels leads to justice. It is only through justice that universal peace can be attained. Just solutions by means of fair negotiations can eliminate social injustice which begets despair and violence. No true physician, worthy of the title, ignores the discords of life and the inequalities within the medical profession.

Cheating

Examination cheating of varying proportions exists at many medical schools. Exact determination as to the quantity of students so indiscreet is difficult to calculate. Another form of cheating in scholarship pursuits is having term papers, theses, and dissertations ghost-written. As an established practice it is not isolated to a few universities but has reached epidemic proportions. Its persistence suggests it is a rescue apparatus to relieve student stress and distress. This serious form of cheating is encouraged by those who have made a lucrative business of rendering this service. They are accomplices in this unethical deceit.

"Students at every major university in the country have access to at least one commercial firm that offers a variety of writing and research services ranging from term papers on any subject for undergraduates to MA theses to PhD dissertations" [Etzioni, 1976]. These paper mills continue to roll on. Many students are ready, willing, and able to buy the second-hand product of learning-work they did not do, making a mockery of the achievements of the noncheaters" [Editorial in Jan/Feb, 1977 issue of The Surgical Team].

Falsity such as this is unethical. It allows succumbing to future blemished practices easy. It indicates the medical student has no respect for intellectual integrity, no sense of the value of learning for its own sake, and of advancing their careers by legitimate means [Etzioni, 1976].

"Those who search for ethical ways of eradicating this betrayal of ethical values feel constrained to acknowledge the decline of respect for such values in many compartments of modern society. Students are alert to the lapses of moral integrity in government, corporate business, and the professions. They are aware also of the cheapening of language communications, in style, applications, sheer volume, and of the weakening of the connection between learning and earning. If at the same time they see degrees as passports to employment—as their derelictions show they do—this is likely to be felt as a contradiction" [Editorial in Jan/Feb, 1977 issue of The Surgical Team].

Deviation from goodness is not only the basis of immorality. It is the acceptance of evil as being the norm. Perennial adherence to truth is the standard for evaluating all human acts. Every person is called to be good but some do not hear its voice. Dialogue between faculty and students is lacking in giving adequate attention to the serious deviation from student probity and its consequences.

Welcomed are the suggestions from Burnham S. Walker at Burbank Hospital in Fitchburg, Massachusetts. Walker proposed "that undergraduates students be passed or failed on the basis of daily laboratory performance and occasional examinations; and that just as every ethical physician makes a daily visit, at least, to patients in the hospital, so should every ethical professor make a daily visit to each graduate student. Both the physician and the professor should spend enough time and make enough observations to know whether or not progress is being made. The physician or the professor should not accept the responsibility for more people than can be effectively observed" [Editorial in Jan/Feb, 1977 issue of The Surgical Team].

"We deplore cheating in learning absolutely, and we are securely convinced that cheating or not-cheating is (and must be) an option wholly within the grasp of moral integrity—the individual's power. The life situations in which the individual confronts this option are almost invariably mild enough that no extenuating circumstance can arise which would prevent the exercise of pure moral integrity. The individual student therefore bears the entire responsibility for cheating or not-cheating. (Incidentally, should there not be praise for not-cheating?!)" [Editorial in Jan/Feb, 1977 issue of The Surgical Team].

Cheating in any form is deplorable. For the medical student it is stealing information or knowledge. Ill-gotten, it is not retained. Tradition has formulated an elaborate, not lengthy, set of canons for propriety and impropriety. These are intended to govern acquisition and use of information during educational experience and in other life situations including the professions. Such canons of information-acquisition-and-use-behavior are not variables that change from one situation to another.

Advancement, achievement, and accolades are available to all in the field of medicine. To obtain them one must be dedicated to learning, diligent in professional actions, devoted to idealism, honorable, and determined to employ to their fullest all acquired talents. These attributes lead to human benefits which bring with them many rewards. Among these is virtue which engenders respect. This appreciation prompted Robert Louis Stevenson [1850-1894] to write *A Tribute To Physicians*:

> There are men and classes of men that stand above the
> common herd:
> The soldier, the sailor and the shepherd not infrequently,
> the artist rarely; rarelier still, the clergyman:
> The physician almost as a rule. He is the flower (such
> as it is) of our civilization.

Chapter 5

Communication Science's Ethical Responsibility

If I do not understand, I pause, I examine."
Michel Eyquem DeMontaigne [1533-1592]

Correction to achieve an ultimate good is laudatory. Vitriolic disagreement for the sake of cacophony or to foster discord is unworthy of either acknowledgement or encouragement. Unfortunately some people in this sophisticated generation are wicked. Often they act or speak without regard for the hurt that may arise from their lack of consideration. Without premeditation the wrong is done before the action is completed or the word becomes an echo.

Many are they who have taken as their character trait bad temperament, repetitious contestation, caustic criticism, and disdainful distance from goodness. Contemporaneously they are cunning, conniving, contemptuous with defection from salubrious virtue that is cloaked in false logic. Such persons are purveyors of evil without recognizing this spurious fault. Bereft of all pudor they continue in a programmed pattern that increases progressively discontentment. This appraisal is applicable to all societal planes. Some whom the world looks upon as being great persons when scrutinized are seen as moral midgets unworthy of the given accolade.

Causality formulating the central doctrine of the laws of ethical conduct was one of the major preoccupations of early philosophers since the era of ancient hellenic glory. Aristotle's four causes (essential, formal, exciting, and final) thrilled the thinking of Western philosophers for many centuries. These four propaedeutical concepts served as reference guides even on those occasions when scholars strayed from this inherited dictum.

With the increase in freedom of thought and the expression thereof, additional vocabulary was applied to the causation of human actions as modifiers. Such adjectives as proximate, intrinsic, contributory, predisposing, and necessary became coupled with cause. Evaluating the cause of an action became less important than the effect obtained. This is the social trap that seduces unethical conduct into achieving a sought-after transitory, publicized, recognized result. Causation as a moral berm against evil is dissolving surreptitiously. It is being replaced by other representations that masquerade behind the fallacy that everyone is doing it. Critics fall victims to vainglory when they cease to be impartial or assume the destructor's role that makes them scorners of truth.

To achieve momentary success, a temporary heroic admiration, or to bask in the diurnal limelight, many in the critic's seat ignore ethical virtues. Morality does not dominate the daily thinking of those in the communication sciences. Many commentators are suspended like a pendulum between the polarities of the limited known facts and those that are completely unknown. Using a part of factual knowledge they metonymize it into the entire gamut of what should be known. Errors of this sort have found their way into medical writings. Thus that which has a multifactorial etiology is dwarfed into a solitary unit. It equates with phenomenon versus noumenon. The former is defined as anything appearing, observed, or sensed as opposed to real essence. Meaning that a phenomenon is that which may be seen but not understood, whereas noumenon is that which is not seen but one tries to understand (God). To avoid being a destructive critic an honest differentiation between the seen and the imaginary must be made. Laxity in accepting the factual from the unreal is noted frequently in reporting the daily news, in lay and medical journals.

The media coverage of national events proves again and again that some commentators are not unprejudiced, but act like wags, often projecting themselves as termagants who beget dissident criticism. Other supposedly erudite persons, medical and otherwise, display the shilly-shally characteristics of those who arrive at a conclusion after a slapdash survey of the subject. The redeeming feature of many television reports is that they have not become scurrilous thus far but a sedulous attribute remains *in absentia*.

In any critical disputation it is an insuperable, immutable reality in all its multivariegated aspects that a pathetic fallacy is supreme only in its own pathos. It remains feeble because it is fallacious. Therefore as both a prefatory premise and a solemn epiphonema the domain of truth reigns transcendentally over "every natural and just state of the human mind."[1]

Criticism in the interpretation of a wrongdoer may not be a canard. Oftentimes it becomes a personal theory, an hypothesis, even a speculation. Sometimes neither the argument given, nor the critical response presents to the inquiring listener a half-truth, a tarnished truth, or a mustard seed of truth. The best of advocating critics and purposeful disputants can be derailed from the truth by falsity minus syllogistic reasoning. Without factual righteousness the mind can be opened to all flighty, imaginative processes. Many well-known medical writers have diminished their image by adopting the iconoclastic philosophy of misinformation to hide lying and falsehood.

Destructive criticism possesses not a smidgeon tinge of origination. Its deportment is consistent with false virtues and gigantic fallacies. Rare indeed is he/she who can say with Montaigne: "If I am talked of, I wish that it should be truthfully and accurately, I should willingly return from the other world to contradict him who should represent me other than I was, even were it to do me honor."[2] These words could serve well as the motto of those in professional medical reporting which sometimes has become subclinical criticism of a colleague's research. The collegiality of communication sciences should cooperate to diminish the psychosomatic sorrow of humanity that fumes out of the burned ashes of vitriolic, acrid criticism which breeds character assassination.

A lesson may be learned by recalling a quotation from Shakespeare's Othello. Act III, scene 3, line 155 [Iago]:

> Good name in man and woman, dear my lord,
> Is the immediate jewel of our souls:
> Who steals my purse steals trash; 'tis something, nothing;
> 'Twas mine, 'tis his, and has been slave to thousands;
> But he that filches from me my good name

---

1. From the last paragraph of John Ruskin's [1819-1900] *Modern Painters*.
2. Michel Eyquem De Montaigne [1533-1592]

Robs me of that which not enriches him
And makes me poor indeed.

Medical Journalism

When ethical manners are dominant there is no need for an overseer to monitor human behavior. A deviation from the accepted moral pattern of human existence usually is instigated by the desire to be successful. This drive can be entrapment. Sometimes the mirage of success becomes a person's religion to his/her own detriment. In this way an intended virtue is metamorphosed into a disguised vice. Ethical strength is a necessity for any harmoniously conceived literary career in medicine.

Exaggerated medical writing is tainted with ethical misconduct. All scientific research requires deportment that is allied to prudent decorum which in turn is bereft of all editorial intemperance. An ethical conscience in all research means integrity and fairness on the part of the investigator. The analyzed results from laboratory efforts must signify that rigidly correct conclusions have been obtained before being presented for publication in medicosurgical journals. Falsification of medical records in any manner or for any reason is an act abhorrent to the innate purpose of science which is the search for truth.

Sad it is to relate that some scientific literature published in medicosurgical journals is tainted. Other material is worthless as an addition to recorded knowledge. Unfortunately there are more than 30,000 scientific printed journals. Eight thousand are medicosurgical. Each is a competitor with the other in the specific specialties for a preferential place in the library magazine racks. The basis for this plethora is to print the voluminous research manuscripts produced by academicians, university scholars, fellows in medicine/surgery, researchers in pharmaceutical enterprises, and by other biomedical disciplinarians. Those who live by the motto, "publish or perish", know that the avenue to peer recognition, academic promotion, university stature, and financial success is the long litany of accepted published articles listed to their credit as a vital addendum to a *curriculum vitae*.

A purposeful review of medicosurgical magazine publications will unfold that many imperfections contaminate literary efforts. Lack of substantiality, insignificant details, insufficient bibliography are flagrantly visible. Mention must be made of obvious didactic flaws, misquotations,

quotations not recognized, research not credited to prior investigators, printed results known to be scholarly false, and many more deficiencies.

Another tactic tinged with deception is partial presentation of research data in multiple manuscripts. The end to achieve is to squeeze as many publications as practical out of one research effort. Another ploy is to publish scientific investigative results in a series of brief articles of minimum length for editorial acceptance. Complying with publisher's parameters permits multiple individual papers on one subject to be accepted by the board of several scientific journals. Another means of publicity is to condense a segment of a manuscript as a letter to the editor. This is a popular entré into the realm of biomedicosurgical literature. Such practices can dilute the intrinsic merit of bioscientific research.

Present-day scientific writings are highlighted by the many names inscribed as authors, plus the notation that gratitude is expressed to several other persons who prepared, corrected, or otherwise contributed to the final completion of the manuscript. Sometimes more than ten names appear on one published manuscript. It is difficult to determine who is the original researcher, who conceived the project, and the name of the team captain.

Half a century ago most scientific articles were authored by one or two persons who did all the investigative work actually composed the graphs, illustrations, and wordage leading to the final written product. With multiple contributors the intimation is piece-work authorship with one individual not knowing what the others contributed. Multiplicity of authors suggests that probably some of those persons whose names appear under the title do not know the entire content of the paper published.

"Ultimately the damage done to science by the proliferation of papers goes beyond the rare case of flamed research. The breakneck pace at which new journals [appear] forces scientists to wade through [mounds] of inflated studies to find the few that contain relevant information" [Allman, 1988].

No member of the scholarly bioscientific community should restrain his constructive or destructive criticism of evil events known to exist. To do so is to render a disservice to his/her profession. The more unethical medical practices are multiplied, the less the medical profession is esteemed. Calling attention to evil can induce humiliation and/or anger. Incipient, smoldering anger can be restrained, contained, or camouflaged.

Humiliation is more difficult to conceal because it is a giving and taking like a two-way street. The humiliator is powerless in the presence of one who does not play into his/her hands. If the recipient of criticism is by choice immune to humiliation, then the critic is impotent. Thus the recipient of criticism is unresponsive. In this situation the intended criticism is devoid of corrective effectiveness and soon evaporates.

Truth stands stalwart on its immovable pedestal. Truth is immutable, and infinite. Truth moves forward, does not reverse itself. It is equally applicable to all writings, reporting, and spoken words. In *lieu* of presenting the facts about the many national and international issues with which the public could make up its own mind, plain truth is often distorted under many disguises.

Truth has become reportorial opinions. These often are the words of not-so-funny comedians and television persons. Other messages are the opinions of writers who blame the middle or upper class citizens for the distress of the poor, the plight of the homeless, the disquietude of the elderly, and the national debt. This prevails even when distorted truth is virtually impossible to counterattack. If truth is unpopular, defending it places the defender in a position that appears to champion that which is wrong. Because a person has a right to publish something does not mean it is the right thing to do, said Mr. Justice Potter Stewart in one of his opinions. Few persons recall that a dozen Galilean peasants by adhering to the truth overthrew the mighty Roman Empire without striking a single blow.

To be admired, communication science has a major responsibility to adhere to the truth. It is not its inherent self-assumed right to extract, to delete, to exaggerate, to augment, to hyperbolize, or to bowdlerize gathered information in the capacity of author, editor, or book reviewer. By these sluttish acts of redaction it takes upon itself the rôle of impartial critic which more often is aggressively destructive than it is intellectually constructive. Scientific speakers frequently have facial grimaces that belie the thespian smile. Without uttering a comment, their facial expressions reveal the inner self—*infelix sum*[3] and not *gaudeamus in veritate*.[4]

---

3. I am unhappy.
4. Let us rejoice in the truth.

Chapter 6

Firmness Versus Weakness In Bioethics

Willy-nilly political terminology is creeping surreptitiously into the lexicon of medicine. Without meowing the advent of this inveiglement, it is the result of outbursts for cost-containment. Added momentum to this involvement emanates from the recurrent bioethical disputes that have been thrust upon the spumed-up people of medicine. Fremescent financial restraint and bogged moral dilemmas have a common nidus of origin. Both are supplementary outgrowths of expensive medical care that limits treatment resources, plus the exorbitant purchase prices for the technological mechanisms and the personnel required to administer this limited therapeutic armamentarium as to frequency of indicated usage.

Cost containment strives for economic restraint with control of medicosurgical care. Becoming the first consideration, there is danger of curtailing the administration of every therapy available. Detriment to the patient is self-evident. Physicians are no longer leaders in deciding medicosurgical treatment. Deprived of this authority physicians remain culpable for mishaps as the responsible agents under the law of torts. As so-called "Captain of the ship" a physician does not have the final say in how the patient is to be managed. Vital decisions are not made by consensus but by an ethics committee. Delicate decisions made in this manner deprive physicians of leadership but does not exculpate them from medical malpractice. Patients suffer when economic forces influence health care. The financial momentum is an imperative that is being advanced more and more with the passage of time.

There are medical enthusiasts who believe in serving all people of all ages no matter the monetary burden, even if it means governmental, corporative, commercial, or individual bankruptcy. Such physicians believe in the liberal, unrestrained use of medical equipment acquiring more and more thereof to supply the accelerated demand. Contemporaneously these advocates propound the theory that the federal government should assume the rôle of paymaster. In the opposite camp are those physicians and public-spirited citizens who would restrict quantitatively limited medical treatment. This policy of restraint would be founded upon either a "first come first serve" basis or place an age cap on those allowed to receive specialized therapy. Thus costly complex treatment would be held in reserve for those patients outside the geriatric age group.

Nolens volens[1] these latter proponents are the restraining element in the medical cadre. The dogmas of conservatism and that of liberalism traditionally are at antipodes with one another. Nonetheless both claim to be the advocates of liberty and equality in a democratic society. Conservatism does not hold that equality is to be sacrificed for greater liberty—especially for an individual or identifiable group. Liberalism is not restrained in its advocacy of increased liberty at the expense of equality.

Distributive justice, socioeconomic freedom, and legal equality do not condone granting a benefit to one group of citizens at the expense of another group in any category whatsoever. If this was allowed, then the destruction of equality as promulgated in our democracy under the constitutional excerpt that "all men are created equal" would no longer survive. With this reason aforethought the financial duress of extravagant medical care is not a unilateral demand but must become a generalized obligation of unbiased distribution. Otherwise a disparity exists in medicine. This conclusion would be founded upon the imbalanced largess of granting equality and libertine rights hastily in medical discussions to a favored social segment of citizens. A grave decision of this magnitude must not be arrived at hurriedly, because

He rules them yet and ranks them in their haste,
For well he knows disordered speed makes waste.[2]

---

1. Whether one likes it or not.
2. Jerusalem Delivered by Torquato Tasso [1544-1595]

As bioethical confrontations increase with changing patterns, the zone of demarcation between conservatism and liberalism is not distinctly separable. In some moral issues medical liberals cross over the demilitarized line to join the conservative forces when they acknowledge the maldistribution of equality or liberty that creates moral discord.

Preservation Of Life

Fungible conservation/liberalism is manifested most adroitly in the unsolved problems of abortion, euthanasia, assisted suicide, selective termination of pregnancy, and the medicolegal conundrum of ordinary versus extraordinary care. These subjects which on the surface seem to be causes that readily would be espoused by some thinkers are not, because their altruism propels them to defend disadvantaged persons. Who is more powerless than the unborn, the elderly, the comatose, or the critically ill patient? Neither medical conservatives nor scientific liberals blether that "certain lives are not worth living." This is the heinous aspect of abortion, infanticide, suicide, and euthanasia because death is the finale of life. It is irrevocable.

The facility of performing legalized abortions is the *zeitgeist* that prodromals legislative approval of euthanasia. If there is no tweaking of the conscience at the killing of more than a million unborn babies annually, then life is cheapened. With the rising sentiment favoring economy in health costs, the financial onus of employing life-sustaining technology for the critically injured, the moribund, and those with chronic diseases can be ignored with ease. Our planned medical economy has an accentuated fiscal parsimony that clamors for diminished expenditures on health care. Thrift in treating long-term infirmities (especially those of old age) is conducive to the acceptance of euthanasia.

The theme of fiscal ineptitude has been advanced for unwanted pregnancies that terminate in abortion. Many babies are destroyed in order to avoid the responsibility for conception. Monetary limitations are potent excuses for abortion. False thinking has advanced its own cause by stating that if a child can not be brought up in economic circumstances of merit, they should not be allowed to be born. A debate on that issue would be interminable. Succinctly, the elimination of the monetary argument for abortion theoretically would eradicate the major indication for this non-therapeutic procedure. Few knowledgeable bioethicists believe this canard. With the mindset favoring abortion another excuse would be offered to destroy the innocent. Abortion has become the *aide-de-camp* of contraception for those whose moral values are bereft of spiritual enlightenment.

Opinions expressed on euthanasia, abortion, and infanticide are influenced more by the desire to be accepted by professional peers than on the intrinsic moral substance inchoate to those actions. Many people of medicine are uncomfortable if they are not part of the majority group or are not included in the quantitatively greater consensus. Other people of medicine fear being ostracized from the main segment of their professional colleagues as an agitator if they become vociferous in challenging the majority opinion. This has been termed "herd thinking." "George Bernard Shaw wrote that you judge a civilization by how it treats prisoners" [Hentoff, 1987]. You also judge a civilization by how it treats the defenseless, the helpless, the inarticulate, and the unborn.

Medical stalwarts were outraged when experiments at the National Institutes of Health were using tissue from aborted fetuses. Investigators at the institutes were testing fetal organs and tissues in their search for cures of diabetes mellitus, blood dyscrasias, and Parkinsonism. The social conservatives were supported by political liberals as they applauded the administration's ban on the use of tissue from deliberately aborted fetuses. Thinking in science and religion does not oppose research on fetuses from miscarriages or stillbirths, but it does oppose research on deliberately aborted fetuses [Griese, 1988].

Contraception proponents as well as some scientists have been indirect propagandizers for "sex without babies." Now commixtures of morally weak people of medicine look upon the laboratory approach to human creation as a scientific achievement of great satisfaction. In their enthusiasm they have not scented that they are proponents of babies without sex. This is pseudo-parthenogenesis, which deletes the word human in any discourse on the respect for human life. These ephemeral flare-ups in medical research result in pandemonium. Scientific exacerbations of this category defeat the probability that a unanimous palingenesis will eventuate in the thought processes on biological creativity by the majority of bioscientists.

"Reducing humanity to a series of problems to be solved in the laboratory would mean the end of human freedom. To make technical feasibility the 'only law of science' is not progress and freedom in research . . . Humanity denies itself, namely denies an uncontrovertible reality, when it refuses to go beyond the horizon of the laboratory. Such a denial would mean what is personal such as love would become nothing more than beautiful fantasies, psychologically useful, but ultimately unreal and unnecessary. This repudiation would become a 'negation of mankind' which would ultimately lead to 'the idea of God' becoming a mythological discourse without any real content. The nature of faith asks to be respected in the generation of a human being who is not a biological or physiological datum unduly sacralized. This nature is the dignity of the human beings involved . . . Through procreation human beings enter the natural creative act of God."[3]

The above dictum is applicable to the new bioscience methods of reproduction. Reference is specifically intended to include surrogate motherhood, frozen human embryos, and fetal tissue transplants. As scientific technology progresses, the laws and ethical conduct pertaining to it are far behind. Anarchy in thinking among the laity reigns supreme as medical thought is stymied with confusion by lack of harmony on this topic infrequently discussed by bioscientists. Meanwhile frozen embryos in Australia have no parents. In America a young lady desires to become pregnant, abort the baby in order to give the fetal tissue to physicians who will use it in an attempt to save the abortee's father who is ill with Parkinson's disease. "The State of Louisiana has enshrined a positive legal view on this enigma. The law states: an embryo created in vitro fertilization is defined as a person whose 'life' can not be terminated—even by the parents. Ironically, that can result in a situation in which an early-stage embryo in the laboratory has more rights than a fetus in a woman's womb, since the woman has a constitutionally protected right to have an abortion under the U.S. Supreme Court's ruling in the *Roe V. Wade* decision" [Horizons, 1988]. Where are the conservative and liberal scientists to unravel this puzzle? Solomon where is thy sting!

Are biological engineers leading medicine down the corridor to iniquity? The good image of a scientist is founded upon research honesty that seeks unaltered, pure truth. Engineering is scrutinized dichotomously as a science that makes things. Therefore it may seem unjust that "when

---

3. Discourse given by Cardinal Joseph Ratzinger, Congregation for the Doctrine of the Faith, Holy See, Vatican City State, Italy, at the Bioethics Congress, University of Bologna, on the 900th anniversary of the founding of this northern Italian university. Quoted in the Long Island Catholic, Page 5, Thursday, May 12, 1988. Published by the Catholic Diocese of Rockville Centre, Hempstead, L.I., New York.

scientists become engaged in making things—that is, when scientists do engineering—the credit invariably goes to science" [Florman, 1988]. This is an ethical question. Is it the purloining of another profession's talent?

The application of engineering skills to medicine has opened new pathways to the understanding of disease, the treatment thereof, and alterations in their production. Thus medicine's vocabulary has been enhanced by descriptive terms and capital letters with new meanings. It is common to read: "Genetic Marker Testing," "Genetic Engineering," "RFLP Mapping," "DNA Probe Testing," and similar phrases. A new world of medical technology is burgeoning in our generation.

"RFLP mapping makes it possible to localize disease—causing genes and eventually to isolate and characterize them. With the understanding of the biochemistry of diseases comes the ability to treat, control, and—one day perhaps—to eliminate them. Testing and diagnosis of presymptomatic patients through tests already available can provide information critical to this process. Such testing could ultimately benefit countless millions of individuals who are at risk of inheriting or developing one or another of a few thousand genetic diseases" [Friedman, 1989].

Attached to this sterling medical engineering is a saprophytic concern relative to the ethical issues indigenous to genetic testing. Unquestionably ethical issues have arisen concomitantly with the emergence of this biomedical technology. In order to arrive at a realistic conclusion on the ethical propriety of this new venture, a restraining versus accelerating viewpoint has emerged. In the latter group are those who adhere to the credo that any ethical question attached to genetic disease testing must be adapted to the advancing pace of medical engineering. This implies that scientific research takes precedence over any ethical objection to it.

Differing thinking is more restrictive in that it desires to preserve human dignity, personal integrity, and social harmony. Contemporaneously these scientists do not desire to berm researchers whose motivation is the solution to sociomedical problems. This may grow into a dilemma that necessitates a realignment in the relationship between what is proper ethical conduct for bioscientists and the anticipated benefits of medical engineering in general.

Security In Bioscience

There arises in medical circles the protective paternalism that promulgates the concept that some scientific research should be classified as "secret" if it has even a scintilla of security value. Here again the advocates of protectionism are lined up against opponents who see no threat to the universal diffusion of scientific knowledge of all biological genre. Initially it must be accepted that "it is increasingly difficult, if not impossible, to distinguish between 'technology of commercial or security value' and 'scientific information'. In optics, materials science, high-temperature physics, and electronics such distinctions can not be made as they are in molecular biology and biochemistry—maybe not today but probably in another decade" [Delicate Balance, 1989]. The reason for the temporary disinclination to be protective is that bioscience issues have the need to maintain a moral propriety. Other sciences have not touched the personal conscience as yet, however the future may unfold ethical improprieties that will demand sensitive consideration in the "harder", impersonal sciences of physics, chemistry, and engineering.

Medical research does not fall into the category of a top priority secret. Nevertheless the current trend is to safeguard new discoveries until they are protected by copyright or secured by legal publication in a scientific journal or elsewhere. Bioscientific discoveries may find their way clandestinely into the territory of a future antagonist. Distortion of a biological study can be used to the detriment of humanity. Both sides of the controversy are at a standstill "because it is uncertain from whom such information should be protected" [Delicate Balance, 1989].

If scientific discoveries have a military innuendo then national security demands a protective silence with logical obscurity placed over pertinent discoveries. Reference is made to such items as agent orange, use of poison gases, and bacterial warfare. Looking upon a medical discovery as a covert enterprise is alien to scientists who have been traditionally international thinkers eager to share their newly gained knowledge with their universe residing colleagues. They are strong believers in the words of Louis Pasteur: "*La science n'a pas de patrie.*"

No one is in disagreement with the concept of the commercial value of medical/pharmaceutical/prosthetic discoveries/inventions in the laboratories of many universities. Such scientific innovations have launched academia into the transnational, multimillion dollar corporate scene. University manufacturing companies that patented their biological/chemical discoveries, do not share its mantra which remains cloaked under a still-strong internationally identifiable security.

A concern for protectionism is becoming more inclusive and vaguely diffused as a rationale for restraining the exchange of scientific information. Under the guise of security, prudential restraint is placed upon almost everything that has a potential for power. Thus secrecy surrounds all technological, medicosurgical innovations that can give supremacy to industrial competitiveness. Under this form of mental orientation, economic goals are confused unnecessarily with therapeutic imperatives. Such factors attack bioethical stamina.

It can be appreciated that some guardians of security might in the future be prepared to suppress scientific information—say, about the incidence of AIDS, the effects of acid rain, or relative contributions to the greenhouse effect in order to protect an international image. In the struggle to maintain freedom of scientific communication, victories are at best temporary. Thus it is that an exchange of views on a national policy becomes out of date before it is transferred to the printed page.

Chapter 7

The Song Of Death

Questions are posed by many of those disconcerted with the too many betrayals and desertions in bioethics together with the obscurity to which it has been condemned. Denial is forceful that any relationship between bioscience and spirituality is needed. The formlessness of the latter in scientific echelons permits no discernment of guilt as a moving directional force to good science. At the crossroads between scientific power and the renunciation of bioethics, the religious knight of morality falls wounded while answering the summons for assistance. The greater the power reached by science the steeper the decline in bioethics. So it appears.

Decisive words engraved in the granite of history stress that science is not able to abolish faith, religion, and God. Medical tradition as it has been understood, bequeathed a legacy that provides criteria for discrimination and evaluation of what is good in the profession with the discarding of everything that is not good. Chivalry in the art and science of medicine finds its champion in bioethics. Whenever the instinct for the nobility of medicine is extinguished, no longer is there the desire for that moral orderliness which respects the great laws of life. "Despite the travails of modern life, the quest for a nobility of spirit continues to embolden the hearts of men" [Von Balthasar, 1997].

Direct Abortion

The chronological history of legalized abortion and the innumerable controversies created by the 1973 Roe vs. Wade decision is a redundant narrative. Added to the multiple perturbations is the anger aroused at the slightest mention of this murderous subject. Any defense for performing an abortion on healthy, normal, unborn babies to please a mother defies human understanding. Physicians studied to preserve life not to destroy it. Involuntarily by dint of an inability to avoid the subject, the world has listened to theorists, economists, sociologists, demographists, and scientists. All their excuses for the need of an abortion are not convincing. Applicable to most of what they have said and written is floccinaucinihilipilification.[1]

Bioscientists' peccant moral flux is unexplainable but is defended as adhering to up-dated theories, hypotheses, and practicality. The most egregious attitudes are favoring abortion and euthanasia which aim at the murder of the youngest and the oldest innocent human beings. Added to the tenuous etiology of this ebbing in morality is the relinquishment of religious belief and the economic imperatives that do not require self-denial and sacrifice. Such thoughts foster a despicable climate of hatred that is deadly when the severity of the odium intensifies.

"Newspapers reported that an Illinois nurse was charged with murder after using prescription medication to put her three children to sleep and then suffocating them. This incident is as equally tragic as the 1996 drowning of two children by a South Carolina woman who then tried to tell the police they had been kidnapped" [Washington Times, 1999].

The legalization of abortion by the Supreme Court's decision in 1973 gave popularity to the phrases: "a woman's right to choose" and "I can do with my body what I want". Both statements became the trade mark of abortion rightists. This foul abhorrence brought about an immoral atmosphere in which women feel free to destroy children with the same ease as those who actively perform abortions. When children become an inconvenience to parents they are abandoned or destroyed. "Murder, child abuse, and abortion have increased about 50 percent since Roe vs. Wade. That is not a coincidence [Washington Times, 1999].

"If that argument seems ridiculous, then it's no less ridiculous than arguments that link the murder of gay student Matthew Shepard to church-initiated statements about the morality of sexual behavior. If these statements help create a "climate of hate," then why don't the numerous

---

1. A word coined by Senator Daniel Patrick Moynihan [D-NY] for the estimation of something as being valueless, useless, and disdainful.

legal and ecclesiastical statements about a "woman's right to choose" create the same climate of hate against born and unborn children? If we're going to make "climate of hate" arguments, then let's apply them equally in all climates" [Sumner, 1999].

Trustworthy conscience demands ripostes to abortion advocates. To enmire them is to emphasize that the Supreme Court ruling on the legality of abortion does not metamorphose abortion into a morally permissible act. It was a damp, dark, cloudy, stormy day of infamy when the majority decision was read. From that date onward the Supreme Court was not worthy to be carried on a palanquin. Hendiadys[2] repeated reminds the forgetful of consummate objections to this execrable decision. Considered by many juridical intellectuals as a trumped up, unfairly aligned basis to the right of privacy the Roe case is falsely founded upon the constitution.

The Supreme Court majority opinion did not adhere strictly to the written maxims of the constitution as authored. Placing abortion and privacy in the same legal pantheon is an absurdity. *De facto* having an abortion may be considered a private matter, especially as to culpability, but abortions are not performed in the privacy of a mother's bedroom. Public facilities, and licensed clinics are the places where the deeds are done. States and the Centre for Disease Control and Prevention keep public records of the number of reported abortions done and the complications pertinent to the procedures.

A former Surgeon General of the United States when questioned on the abortion issue made an imprudent statement that abortion was a backup for failed contraception. "Nearly half of all pregnancies in the United States this year, excluding miscarriages, will be unintended, or aborted . . . many insurance plans still do not cover contraceptives . . . 49 percent of indemnity plans have no coverage for contraceptives . . . only 15 percent of indemnity plans cover all five of the leading reversible methods which are oral contraceptives, intrauterine devices, Norplant, Depo Provera, and diaphragms. All five approved prescription methods would be covered under the Equity in Prescription Insurance and Contraceptive Coverage Act which was re-introduced recently in Congress.

---

2. Hendiadys is a classical figure of speech common in the Bible, Greek, and Latin literature in which 2 words are employed to convey one idea—a favorite style of consummate classicists.

The act would require any insurance plan that covers prescription drugs to cover these birth-control methods" [Melani, 1999]. "It does not take a rocket scientist to figure out that pregnancy . . . costs far more than a pack of pills" [Reinisch, 1999]. Such is the state of moral affairs in this unenlightened age of negative morality.

If payment for birth-control modalities is being advanced, unnecessary surgery to accomplish the same results is not far behind. Specific reference is made to vasectomy and Fallopian tube ligation/resection. An example is found in the privately funded program that pays $200 to drug-addicted women to get their tubes tied or use some other long-term means of birth-control [Irvine, 1999].

"The California-based program has drawn the wrath of critics, who call it short-sighted, racist, and a source of drug money for users . . . [supporters] say this is a response to a system that often fails to punish women who give birth to drug-addicted babies. Inquiries have been made by men who seek vasectomies with similar request for payment. The program does not pay for male procedures, although they are often covered by state-funded health care programs" [Harris, 1999]. "Coercing women by bribing them with cash is not the way to go about it" [Trombley, 1999].

As an addendum, there are advocates of the morning after pill which is not a safeguard against pregnancy. This hormonal pill is prescribed to be taken within 72 hours after coitus to prevent fertilization of the ovum or, if it occurs, prevent implantation of the embryo in the uterus. Fertilization of the ovum in the fallopian tube is pregnancy. Five to seven days after fertilization, the new human being arrives in the cavity of the uterus where it is implanted in the wall. As to the "morning after pill", when it blocks implantation, its action is the same as any other abortifacient. Therefore this drug is not a secure preventative against pregnancy. It does not reduce the number of abortions but by its failure it increases them.

Selective Termination Of Pregnancy

"We all know that it was not an apple that was the core of the problem for Adam and Eve. They ate the fruit of the Tree of the Knowledge of Good and Evil on the serpent's promise that they would be like God

"Not enough of us remember, though, that there was another forbidden tree in the Garden—the Tree of Life. It was precisely to prevent

Adam and Eve from snatching the ultimate prerogative—the power over life and death—that occasioned their expulsion from Paradise.

"Today's Adams and Eves still want to be like God, determining who shall live and who shall die. They snatch at the tree of abortion and euthanasia, of war and violence, accepting too readily the killing of one human being to solve the problems of other human beings.

"Each day, the Christian community turns its attention to these age-old attacks on God's gift of life. This attention is not something new in our faith, but it has a special urgency as millions of children's lives are sacrificed to abortion, as more nations and states in our nation justify the killing of the elderly and ill, and as nations seem intent on squandering, through the re-emergence of ethnic and mercenary armed action, what might well be a wonderful opportunity for a peaceful order in the world.

"In light of these two trees in the Garden—or perhaps in the thoughtfulness and prayer of their shade—we have reflected on our successes in the re-establishment of respect for human life. And successes there have been, in the courts, in state legislatures, and especially in the hearts of people" [O'Donnell, 1991]. With the commencement of 2001, it is estimated that 45 million abortions have been performed. Many more are unrecorded.

Even the calm, stoic, imperturbable British were shocked, angered, and bewildered when newspapers published the account of a young, supposedly mature, English woman who desired to have a selective abortion of one of two babies in her womb [Chicago Tribune, 1996]. Her excuse was that she could not afford to raise more than one child [Aitkinhead, 1996]. A few days after the announcement the Queen Charlotte's Hospital in London disclosed that the announced termination had been performed over three months ago [Herald, 1996]. This has given vent to anger of the abuse of abortion under the law [Ibrahim, 1996].

Elective Fetal Reduction is also termed Selective Social Termination.[3] Called by any name it is an elective direct abortion. It is a procedure by which one or more fetuses are aborted with the other or others allowed to remain in the uterus [Rorty, 1996]. The indication for the abortion is primarily a socioeconomic, nonmedical excuse. "Most multiple pregnancies, especially those in which there are three or more fe-

---

3. Known as multi-fetal pregnancy reduction when multiple fetuses are present.

tuses are iatrogenic as a result of the use of infertility drugs and/or insemination or *in vitro* fertilization and the transfer of multiple embryos" [Crossley, 1996]. Such multiplicity is a complication of the interference with the normal physiological process of biological reproduction.

There is no ethical difference in performing an abortion for multiple pregnancies and a single abortion procedure. The number is irrelevant as to the intrinsic evil of abortion. This continues to be an immoral, unethical obstetrical operation even if it contradicts some spokespeople representing medical specialty organizations. Using expressions such as "not the result of negligence or poor planning as are most abortions. Moreover, the high cost and risk associated with attempting to carry a multiple pregnancy to term distinguishes the issues involved from those in a single abortion procedure" [ACOG, 1992]. No ethical struggle involving selective termination of life is needed to arrive at the conclusion that, even with an approbation of a sympathetic public favoring it, abortion is immoral and is not to be performed by any physician.

Brain Death: Coma

Controversy persists and doubt exists when a comatose patient on life-support apparatus is declared brain-dead. Is the patient truly dead, dying or alive? There are neuroscientists who contend that cessation of brain function is not the equivalent of somatic death. "Because one of the reasons for determining death based on brain-related criteria is to allow organ removal and transplantation. It is imperative from the moral point of view to be able to determine beyond any doubt that the person from whom vital organs are to be removed is truly dead. For someone who is not dead before vital organ removal will surely be dead after their removal" [Evers, Byrne, 1990].

The emergence of organ transplantation requires new criteria for death certification. The basic problem centers on irreversible coma. In defining this pathophysiological state criteria are needed for its recognition. The definition of irreversible coma was translated into brain death [Harvard definition, 1988]. Most medicolegalists accept brain death as being identical to death of the person. The Uniform Determination of Death Act [UDDA] is specific in its definition of death. "An individual who has sustained either irreversible cessation of circulatory and respiratory functions, or irreversible cessation of all functions of the entire brain, including the brain stem, is dead. A determination of death must be made in accordance with accepted medical standards" [UDDA, 1990].

Brain death is not euthanasia. It is a medical diagnosis made by physicians in accordance with strict medical requirements. Legislatures and courts, while adopting the concept of brain death, have left its determination to the medical profession. Ultra-sophisticated medical technology and fine technique in vital organ transplantations have added a moral dimension to life's final certainty. Physician-members of organ transplant teams are not permitted to pronounce dead a patient from whom anatomical organs are to be removed [Colburn, 1985].

Neomorts

Medical challenges and newer surgical opportunities are foretold for the third millennium. Accompanying expectations will raise moral questions now unknown. With these awaited medicosurgical blessings no veiled, undefined ethical misalignments are to be minimized. Needed ethical guidelines must be available for those engaged in these brave, brazen, formidable professional enterprises. Reinventing ethical codes to special events may not be needed. Alliance of old codes and existing regulatory doctrines to meet the unseen situations can be synthesized into a formula that is a model for the future.

This proposal should produce adamant responses that will deluge negative reactions. The ethical, educational module can be customized to address and solve specific moral issues. Hopefully, commencing a new millennium augurs favorably for a perpetual vitality that will infuse into the biosciences the best of everything pertinent to professional conduct.

Medicosurgical technology by its importance must assist in widening the range of influential bioethics. As technology delivers more kinds of medical services, the greater the necessity for its adherence to acknowledged ethical documents. From this attachment to ethics comes the tranquility and equanimity that gives quietness to professional composure which is conducive to superb medicosurgical performances.

The above three paragraphs are suggestive of a prologue which they may be to the discussion of neomorts. Ethicists have given profound thought to the confrontation on the medical use of brain dead patients. Dramatically a patient is pronounced dead. The body is not taken to the morgue but it is rushed into an operating room where artificial life-support systems are in place to receive the "deceased". Here the heart and lungs are revived. The body functioning, the person is not alive but brain dead.

"These 'living' dead, called neomorts, can exist for up to two weeks while researchers use them to test new medical procedures and to store organs for transplantation. Neomorts, however, must have died recently, and their bodies must be relatively undamaged and disease-free, to be of any use. Doctors call the wards 'neomortoriums'—a cross between a morgue and an operating room. The idea of neomorts has raised ethical and religious concerns that doctors now are beginning to discuss. Opponents have likened the process to a Frankenstein movie, envisioning mad scientists bringing the dead back to life.

"Doctors say there is nothing sinister about it. Neomorts are people who legally have died and have no chance of being revived, unlike comatose patients. People wind up as neomorts only if they grant doctors permission before their death to use their body for science or if their families give permission when the patient has not specified any wishes.

"Scientists say neomorts give doctors a chance to test new drugs and medical procedures before they use them on living patients. Neomorts are a source of transplantable organs and provide storage place for organs until a recipient can be found. They also help surgeons learn new medical techniques as well as substitute for some of the more than 90 million animals used for scientific research each year.

"Dr. Willard Gaylin, president of the Hastings Center in New York, a think tank of medical experts which debates ethical issues, proposed the idea of using neomorts in medicine in an article he published in 1974. The proposal was so controversial experts swept it under the rug, hoping to avoid any public outcry. But in 1981, surgeons at Temple University in Philadelphia put the Jarvik-7 artificial heart into the functioning bodies of five brain-dead people to test ways to implant the device.

"Dr. Jack Kolff, chief of cardiothoracic surgery at Temple and principle investigator during the neomort surgery, said doctors probably would not have been able to successfully implant the artificial heart in Seattle dentist Barney Clark in 1982 if they had not practiced on neomorts" [Salamone, 1986].

The director of the University of Florida's Medical Humanities Program who teaches bioethics to medical students said: It is no different than giving a body to science [Moseley, 1986].

In cases where a pregnant woman is brain-dead, doctors have kept the body functioning with life support systems so the fetus can develop. Surgeons preparing for organ transplants also have kept neomorts' bodies functioning until doctors could remove the organs [Salamone, 1986].

Added to the bioethical propriety are some medicolegal questions. Do neomorts fall under the restrictions of the existing laws regulating organ donation as the Anatomical Gift Act? Some states have property rights over a deceased relative which entails signing documents that legally transfer ownership. Analytical questioning leaves unanswered who is to balance family wishes and society's needs for human organs?

Euthanasia

The etymological origin of the word euthanasia is found in the Greek *eu*, good + *thanatos*, death. The good death theme is common knowledge as a result of the publicity it has received universally. Obviously all physicians do not agree on this good death plan. As usual there are two camps: advocates of euthanasia and its opponents. Opinions may vary but it is reasonable that this word should not be applied to the dying when the question of medical intervention or surgical non-intervention arises. When medicosurgical treatment is known to be futile and it is not given justifiably, the words passive euthanasia are applied inappropriately.

"Euthanasia is the deliberate action to terminate life by someone other than, and on the request of, the patient concerned" [Definition given by the Netherland's State Commission on Euthanasia in 1985. Cited in H. Rigter]. Pro-euthanasia argument based on decisions not to treat a dying patient has been termed aid-in-dying. It disguises more than it reveals. There are lawyers and physicians who state that there should be immunity for the physician that kills a patient, when the action fulfills certain conditions [Harvard Law Review, 1992]. This is to preserve the medical professions ethical image.

Momentous public debates on euthanasia has not only an ethical concern but legal, religious, psychological, and medical implications. Bioethicists are in the lead command to reach every audience they can to convey arguments against euthanasia effectively. It is the obligation of bioethicists to encompass all who should participate in the euthanasia debate which must include the public [Wolf, 1992]. The message is that euthanasia is wrong, morally abhorrent, and physicians who advance it are Hippocratically unethical.

Some professional people perceive the need for euthanasia as being a part of or the result of modern medical technology. To keep alive patients who in past generations under the same circumstances would be dead may be a medical challenge. Others may have the sensation of power over life and mastery over death [Fenigsen, 1989]. Using complex technology to prolong life may have some hidden desire to use it to shorten life. There is no need for any medical technology to kill. It seems to use anything medical for this purpose is to foster an ironic, incongruous oxymoron.

Magnificent developments in medical technology have given rise to the secularization of humanity and perhaps to a distorted vision of human beings as created by God [De Wachter, 1992]. "For instance, transplantation may mean that we no longer each see our self as one, integral whole, but as a collection of interchangeable parts, which translates into a modular theory of human identity" [M.A. Somerville in Shea and Spadafora, 1992]. This theory has mechanistic connotations which may also be linked to the increasing number of persons who regard euthanasia as acceptable. "We are, in general, unsentimental about disposing of out-dated, worn out, or no-longer-efficient machines, at least in some respects, we may apply this same attitude to ourselves and others. Euthanasia could be an expression in practice of such an attitude [Somerville, 1992].

The theoretical, not impossible, pragmatic connection of euthanasia with a mechanistic approach to persons is related to irresistible consumerism which characteristically disposes of worn-out mechanical items or useless products. What is not discarded results in a net overall economic loss. "If we see ourselves simply as products or cogs in the wheel of production in a consumer society, then, once we are no longer valuable products or producers, according to the dictates of a strict consumer philosophy we would need to be disposed as cheaply and efficiently as possible. Although euthanasia is promoted as a merciful response and most of those who advocate it have this as a primary aim, it does not fit within this consumer philosophy" [Somerville, 1993].

Furthermore, the practice of euthanasia, itself, could be seen as consistent with the philosophy of a consumer society, because it means that "death becomes a matter of management" [De Wachter, 1992]. Associating euthanasia with consumerism is faulty and illogical. The economic analogy referring to discarding the old for the new is forged in frailty. Killing dying patients leaves a void that is not filled with new-born babies. Abortion is the berm against replacement. Death reaps its harvest at both extremes of the human spectrum because of human selfishness, negligent vigilance of bioethics, and flawed law.

This is why and how Dr. Kevorkian resorted to a suicide machine which was given a trademarked name, the Thanatron [Hister, 1991]. After several successful uses of the patented Thanatron, legislation has been passed in Michigan making it a crime to assist a person to commit suicide [Act 84, *Public Acts of 1992*, 1992 Michigan ALS 84, 1992, P.A.84; 1992 Michigan HB5501]. Even when continued life is devoid of any enjoyment, the physician/surgeon has the ethical responsibility not to assist in terminating it. Euthanasia contributes to more of the moral decline so diffuse in this age of scientific pride. Nothing in this death wish is a moral advancement. The melody of life has lyrics of love. The song of death is cacophony.

Redefining treatment protocols has its proposers and protagonists. When presenting physician-assisted suicide as therapy, it is advanced as an ethically justifiable form of care for the terminally ill. Such is the assault on traditional ethics which once assumed that the saving of every individual's life was medicine's highest concern. A priority that was primary from the baby in the womb to the elder at his tomb.

Publications, discourses, rhetorical outbursts against this ancient ideal are repetitious. The constant continuance of which remains a parody. Hypocrisy arises from these diatribes that pays tribute to vice and erases virtue. If bioethics is thrown away, the culture of death will be accepted easily. Then medical care givers will cease to be angels of mercy and metamorphose into apocalyptic agents of death whose redemption is uncertain.

Chapter 8

Bioethics In Practice

Morality is the nucleus from which bioethics grows and multiplies. Out from morality comes trust, reliability, and the faith that nourishes the physician-patient relationship. Ethical demeanor is never irreverent to moral codes. No matter the professional talent which enables a bioscientist to acquire fame, public adoration, and material honors, if the work-done is tainted, it has neither merit nor value.

Immoral mischief is repetitious not a solitary fleeting innovation. These annoyances can disturb the keenest mind. Appropriate usage of the brain does not mar it. Contrarily, misuse disturbs its gray matter. Veering away from ethical perfection may not derail competency but it is conducive to factious heresy against morality. Making correct bioethical decisions is more than a probability. Especially when deductions are derived from lucent, logical reasoning arrived at by precise knowledge learned by extraction from scientific information. Thus is avoided rendering a decision that seemed correct at the time made but actually was wrong. Inaccurate, poor decisions are derived from misinformation, miscalculation, miscommunication, and misdiagnosis.

Intellectual bioethical decisions are the symbol of excellent moral achievement. Which by its moral force provides a *stare decisis*[1] in the

---

1. *Stare decisis* is a Latin phrase for: to abide by or adhere to decided law cases. Policy of courts to stand by precedent and not to disturb a settled point [Neff vs. George, 364 Illinois 306, 4 NE 2d 388, 390, 391]. It is an established legal doctrine that, when the court has laid down a principle of law as applicable to a certain state of facts, it will adhere to that principle, and apply it to all

right direction away from deviant philosophies. Mental, emotional imagery is the manufacturer of the agglutinins that make susceptibility to immorality very facile. Avoiders of maleficence develop traits of passel boldness, independent brio, and vigor against bioethical infringements. Contemporary social structure challenges moral values, ethics, and time-honored principles. Congeners for veracity are the staunchest supporters of wholesome bioethics.

Transgressions In Bioscience

Within the purview of biology there is an increasing trend for the acquisition of chemistry and engineering into its ranks. These new arrivals are now ancillary disciplines to bioscience. Autogenously in their own spheres each did not have the same need as the biosciences to decide ethical problems. Chemistry and engineering have no serious encounters with magnitudinous ethical contretemps that impede their advancements and performances.

By comparison it is factual that mathematical disciplines are not threatened by the same moral hazards as confront bioscience. All sciences give intellectual vigor to society as each contributes to the culture of the world. In this way ethical ideals are assimilated perfecting a nation's refinement. An opposite influence results when ethics is weakened, impoverished or mortified.

An undetected ethical ploy in bioscience is replicated with ease when dour accountability is lacking. Repetitious reduplication hardens the conscience against the sensitivity aroused by wrongdoing. Dreadful acts detour from guiding signals against them. Not ruing the evil day, the aptest perpetrator believes corrective criticism is a form of envy or is the product of rancor and vindictiveness.

In the philosophical region of medical judgment, particularly those involving ethical solutions, the reports and opinions presented are not always exceptional archetypes. A physician may not consistently rely

---

future cases, where facts are substantially the same, regardless of whether the parties and property are the same [Horne vs Moody, Texas Civil Ct. Appeals, 146 S W 2d 505, 509, 510]. *Stare decisis* is the authority, or binding precedent in the same court or in other courts of equal or lower rank [State vs Mellenberger, 163 Oregon 233, 95 P 2d 709, 719, 720].

upon his/her own educated conscience in arriving at bioethical conclusions. To be accepted by colleagues, to maintain an academic position, to secure hospital staff appointments/advancements, and innate weakness of character some physicians stray from their consciences' directives. Without a highly acclaimed bioethical code of honor a physician becomes a shopkeeper of medicine minus the *imprimatur*[2] of professionalism.

> Which may be called the ethical process, the end of which is not the survival of the fittest of those who may happen to be the fittest . . . but of those who are ethically the best.
>
> Thomas Henry Huxley [1825-1895]

Moral Medicine

In the time of Hippocrates morality for the physician was simple, concise, and didactic. He stated its essence in one sentence: "I will preserve the purity of my life and my art." For the physician of today, a question of conscience is involved in his professional life more often than is recognized. Many results of a medical decision may be remote as to time but the effect may be vast. Major questions to answer emanate from earnest efforts to do what is good—the best for the patient. The problem to be solved is not only a matter of avoiding an evil action but also of fostering good. Because of current malleable morality the net good or bad effect may be so remote, the present generation neither sees nor presages it.

With its indigenous ethical restrictions the art of medicine has in it from the time of origin an eternal quality for good derived from its selflessness. Physicians while obtaining a medical history look into the hearts and minds of patients at a time when they are most vulnerable. Even as Hippocrates brought into his practice of medicine a code of ethics, so all his descendant, modern-day colleagues must bring into their rushed professional lives a reasoned, faithfully accepted morality. Without which the aura of medicine will evanesce into nothingness as a highly respected discipline.

---

2. *Imprimatur* is Latin for: let it be printed meaning an official sanction after censorship and redaction [an approval].

Understandably, the physician's life has many complexities inchoate to the acquired knowledge of medicine, surgery, and its various specialties. Doctors of medicine are encased in many restrictions labeled standards of practice. These have arisen from within and without their profession. Legal rules and regulations add additional *caveats* to the labyrinthine maze. Although confined in this globe of reservations every act is visible to the world. A doctor's responsibility extends not only to individual patients but to their families, and civil society. Each has placed their own demand for the performance of professional duties as well as expecting his/her full cooperation. Physicians are expected to follow the *mores* of humanity and to participate in those activities which improve the health, welfare, education, and the social growth of society of which he is a respected component. The moral physician is not three people as described by the French poet La Fontaine[3] who wrote: "A man is three people: what people think he is, what he thinks he is, and what he really is." Bioscientists must be what they have been trained to be.

Unnecessary Surgery

By training and daily activity in the operating theatre surgeons see what they are doing supposedly with clearer eyes than non-surgical physicians. This objectivity teaches the moral superiority of honesty to reality which if they do not perceive with integrity can bring about morbidity and mortality to patients. For surgeons, moral-based ethical performance appeals to golden immortality. As a specialty surgery does not usually clash with regularity. It is harmonious with the reverent, old-fashioned scenes in its historic drama. The splendor of surgery is not deceived for long by the foo-fa-raw ornamentation that entices temporarily.

Once surgeons were led down this pathway by psychiatrists. Both had good intentions. The end-result was not. This sad misadventure ceased in the 1950s. Known as psychosurgery the promise of its value was turned into a sorrow for many patients. The term psychosurgery was the amalgamation of psychiatry with surgery. It meant brain surgery done primarily for behavior control rather than for removal of pathologic tissue. "In Oregon . . . the law defines psychosurgery as 'any operation

---

3. Jean De La Fontaine [1621-1695] poet attendee at the court of Louis XIV

designed to irreversibly destroy brain tissue for the primary purpose of altering the thoughts, emotions or behavior of a human being'" [Zakowski, 1976]. Neurological surgery does injure brain tissue when procedures are done to remove brain tumors. Other neurosurgical operations destroy tissue when treating epileptic foci, Parkinsonism, and certain other syndromes.

Annals of history records the first published account of a similar procedure that appeared in 1891. Modern psychosurgery is considered to have begun in 1935 at the instigation of Egas Moritz, a Portuguese neurologist, who was awarded the Nobel Prize. He was credited with the discovery of prefrontal leucotomy [lobotomy] as having therapeutic value in certain psychoses [Zukerman, 1977].

The popularity of this procedure declined from 1935 to 1950. By 1960 it was unnecessary and disappointing. Increased awareness of the side-effects, combined with the advent of the psychoactive drugs, tranquilizers, and other medications hastened the demise of this procedure leading to its eventual discreditation. Even during its brief sought after acclaim public outcry questioned the uses of psychosurgery. The protests made it an extremely controversial technique which was marked as useless, dangerous, fraught with perilous complications, and unpredictable side-effects. Demands were made for governmental control of the procedure because of its social and moral implications that were outside the realm of medicine.

Currently there are discussions on influencing brain activity. This is by implantable brain chips which has aroused ethical issues of deep concern. The plan is to insert computer chips in the human brain. They would act as sensors or actuators. These would assist the blind, those with momory loss, and others with hearing impairment. Working in concert on this development [termed nanotechnology] are bioengineers, computer scientists, and neurological surgeons. The basic plan is to connect designated properly, neural tissue with microcomputers. An artificial vision system is contemplated by using an ultra-small television camera with an ultrasonic distance sensor [McGee, Maguire, 2001].

To the selected segment of the brain that pertains to anatomic specific function, platinum electrodes are implanted on the surface of the brain's visual cortex that are attached to a microcomputer which triggers impulses. Implantable brain chips are not undesirable assets to the disabled. Such mechanical interventions are not controversial as therapeutically permissible. Bioethical questions may arise when selection is necessary regarding who is to receive the apparatus. As well as questions of equity costs for the technology and its surgical installation. Misuse of implantable brain chips is a threat to personal dignity if the results impair the intellect and control free-will which can take place. Under the control of unethical and immoral people this technology can bring havoc to a person so wired and victimize other persons. The sinister prospects for invasion of privacy and restriction of liberty are alarming [Headlam, 2000] [Thomas, 1996].

Some surgeons have the reputation of being quick with the scalpel. Justified or not there is no exact method of determining the validity of the allegation. Surgeons are guided by ethical parameters. Violations of which have their own means of adding more distress to a troubled conscience. Not to mention the blemishing of reputation and the tarnishing of character.

Unnecessary surgery is self-explanatory. It is performing a surgical operation that was not needed or removing a normal anatomical organ with knowledge aforethought that no disease existed as an indication for the surgery undertaken. Such actions are morally wrong. Gynecologists are in that position when a hysterectomy may not be indicated for uterine fibroids. A responsibility arises to preserve a uterus whenever possible rather than be hasty to remove it.

For publication there are surgeons who amass a volume of procedures to sanction conclusions founded on statistics. This desire may persuade judgment in the wrong direction when deciding to do or not to do a surgical procedure. By the number of procedures performed the surgeon can claim his accumulated experience allows him to certain conclusions which may be presented as a contribution to bioscience. If it is an experience based on errors it is an unethical conclusion. Only experience founded upon true knowledge, gained honestly, is commendable. Experience supported by error and repeated erroneously is false experience clouded with danger. No surgeon should perform unnecessary surgery purposefully. Liability is not directed at operations resulting from an honest mistake in diagnosis. Diagnostic error with honesty does not condemn surgical intervention especially when an acute abdominal disease is suspected.

Qualifying certificates attest to a surgeon's training, but it does not verify that he is, but should be, a morally upright person who strictly upholds the highest esteem of bioethics. A surgeon is tested at the operating table where his two hands and one mind are united synergistically to form the trinity of perfections which imprint with the seal of approval the mark of surgical excellence. These are the mental, moral, and mechanical attributes which are the instrumentalities of surgery. The first is knowledge, the second judgment, and the third surgical technique. Fortunate indeed is the surgeon who possesses these three attributes. This triune perfection with an incorruptible conscience is the badge of courage and skill for all surgeons to wear [Ficarra, 1968]. Because a "[g]ood name in man and woman dear my lord, is the immediate jewel of their souls: Who steals my purse steals trash; 'tis something nothing; 'Twas mine, 'tis his, and has been slave to thousands; but he that filches from me my good name robs me of that which not enriches him and makes me poor indeed" [Iago in Shakespeare's Othello].

Unneeded surgery is a luxury undergone for career reasons. A classical example is found in the *castrati*. These are boys whose testicles are removed [orchidectomy]. Castration is performed to preserve the purity of their voices into adulthood. Also called countertenors, a preferential designation in the operatic world, they are men who train their natural tenor or high baritone voices to sound like a woman's soprano or high alto voice. Although a falsetto sound, it is more supple and functional as a musical instrument.

Countertenors originated in the ancient Church's structure that did not permit women to participate in its religious services. High notes had to be sung. Boys could reach them but not when adulthood arrived. To preserve the soprano cantor, removal of the testicles was the solution. Strong, flexible high voice was preserved.

Castrati became well-known opera stars. At age-fourteen, Wolfgang Amadeus Mozart [1756-1791] wrote his opera *Mitridate re di Ponto* for three superstar castrati of his day. Even when women crossed the barrier that kept them out of the music world, there were composers who continued to write for countertenors. "The current vogue for countertenors is like many trends based on historical practices. It owes more to overzealous musicologists than real music lovers. The great Johann Sebastian Bach's *Passions* and other baroque music rendered by boys yelping have sounded a lot better when great female singers sang them. It remains true today, despite the high quality of the male voices available to sing them" [Innaurato, 1999].

Castration is invasive surgery. When done for economic reasons it is quasi-mutilation. The procedure is not done as a therapeutic measure. Hence it is not necessary either to preserve life or regain health. Most surgeons would not remove normal testicles. This decision resides in the intellectual, moral stamina of the surgeon who with right reason and honest conscience believes it is not necessary.

The same dictum is applicable to interventional cardiology. Many physicians wonder if all the cardiac procedures are pathophysiologically indicated. "In the last seventeen years cardiovascular procedures have increased 355 percent" [Lahey Clinic Magazine, 1999]. Cardiac catheterization is central to interventional cardiovascular medicine. But is it being overdone?

Introduced in 1977, balloon angioplasty uses a catheter to reach the obstructed section within the coronary artery. A second catheter with a balloon tip is passed inside the first catheter. The balloon is inflated to enlarge the artery and increase blood flow. Then the device is deflated and removed. Each year approximately 650,000 angioplasties are done. Are they all justified?

Stent procedures are increasing in frequency. A stent is a small expandable metal tube that is inserted like an angioplasty balloon catheter. It is advanced into the area of the blockage within the artery. When it is deployed, the stent is expanded, locked in place forming a rigid tunnel that keeps the artery patent. In 1996 in this nation 177,000 stents were inserted into human hearts [Lahey Clinic, 1999]. All were said to be necessary.

When arteries in the heart are diminished in caliber or blocked by cholesterol and other fatty substances, high-speed rotational atherectomy has been advocated. Approved about ten years ago by FDA it uses a rotating burr device. It is a catheter-apparatus threaded through the body to the blocked artery where it grinds the plaque into minuscule particles which pass out of the artery with the blood circulation.

Many other cardiovascular procedures are available for treating patients who have heart diseases. The seriousness of these illnesses frightens the patient who places all trust in the physician. Hence it is easy to induce a patient to consent to a cardiac procedure that is not necessary. Conscience must not become hardened to eliminate what is right due to pressure from haste and to keep productivity moving. When medicosurgical competency embraces a high respect for morality, bioethics is not impugned but is part of a therapeutic regimen.

In relationship with unnecessary surgery are excessive consultations and laboratory studies. More than is required of both often is a safeguard against malpractice. Easily this becomes an excuse not a valid reason. Multiple unwarranted consultations and repetitious laboratory procedures is an unethical practice by the physician who requests them.

Obstetrics And Gynecology

The study and treatment of diseases in women have become a highly specialized field in medicine. Since 1973 their legal right to perform abortions has disunited this specialty. It seems to some that obstetricians have defeated their own purpose as a specialty which is to deliver babies. Abortion dismisses empirically the procreative nature of womanhood as the fullest expression of femininity. Simultaneously it deprives women of their natural ability to participate in this feminine gift that is the continuance of human society.

Obstetricians and gynecologists should not encourage patients to do anything that violates her conscience. It is the moral obligation of these specialists to have primary regard for the patient than for his/her own opinion concerning a person's personal problems and illnesses.

Sound obstetrical and moral teaching prescribes that the pregnant woman must be supervised during her prenatal period. Although studies are well documented to indicate the safety of surgical procedures during pregnancy, there remain many fears regarding doing surgery. Procedures should not be advised hurriedly during pregnancy. Among the procedures performed with safety during pregnancy are cholecystectomy, appendectomy, cystoscopy, mastectomy, and thyroidectomy. Added to these are many cardiac procedures. Xrays with adequate protection have been taken during pregnancy. However this is not to be encouraged as innocuous. Xray studies are to be performed with strict circumspection. This recommendation has been given by the American College of Radiology since 1958 when this society of specialists published *A Practical Manual on the Medical and Dental Uses of Xrays With Control of Radiation Hazards*.

An attending obstetrician and gynecologist must be aware of the possibility that extrauterine pregnancies occur. The serious nature of a pregnancy outside its natural habitat when undetected can be lethal. Specialists have sufficient knowledge and experience to diagnose extrauterine pregnancy. Such pregnancy can occur in the Fallopian tube, within the abdominal cavity, even in the ovary. The most common site is in the Fallopian tube. Presenting itself as an acute surgical condition within the abdomen usually leads to proper diagnosis and treatment.

Abdominal pregnancies may be either primary or secondary. Usually an abdominal pregnancy is a migration from a tubal pregnancy. As the pregnancy progresses a sonogram will identify the unnatural location of the pregnancy. Cause of maternal death is massive hemorrhage. In view of the seriousness of this abdominal pregnancy associated with high mortality when not identified, what are the moral implications?

Whenever it is possible, the woman should be allowed to carry her pregnancy to the trimester wherein neonatology can come to the rescue of the infant. The baby can be delivered surgically similar to any other patient who has been carried along in her pregnancy and then subjected to caesarean section. However, if any complication develops before the period wherein it is known the fetus is viable, the complication can be treated even if it results in the death of the unborn. The most serious complication in either a tubal or abdominal pregnancy is bleeding. Surgical intervention is permissible because the primary intention is to arrest the hemorrhage. If, secondarily the fetus is harmed, neither a moral nor a legal wrong is committed. The rationale is that a pathologic state exists which can be corrected only by removing the cause: an ectopic, ovarian or abdominal pregnancy.

The unfortunate event of anatomic malformations [congenital anomalies] in infants following the use of the hypnotic drug thalidomide during the early term of pregnancy was a warning to the necessity for caution in prescribing drugs during pregnancy. Since the early 1960s women have been advised against taking drugs during pregnancy. Physicians are alert not to prescribe medication to pregnant women. Attending physicians have a moral obligation to discourage pregnant women against self-medication.

Modern discussions on pregnancy bring forth the topics of surrogate motherhood, frozen embryos, artificial insemination, and cloning. Ethical objection to many and all these mechanical artifices has not altered their practices. Ignored is the dictum that what is technically feasible is not always morally permissible. The biosciences have many impurities that threaten the moral order by which it should stand firmly. Many more will be generated by entrepreneurs who have forgotten medicine is a profession not a business.

Chapter 9

Life And Death Ethical Decisions

Although everyone on earth is invited to the resurrection into heaven each one must walk through the sorrow of Golgotha. Pain and suffering is the rent paid for residing on this planet. All this is real and present even when excellent medical technology is available and applied.

In earlier years the socioeconomic aspect of medical practice was absent or dawdled behind the hastened medicosurgical advancing progress in a *pas de trois* manner. Today the multiple governmental overseers and the self-appointed ombudsmen observe physicians/surgeons *via* a combined telescopic and microscopic scrutiny in a formidable, sometimes contractual, partnership. This overlooking presence has made its indelible mark on the medical profession.

The ever present technology fomented the theme of a fallacious promise that medicosurgical efforts were approaching infallibility in the competition to preserve life with heroic, mechanical, technical, and manual procedures. This concept introduced radicality in surgical treatment that gave a prolonged life to the maimed patient. Many therapeutic measures lengthened human existence quantitatively simultaneously diminishing it qualitatively.

In this era of stressful medical emotionalism of multiple origins, it is valid for all concerned to analyze with meritorious or demeritorious assessment the past medicosurgical experience in the administration of extraordinary therapy. Without circumlocution or enantiosis the deficiencies, blunders, and social foolishness attended thereon must be given a second, even a third, review. A reevaluation must not be influenced by the non-medical society. New social ideas on the amelioration of diseases, the elimination of disfiguring deformities, and the retardation of death have an evangelical appeal even an angelic charisma. However with the passage of time they are usually denied, discarded, deposed, disproved, or disavowed. Most proponents of unrealistic therapeutic achievements, whose inexperience coupled with inadequate knowledge lead them astray, eventually fall into the abyss of oblivion.

The medical realism of impossibility for miraculous performance has become repugnant to some levels of modern society. Ready acceptance of medical limitations is not credible. An erroneous belief in the power of medical excellence arrives at no negative acceptance in the prowess of the physician aligned with an intricate medicosurgical armamentarium. The laity attributes nonexistent spiritual healing powers to the people of medicine because of the continual advancement in the progressively improving diagnostic capabilities. The marked sophistication encompassing radiology, radiation therapy, the laser beam, newer diagnostic, therapeutic instrumentations, the salubrious magnitude of current pharmacopeia, biochemical, genetic engineering, and oncogenesis has instilled false hope that medical talent is omnipotent, unfaltering, and conquerable of all maladies.

The dint of public pressure has erupted into a disputation between ordinary versus extraordinary medical treatment. This argumentation has eradicated the vexatious and isolationistic facade of medicine. As a learned, formal discipline the art of medicine from its very essence is concerned with every aspect of humanity including the philosophic, socioeconomic distresses inherently immanent to human interpersonal and societal relationships.

In turn the professional medical person who practices this art is one who has benefited from a collegiate education and a strenuous university vocational process. As such, in addition to his/her own philosophical development, he/she stands firm as a barrier or challenger to falsity, half-truths, faulty theories, and unsavory medical clamor. This attribute is the quintessence of ethical behavior. Principles of ethics are not a professional extravagancy. Because their ultimate purpose is balanced as to the value of human life. Moral principles are an indispensable *via vitae* for the survival of medicine as a noble profession even as they are necessary for the survival of mankind.

Ordinary And Extraordinary Care

With a positive ethical viewpoint, it is appropriate to distinguish between the term ordinary and extraordinary as to their etymological meanings. As a prelude it is acknowledged that the definitions or synonyms descriptive of these words are taken from diverse standard English American dictionaries.

Ordinary is employed usually to indicate "of common or every day occurrence." It refers to that which is customary, usual, regular, or normal. As interpreted it is "according to an established order." Other usages indicate that ordinary is common in rank or degree; of average merit or consequence; and that which is common-place.

The word extraordinary is derived from the Latin prefix *extra*, meaning without, and the noun *ordo*, which is translated into English as order. Thus it means "being beyond or out of the common order." It implies a course or method not pursued customarily. Anything is extraordinary if it exceeds the ordinary degree or is unusual. Hence it is something or that which is singular. It indicates what is employed for an exceptional purpose or on a special occasion. Among the synonyms listed for extraordinary are: amazing, marvelous, monstrous, peculiar, preposterous, prodigious, remarkable, strange, striking, unprecedented, unwonted, odd, or rare. Another most pertinent definition of extraordinary is "not according to what is used or done habitually."

As applied to the medical profession, ordinary means are those human endeavors, medicosurgical techniques, laboratory procedures, diagnostic modalities, and utilized mechanical contrivances that are employed daily in the course of standard medical events. It does not imply the utilization of untried medical experiments, activity contrary to nature, or improperly arrived at judgmental decisions. Neither ordinary treatment nor extraordinary care accepts euthanasia as part of their therapeutic assets.

Even under the umbrage threat of human displeasure, persons in medical practice should never write nor say anything concerning which they know nothing or is tendentious. Invidious, untaught persons are absolutely invulnerable because they are protected by the armor of ignorance. What is important in the hallmark of medicine is not the marble corridors of hospitals with walls lined with portraits of wealthy philanthropists but the quality of the physicians who walk through them.

Only the medical profession has the intellectual, scientific, and deductive judgmental capacity to mold into an integrable, fungible unit the criterion for a decisive, determinative conclusion as to the clinical evaluation of human life. This appraisal is the indispensable ingredient to the complex constituents of medicine, law, and philosophy that are intermingled with the thanatological thesis of when to terminate artificially sustained vegetative life.

Medicosurgical expertise alone can express with cognitive scientific probability the efficiency of proposed medical or surgical therapy. This final analytical conviction is founded upon predesignated medical judgment which is a major attribute of the educated, well-trained, experienced physician.

The distinction between ordinary and extraordinary medicosurgical treatment remains the prerogative of the attending physician as an individual, as a member of a hospital staff or by a designated ethics committee authorized to decide disputes on pastoral medicine. In a widely publicized California medicolegal inquiry, "the court sidestepped the common perception that because a respirator involves a large and invasive machine, it is extraordinary and intravenous feeding, because it is common and less invasive is ordinary" [Rust, 1983].

Neither attorneys nor physicians have an intellectual Ophir[1] from which the wisdom of Solomon can be obtained to solve the variegated medicomoral perplexities that confront humanity. Both do have an inerrancy and a non-erratic ethical intransigency that are the inherent positive symbols of medicine and morality.

As a consequence, in the mental balancing between the worthiness of ordinary versus extraordinary medical therapies, the quality of life must be measured against the quantity of life. Without intrinsic merit there are those disputants who place a crape on intelligence as they stir up social distress, medical upheaval, legal eruption, and ethical discord. In order to eliminate the threat of these invectives, no mistaken conclusion is to be drawn from what has been written in the historical past.

Reaffirmation is made of the enunciated moral teaching that is consonant with medicosurgical progress. For almost three decades the philosophic explanation has been that neither patients nor physicians are obligated morally to initiate or continue extraordinary means of preserving

---

1. Ophir is a land rich in gold, I Kings 10:11

life [Declaration from Vatican, 1980]. Means are extraordinary when they are unduly burdensome in the patient, unduly expensive (medical cost containment has become an economic necessity for the continuation of adequate hospital care), and ultimately useless, either singularly or in combination.

Hence if a person is in the process of dying, he/she is not obligated morally to use, continue to use, or accept extraordinary means of prolonging life. When the dying person is incompetent, neither the guardian nor the attending physician is required to instigate, to use, or continue to use extraordinary means of prolonging life. Certain unusual circumstances could make the use of extraordinary medical therapeutic measures desirable or even mandatory. An illustrative example is in the situation of a brain dead mother whose unborn infant can be brought to viability and saved if the mother is kept biologically alive by means of respirators and intravenous feeding [Ethical Directive, 1991].

Decisions about the initiation or continuance of extraordinary means of preserving life are made regularly on a daily basis in hospitals throughout this nation by patients, their guardians or their treating physicians. This does not infer that difference of opinion on this subject does not flourish.

Arthur Schopenhauer [1788-1860] the German pessimistic philosopher once said: "Opinion is like a pendulum and obeys the same law. If it goes past the center of gravity on one side, it must go a like distance on the other. And it is only after a certain time that it finds the true point at which it can remain at rest."

Misinformation is sometimes presented as fact when in reality it is a conjecture scientifically unverified. An example in point was a new management of premature infants in the 1950s. "To counteract the high prevalence of pulmonary edema in premature infants and concerned secondarily with the possibility of aspiration pneumonia during feeding, some experts proposed that all premature infants be deprived of food and water for several days following birth" [Hansen and Smith, 1953]. This proposal was adopted in many countries throughout the world. Hundreds of thousands of premature babies were fasted and thirsted for several days after birth causing these innocent infants to die needlessly. This is ordinary care disallowed under false bioscience's erroneous proposal.

Life support is a disputatious subject that arouses ire in scholars within and without the medical profession. A physician who was director of a hemodialysis unit applauded a judge's effort to bring the issue of technological prolongation of the terminally ill from "the isolation of ethical contemplation to the public arena. [W]ith a plea for society to institutionalize its moral verdicts by legislation [Kaufman, 1985] . . . The major bioethical question to be answered before the next century arrives is 'Under what circumstances may life sustaining therapies be withheld from a severely deformed, seriously injured, comatose or terminally ill person?'" [Scher, 1985]. The implications are individualized according to each readers mental image.

But it does raise the question as to what does life support support? To many people it is strange for a physician to continue a useless treatment. To perform what is useless is senseless. Startling as it may be, technologies are ordered for patients described as life support when life is questionable. Then there is the question of temporary support to permanent support systems.

The word permanent shrinks in terms of longevity as the inevitable hour arrives when death conquers the most powerful machine. Yet all the artificial modalities that sustain life are desirable. Finely tuned, highly developed life support systems have led to the situation in which personhood, the participation in life's interchange with fellow human beings is either totally or partially lost, while organ function is maintained. This is a daunting challenge that defies total answering.

"So each new technology presents new clinical and technological problems; continual improvement and refinement goes on with all of them. But we say that these technologies also pose ethical problems. Indeed, it is commonly suggested that the concern about ethical problems in medicine is stimulated primarily by the advances in medical technology. So, there is a general impression that this enormously positive and quite beneficial development creates ethical problems. It may be useful to be more precise about the nature of these problems: in our civilization, we have gotten very good at defining technical problems and remain fairly primitive in defining ethical ones.

"Two features of life support or, better, organ support technology give rise to the ethical question. Both are features not so much of the technology but of its historical development. One is that the technical developments have moved from partial support to total support. We speak of a 'support system.' The Drinker Tank was a mechanical device able to exert mechanical pressure sufficient to substitute for the loss of the intercostal musculature. It performed one function only: it moved air in and out. But, as technologies for support of other organs were invented, machines came to be added.

"It is relatively rare that patients end up on a total system, although some patients get fairly close to it. Yet, as the steps toward total system are taken in an intensive care unit, signs of concern appear among those responsible for the care of the patient. Intubation is almost routine. When dialysis needs to be added, some questions are raised, and when the need for hyperalimentation arises, people begin to argue. As steps are taken toward a total support system, the suspicion appears that an ethical problem is brewing. Of course, we must recognize that the total system is not really total. It is only quasitotal. And here we glimpse one of the genuine reasons why we have an ethical problem. The system is quasitotal because we have no direct brain support system. The brain can be perfused by supporting ventilatory and circulatory systems, but that is indirect brain support. When the central nervous system is seriously damaged, particularly in its higher cognitive functions, we have no direct intervention. Thus we confront the sort of patient about whom ethical questions are most frequently raised: one whose heart and lungs and kidneys and circulatory system are being supported but whose cognitive functions are profoundly and permanently destroyed.

"We talk about the maintenance of life; we don't often talk about the maintenance of personhood. It interests me little, indeed, not at all, to be alive as an organism. In such a state, I have no interests. It is enormously interesting for me to be a person. With my history, with my place in life, doing the things I enjoy doing, loving those I love, causing the problems that I like to cause, I live my life. It is the perpetuation of my personhood that interests me; indeed, it is, probably, my major and, perhaps, my sole real interest. Life support development or organ support development, however, has led us to the situation in which personhood seems either totally or partially lost, while organic life is maintained. This is, of course, a profound philosophical problem; the very nature of human life and personhood. The profound philosophical problem, which has been pondered by savants since the beginning of our culture, need not be answered in full in order to reach some acceptable resolutions of particular problems" [Jonsen, 1987].

"It is now almost cliché to say that contemporary medical ethics races almost breathlessly to put the words with the music of contemporary medical technology and progress. Medical technology has advanced remarkably. Oddly enough, much of this progress evolved in conjunction with the exploration of outer space and its incumbent quest for specialized synthetic materials and machinery. The horizon of medical capability in this period has widened explosively from surgical intervention, diagnostic modalities, laser technique and much more.

"Progress, however, is not without its problems. The same technology that restores health and prolongs life in most instances, can be of questionable value by prolonging, not life, but dying. And this dying can be as horrifying and tragic as a traffic wreck. Today's questions are familiar to everyone and are quite perplexing. When do we pull the plug? When is enough enough? Are we morally obliged to do everything we are technologically capable of doing? No matter how often we have encountered such questions or helped others do so, they are always current and hauntingly novel.

"Guidelines on the Termination of Life-Sustaining Treatment and Care of the Dying from the Hastings Center 'offers comprehensive ethical guidelines for decisions on whether to forgo life-sustaining medical treatment.' It addresses 'not only the care of patients known to be dying or terminally ill but also the care of patients who are critically or seriously ill or simply facing a decision about the use of life-sustaining treatment.'

"Four values are central to the articulation of the guidelines:

1. The patient's well-being (often called the "principle of beneficence").
2. The value of the patient's autonomy or self-determination (which establishes the right of the patient to determine the nature of his or her own medical care). This is the moral basis for the principle of informed consent (which itself includes the right of informed refusal). The guidelines are to put the patient always at the center of the decision-making process. This in turn leads to the issue of decision-making capacity and proxy consent (called surrogate consent).
3. The third significant value is the integrity of health care renderers. Which means they are bound by stringent ethical obligations to the patient by virtue of their professional status and rôle. But they have a right to remain true to their own conscientious moral and religious beliefs. In a situation of conflicting consciences, the health care professional should be able to transfer the patient to another's care.

4. There is the value of justice or equity. This entails the balance between the patient's right to adequate, appropriate health care, and the distribution of available health care resources. Specifically, regarding the termination of life-sustaining treatment is the added value called the sanctity of life. This moral value places the burden of proof on those who would foreshorten life or fail to forestall death.

"With the articulation of these four values as an introduction, the Hasting Report is divided into six parts. Part One examines the four basic values in light of the specific issue of deciding for or against life-sustaining treatment. For example, the principle of beneficence becomes a question of whether the burdens of treatment justify the benefits the patient receives from it. If the burden outweighs the benefit, the treatment may be withheld or withdrawn

"Second is the principle of patient self-determination which stipulates that such a life-sustaining treatment decision belongs to the patient. In the absence of decision-making capacity, the right belongs to the patient's surrogate. Thirdly, the health care professional should respect the decision of the patient. Fourthly, in justice, the health care professional's first obligation is to the patient, not to the budget nor to potential other patients.

"Part Two applies the more general presentation of life-sustaining treatments to specific types of treatments: the long-term life-supporting technologies (ventilators and renal dialysis), emergency interventions, guidelines for antibiotics and other life-sustaining medication, palliative care, and pain relief, and administering nutrition and hydration. Part Three considers advance directives for one's future possible treatment. This is of particular interest to those who may help others consider what to do—or not do—in the event of a medical crisis.

"Part Four presents guidelines on the declaration of death. The contributors propose uniform national legislation—proposed, in fact, by the President's Commission for the Study of Ethical Problems in Medicine and Biomedical and Behavioral Research (in July, 1981). This is called the "Uniform Determination of Death Act" which states: 'An individual who has sustained either (1) irreversible cessation of circulatory and respiratory functions, or (2) irreversible cessation of all functions of the entire brain, including the brain-stem, is dead. A determination of death must be made in accordance with accepted medical standards.' The Guidelines urge that this be adopted as law—despite the resistance of certain religious minorities and those medical professionals who would argue for only higher brain death as opposed to total brain death.

"Part Five centers on policy considerations. Specifically guidelines on the formation and functioning of ethics committees within a given health care institution, guidelines on institutional policies regarding patient admission, transfer, and economic considerations *vis-a-vis* life sustaining treatments. Part Six discusses special problems of varying degrees of interest:

1. terminating treatment, active voluntary euthanasia and assisting suicide;
2. withholding and withdrawing treatment;
3. decision-making capacity and competence;
4. quality of life;
5. age as a factor in decision-making; and
6. accommodating religious values and beliefs.

"This is a comprehensive document emphasizing every aspect of the critical problem of making a decision about life-sustaining treatments. While it is addressed primarily to the personnel of health care facilities, it is aimed at the patient who is always central in health care decisions or the patient's surrogate who is chosen by the patient and executes his/her wishes" [Smith, 1985].

People of medicine are licensed to do procedures on human beings that can be helpful, harmful, and murderous. They must always choose the better ones. Professional persons should be the recipients of the accolade Aristotle gave to Socrates, "This is the man whom evil men do not have even the right to praise, who taught us to be happy, while being good." When bodily life no longer has the capacity of higher good to self and to others, to preserve that life artificially does not contribute to the possibility of higher good[2] capability. Human beings must face the

---

2. Higher good is stated also as the highest good, the greatest, and supreme good which in Latin is the *summum bonum*. It is that good which transcends all other goods but includes them. St. Thomas Aquinas defines the highest good as obedience to and oneness with God. Plato defined it as the supreme idea, the totality of being. For Aristotle it was eudemonism which consists in

dogma of their own mortality: that suffering is a firm facet of human life and death is unavoidable.

Concisely and compactly it is proper to write that an ill patient whose biographical, personal active life is gone may refuse or discontinue treatment: when they are disproportionate to any foreseeable benefit or which treatment imposes stress, strain or suffering out of proportion to any anticipated biological well-being, improvement or enhancement of body physiology. When inevitable death is imminent in spite of the means used, it is permitted in good conscience to decide either to refuse or not to administer forms of treatment that would secure only a precarious and burdensome prolongation of life. The attached proviso thereto is that normal ordinary, required care due the sick person is not interrupted.

No-Code Order: Do Not Resuscitate

In the past many years, significant strides have been made in the developmental evolution of medical and ethical concepts in the treatment of the patient who has experienced a cardiopulmonary arrest. The widespread application of available technology has produced a number of success stories, and, unfortunately, some patients whose cardiac function was reestablished had no return of cognition. Reports of patients who remained post-resuscitation in a permanent vegetative state, on or off a ventilator, prompted their families, attorneys, judges, and legislators to permit patients to be directly involved, before the fact, in asking that no resuscitative measures be employed upon them [Gregory, 1985].

Following the positive statements and recommendations of the President's Commission, medical staffs and hospitals throughout the country have been implementing policies to permit the writing of No-Code Orders. With a few minor exceptions, these have been well-accepted by patients, their families, the legal, medical professions, and the lay public. In rare instances, the perception of a threat of civil action or criminal prosecution against those who write or implement such orders has served to retard the recognition of what many understand to be the

---

the harmonious satisfaction of all rational powers. Eudemonia is happiness or well-being, acclaimed by Aristotle as the universally recognized chief good, and described by him as consisting in the active exercise of the soul's powers in accordance with reason.

patient's right to accept or refuse this treatment in the ultimate care setting [Gregory, 1985].

Massachusetts' highest court ruled that a juvenile court was authorized to issue a no code-order on an infant who was terminally ill and had been abandoned by his mother. The infant was abandoned by his mother at birth and was a patient at a hospital. The child, a ward of the Dept. of Social Services, had cyanotic heart disease; pulmonary atresia; hypoplastic right ventricle; hypoplastic pulmonary artery; and small patent ductus arteriosus. The court noted that there was no treatment proven or experimental, that was available, and that death normally occurred within the first year of life, regardless of the course of treatment. When the child was three months old, his physicians recommended that a no-code order be entered into his medical chart, providing that no heroic medical efforts would be made to resuscitate the child if cardiac or respiratory arrest occurred. Heroic efforts included intracardia injections of epinephrine, heart massage, or electric shock treatment. Medical testimony indicated that a heroic effort would not be in the child's best interests and would offend medical ethics.

Both the social services agency and the child's guardian *ad litem* declined to consent to the no-code order. The hospital then requested the juvenile court to decide on the order. The court entered the no-code order, and at a later hearing confirmed the physicians' recommendations to discharge the infant to a foster home. The court said that discharge was the equivalent of a no-code order because the child probably would die at home if cardiac arrest occurred.

On appeal, the high court said that the Juvenile Court had ample jurisdiction to enter the no-code order. The hospital had a right to seek such an order, and the judge's findings were amply supported by the evidence. Noting that the juvenile court judge at all times was willing to reconsider his order if the child's condition changed, the high court affirmed his power to issue such further orders as might be appropriate.

The appellate court added that the issue was not one of right to life. In a no-code case, the question is not of life or death but of the manner of dying and what measures are appropriate to ease the imminent passing of an irreversibly, terminally ill patient, the court said [Custody of a Minor, 434 N.E. 2d 601 Mass. Sup. Jud. Ct., April 5, 1982].

An advance answer can be given to the question of life prolongation. By beforehand realization, consideration of the question answers it. To the last will and testament and the living will the testator adds the penultimate will. Unlike the living will which addresses the right to die, the penultimate will stipulates an individual's desire in event of mental incompetency when a decision is required pertinent to illness, injury and/or coma.

The testator may designate a legal guardian for this purpose who generally is an attorney or the attending physician. An addendum to a penultimate will may be indicated as to a preferred place of residence should it become necessary for incompetency and/or inability to care for oneself. Also stated may be financial limitations placed on health care and the amount to be expended on nursing home/senior housing facilities, *et cetera*.

While some of these items may be contested in a court of law, they would be considered adequate and useful guidelines when family and physicians disagree on the course to be taken. The penultimate will may have considerable persuasion when the decision is to be made as to definitive treatment rests more on whether a younger person is competing for the same mechanical assistance than on whether the older person would benefit from the treatment plus the elder patient's wishes in the matter [Pollner, 1980].

A proposed example form of a penultimate will that provides for contingencies that may arise in which the testator may become incompetent and another person may have to make decisions is illustrated.

Form of Penultimate Will

I, RICHARD P., residing at 700 East 72nd Street, City, County and State of New York, being upwards of 18 years of age and of sound mind, pursuant to §78.05 of the Mental Hygiene Law of the State of New York, or any similar or successor statute, do hereby make, publish and declare this to be my Last Designation of Committee hereby revoking all other designations of persons to act as the committee of my person and/or property heretofore made by me.

1. I hereby designate my brother, PHILIP, who presently resides at 3200 Riverside Drive, New York, New York, as the person whom I desire to be appointed as the committee of both my person and property in the event that I shall be declared an incompetent pursuant to Article 78 of the Mental Hygiene Law of the State of New York, or any similar or successor statute.

2. I hereby request that my said committee and any court which will have to make decisions with respect to my person and property in the event of my incompetence consider my following wishes:

    (a) That Dr. Irwin Laven be my physician whenever medical care or advice is needed:

    (b) That if at the time of my incompetence, my said wife is deceased, I request that all of my possessions be given to . . .

Chapter 10

Malevolence In Bioscience

Born of necessity, medicine originated in response to humanity's distress from illness brought on by unknown diseases. Nourished by the ingenuity propelled by philosophic intelligence it has multiplied in efficiency to become a major benefit to all mankind. Many physicians do not think in terms of bioethics. Being entranced by the vast amount of scientific knowledge available and continuing at an unprecedented rate, their concentration has no time to challenge the propriety of the research products derived from the startling super-modern technology.

Science today does not enjoy the certainty that was invested in it years ago. Sensational scientific discoveries that blazon the front page are not always correct. Fraudulent intent may not have been the primary purpose. It may be the prompting of heady, hopeful self-deluding enthusiasm that inveigles even the mentally alert. Anxiety to be published first, to gain pioneer credit, academic acclaim, financial advancement, and/or an achievement award can dismantle integrity under siege. Manipulation of biomedical findings, tampering with statistics, miscorrelations, faulty calculations, mathematical miscounting, and other manufactured machinations that deceive purposefully are a devised deterioration of bioethical appropriateness.

Posthumous Reproduction

"While the technology involved in the cryopreservation of gametes and embryos is almost commonly accepted, the ethical and social issues raised are complex and controversial" [Shuster, 1994]. Posthumous reproduction is the production of a child after one of the would-be parents die. Virtually any man may have his sperm frozen and stored for later use [Bunge, 1953]. Women have used donated sperm for insemination without knowing the source from whence it came.

The cryopreserving of sperm makes possible to conceive children after the genetic father dies. Legal disturbances arise without any *iota* of thought given to morality when one partner or both die before the embryo is implanted. Added to this confusion is another as to the survivor's desire to establish a pregnancy with a third person to whom the dead partner did not give consent to, can not do, or has expressed orally and/ or in writing an objection [Smith, 1995]. These questions arise when parents do not specify in writing what they desire in the event one or both die [Ibrahim, 1996]. What are the legal, ethical, and medical concerns of these orphaned embryos who have been abandoned? [Robertson, 1994]. Should the embryos be kept in storage, used for research, be donated to infertile couples, or discarded? [Kolata, 1997]. Each of which has a bioethical complication added to the original prohibition. Postmortem insemination allows fatherhood from the grave that adds to the ethical problem already in existence [Gilbert, 1993].

Although procreative decisions are guaranteed by law under the right to privacy [Griswold vs Connecticut, 381 US 479, 485-86, 1965], this fundamental right does not make it morally honorable. Court decisions are not uniform adding to rather than alleviating the quandary on the posthumous reproduction complexity [NY State Task Force, 1998 and Sherman et al, 1987].

History, tradition, culture, and heredity have contributed to the majestic value of reproduction. The experience of human birth, rearing children, the cohesiveness it brings to family enrichment are blessings of natural living. Children born of gift-exchange have no congenital honor to their births. An inborn relationship is halved which is not fair and equitable to the child conceived as a biological product. Even the good intention of wanting a child is not a sufficient, valid reason to justify using the available, feasible reproductive strategies. Accessible technology readily at hand for usage does not automatically sanction its ethical conformity to appropriateness. Man-made, artificial reproductive options are morally and socially offensive without being ethically acceptable.

Scientific breakthroughs, bioengineering innovations, and many more achievements may have elevated the quality of life and prolonged it.

However these advancements have brought forth ethical embarrassments that are not avoidable. A serious one centers on the thousands of human embryos, so-called leftovers, from in vitro fertilization procedures encased in liquid nitrogen. These in limbo embryos are residuals from multiple ovulations instigated by drugs. Having been "captured" surgically they were combined with sperm and are imprisoned in a petri dish for one to two days and then inserted into a woman's uterus.

Very often a couple produce large numbers of embryos using only a few leaving the rest in storage floating in liquid nitrogen. This is the residue of a manufacturing process that uses biology to make a commodity that is personal property under refrigeration. Many women donate their property to medical research for payment. Stem-cell research is very popular and purchasers of embryos for this purpose are many [Charen, 2001].

Pregnancy In Brain-dead Woman

Posthumous pregnancy is using a woman's corpse as a fetal incubator. This is the situation that involves a deceased brain-dead pregnant woman whose artificially maintained body is used to support her fetus until it becomes viable [Field, 1988], [Dillon, 1982]. The woman's wishes may not be known but this life-sustaining regimen has been contested but not denied. Decisions to sustain a dead pregnant woman for the sake of her baby have been ethically justified on utilitarian principles [Field, 1988]. A deceased woman's explicit refusal to be maintained as a fetal incubator, expressed before her death, does not in itself carry moral weight against the possibility of fetal survival. The utility concept demonstrates the mother is unharmed. None of her rights are violated and great good can be done for another [Dillon, 1982]. This doctrine is compatible with the time-honored, long-standing tradition in Western society, named appropriately: the medical rescue of the fetus from death.

The rescue hypothetical defense does not eliminate objections from many sources. Legally the woman has no duty that would require her to have her body used as a fetal incubator without her consent. Up to this time no person has been required to give up a vital organ to save the life of a family member because of a special family relationship. Physicians are not permitted to remove organs from a dead patient without consent from the deceased ante-mortem, or next-of-kin, no matter the good intention to save another life. To use a woman's corpse as an incubator without her prior consent would be analogous to stating a woman loses her right to refuse to donate organs upon her death by becoming pregnant. This is a legal theory: a comparison that has flaws. It is well-established that women do not lose their constitutional or common law rights by becoming pregnant [Annas, 1995].

It is written that female incubators establish a perilous precedent that may justify using such somatic life-support when a woman is comatose or in a permanent vegetative state. This is not the same as using the woman's body as an inert receptacle for artificial insemination. This is a grotesque suggestion unworthy of any consideration even by a corrupt demon of iniquity. Such moral depravity is alien to bioscience. It is destructive to the human element that glorifies pregnancy a valuable, worthwhile, holy experience.

Aborted Fetus As Genetic Mother

Transplantation of fetal germ cells has been presented as assisted reproduction [Shoshone, 1992]. It suggests aborted female fetuses might be used as a source for oocytes in donation programs. The proposal is to remove oocytes from ovaries of aborted fetuses, mature them in vitro. Then use them as donor oocytes for couples who need eggs as part of their in vitro fertilization effort. Another method would remove ovaries from aborted fetuses and transplant them into women who lack ovarian functions. The transplanted tissue would be an adjuvant contributing to the recipient's normal reproductive cycle [Gosden, 1992]. At present, utilizing fetal eggs for conception is hypothetical, speculative but not an impossibility [Ethics Commission, 1997]. "Its rationale has been that, if sperm from a dead man can be used for posthumous insemination, so too should eggs from an aborted fetus" [Schuster, 1999]. *Non sequitur*[1] that one immoral act can be used to justify a subsequent eviler act.

A dead fetus can never be an independent living person. To use eggs from an unknowable person is wrong as it undermines the moral precept

---

1. *Non sequitur* is Latin for: it does not follow. In logic it is an inference or conclusion that does not follow from established premises or evidence. Hence it indicates a statement to which no answer seems either appropriate or reasonable.

of procreation as a voluntary choice. Moreover, it is problematic that the woman, who has an abortion, may also have the ability to make a right decision for her aborted fetus. "Whether a child's interest is served by having an aborted fetus as a mother is highly problematic. It would be shortsighted to view the harvesting of dead fetuses' bodies in isolation from our moral attitude towards ourselves and our notion of human dignity" [Schuster, 1999]. The fact that the child would not be born, but for the use of fetal eggs, does not justify their use, any more than it would justify using cloning, animals as gestators of human fetuses, or the creation of human-animal hybrids that would not otherwise be born" [Annas, 1998].

Reproductive choices can run rampant if not halted by a morally trained ethical conscience. The likely result could be destructive social behaviors and unnatural procreative habits that would foster a culture that tolerates the unthinkable in human reproduction. It would encourage "a radical genetic and technological control over life itself and the making of human beings" [Bioethics Law, 1994].

Examples of domination over procreation has been noted in past years. Like using technology by would-be parents to engineer children to their specifications. In 1999, one online auction offered bidders a chance to own designer genes by purchasing ova from young, beautiful models [Kennedy Institute of Ethics Journal brochure, 2001].

The United States, like most western countries, has witnessed an increasing demand for reproductive technologies. Experience reveals sperm retrieval from dead men is among them [Fishman, 1994]. Infertility has accented the public desire for more information on solving the procreation deficit. Then there are a limited number of people who find it acceptable to desire children after death. Most proponents and advocates of these imitations of nature reduce human reproduction to a utility without any thought given to bioethical devaluation. Lacking are values of family relationship, parental responsibility, human dignity, and the immorality of the acts pursued [Nelson, 1994]. The adults who engage in highly questionable practices are suspect as well as the society that permits them [Shuster, 1999].

Although the evolved technology in the manipulation of gametes and embryos is an accolade for bioscientific technique, ethical and social issues are appurtenances that are not avoidable. These are not innocuous but complex and controversial. They importune morality and are unethical. Procreation under these circumstances as a human mechanism and one of the ten normal biological functions is deprived of personality. Becoming a commercial enterprise the consumer pays for services in a business-like manner. The supply is generous to meet every requested demand. No legal restriction is placed on spermatozoa that can be bought, sold, stored, and discarded.

Reproduction technologies are factory fabrications without any intimate, affectionate, personal biological kinship. Unnatural conception is an immoral, non-physiological device that insults the poise, self-respect, and deportment of humanity.

No psychological speculation is required to either seek or acknowledge that biographical history places physicians in the cynosure category marked by dignified performance, integrity of character, and skilled competency. Collectively these assets produce the admirable and substantial figure of the conceptualized medical doctor. Ingrained bioethical high requirements are intrinsically innate to the medical profession. This theological moral element heightens the esteem physicians have enjoyed so long. Participation in any artificial reproductive techniques detracts from their honorable glory, drowning hard-earned reputations in shallow still waters.

Chapter 11

Respect For Human Life

The origin and dignity of procreation is instinctively preserved by domesticated tamed, and savage animals. Because of divine given intellect and incomparable free-will human beings should have a more forceful protectiveness for human procreation founded upon fundamental moral judgments formulated through these animated attributes of the soul. No physiologist, research anthropologist, and other bioscientist can claim by any philosophical reason that by the acceptance of his/her scientific competence and recognized expertise to be able to decide on another person's origin and destiny. Especially is this an applicable norm in the medical subphylum of sexuality and procreation in which is actualized the fundament recognized values of love and life.

Medical science, technology, and bioengineering are to be at the service of the human person. Functioning for any other purpose questions their existence. Some of their research programs threaten to decivilize human love. Science without conscience leads to the ruination of moral research which should not disturb, disrupt, or destroy the concept of *corpore et anima unus* [the body and soul are one].

This is a moral mandate for scientists to preserve the nature of the human person. This includes his/her bodily dimension as a unified totality with a true, realized nature which is corporal and spiritual. Because of its substantial union with a spiritual soul [the life principle], the human body is not to be evaluated as a complex commixture of cells, tissues, organs, and other anatomic components. Even though the constituent parts collectively manifest themselves through one organic structure.

By comparison with the conveyance of other forms of life in the universe, the transmission of human life has a special character of its own, which derives from the special nature of the human person [Origins, 1987]. "The transmission of human life is entrusted by nature to a personal and conscious act and as such is subject to the all-holy laws of God. These are immutable and inviolable laws which must be recognized and observed. For this reason one can not use means and follow methods which could be licit in the transmission of the life of plants and animals" [Pope Pius XII, 1950].

Selling And Auctioning Ova

Auctioning, buying, selling, and other commercial ventures of human ova to produce designer babies, select gender, and to industrialize surrogate motherhood are volcanic bioethical eruptions. Such scandal is in very bad social standing, unethical, but not illegal. No law bans the sale of human sperm and ova. Individual human rights is the protective covering guaranteed by the American legal system. This endows an individual with ownership and master of his/her own body. This is commodification of the human body—especially the female body.

Business has crossed the last frontier of decency by dealing with potential human life. The cycle of interference is proved by the sale of human reproductive elements: ova, sperm, and reproductive capacity [surrogate mothers]. An ovum is expensive the contemporary price is $3,000 and more for a healthy specimen [not guaranteed]. Payment is justified for the cost of the procedure to obtain the ovum and for the female donor's time and inconvenience [taking superovulation drugs and surgical intervention to retrieve the egg].

This is another expression of the eroding legal principle that banned the buying and selling of human bodies and organs. American courts have been expressive in declaring property rights in genetically engineered products created from genes to cells. Repugnance is inherent in the ghastly notion that human life can be bought, sold, auctioned, bartered, patented, inherited, and be part of a legacy.

Gone is the belief in the common good. Favored is the more self-centered principle of individualism with its rights above all else. This is the choice of the modern value system which is found to be most useful as it focuses on profit, trivialization of human life, redefinition of commercialism, and to be part of the globalization of bioscience. No consideration is given to the blurring of bioethical norms, that everything human has a price, and no consideration is to be given to the children born out of this manufacture. A biotechnology firm in Maryland has applied for over 6000 patents. Not only are they trying to protect their methods, they are seeking ownership of the results of their research—human genetic information [Kennedy Institute of Ethics Journal brochure, 2001].

"Reproductive and genetic technologies give us the unprecedented power to create, manipulate, and alter human life in the laboratory. That power has to be tempered by key restraints . . . our laws must state clearly that the human body, its parts, and processes are not property or objects of commerce and are not to be bought and sold.[1] Second, in any situation where a new human life is to be created, the interests of the future child must be paramount . . . Auctioning ova, designer babies, sex selection, and commercial surrogacy are just the tip of the iceberg. We need a way to look at these issues every day, and to instill a mechanism to both protect the public and ensure that society's best interests are respected" [McTeer, 1999].

Infertile couples and others who streamline reproduction to their own pattern have used the web to shop on line for cyber-donors' ova. Web sites are expanding this practice with anonymity of the sellers. In the unwired world the purchaser can select from a list of 1,500 prospective donors. The selective women under the Web site program called Creating Families is indoctrinated into a period of preparation. This includes a series of parenteral hormone injections to encourage ova production. As an aside, the Creating Families Web site provides the surrogate mother if requested at a cost of $15,000. The novelty of all this is that this reproductive process has found its way onto the World Wide Web giving tremendous publicity to immorality that wounds again and again the crumbling bioethical standards that once were stalwart. Commercialization of reproduction insults human creation [Deam, 2000].

Instances of commerce in human ova continue to be reported in the news media. Since it is legal, there is no stopping its recrudescences. Infertility organizations have been the most vocal in its vitriolic criticism. Representatives of these groups are concerned that it will bring

---

1. European law is based on the Rousseauean principle that no one owns his/her own body.

about an unfavorable reaction against egg donation in general as an immoral procedure. No European country allows the buying and selling of human eggs. Most foreign nations forbid the donation of human ova. European bioscientists do not have an affinity for professional activities that could be perceived as eugenic. Cognizant of the Third Reich experiments they are selectively wary of genetic engineering as well.

A distaste for ova commerce is reflected in European dislike for manipulative capitalism. Even the aversion for the economic connection does not answer completely why many European nations are banning ovum transplantations even when no money is exchanged. Credit must be given to them for not being so liberal on sociomedical issues as some Americans would have us believe. Europe and Canada have their own moral scruples which they follow without notice.

"Many issues are at stake in the egg donation debate. Canadian Patricia Baird warns, "These [fertility technologies] have the potential to turn children into a commodity, to commercialize them, and that diminishes human dignity." Europeans and Canadians who see human dignity at stake both when fetuses are aborted and when human eggs are sold bring a more morally coherent outlook to bear on decisions in areas like genetic engineering" [Schaefer, 1999].

In selling and auctioning ova selfishness prompts the buyer and greed propels the seller. The immoral business of selling ova with its profit for eugenic excuses and the purpose of having beautiful offspring is an insult to human reproduction as a natural physiological function ordained as a consummate fulfillment of love designed for marital bliss.

To have physically beautiful children is a blessing, a parental desire that is commendable. However to purchase ova for the primary purpose of beauty alone is a hazy, cloudy negation of other attributes. Ignoring the creation of a human soul accentuates the physical over the spiritual. Making the body more significant than the spirit forgets that every living person grows old, even ugly, and dies like all living plants and animals. Only divinity lives in perpetuity.

Forgotten is the observation that all beautiful people are not the moral best. That personality may be lacking in them and good character absent. Beauty is deceptive, can conceal an evil conscience, does not guarantee good health, longevity, and a happy death. Beautiful bodies do not have a monopoly on attractiveness. Those considered less than beauteous may have other character traits that outshine physiognomy. Their spiritual magnificence may not radiate this invisible attribute but it is revealed when the person is known. Recognition of spirituality outshines any physical attraction. Whatever is physical is temporary. That which is spiritual lives on and on into eternity.

Frozen Embryos

The fate of seven embryos frozen in liquid nitrogen was determined by a judge [Dale, 1989]. His decision involved a disturbing ethical impasse.

"A couple had begun a process of in vitro fertilization, but were divorced before the embryos were placed in the womb of Mrs. Davis. Her ex-husband wished to destroy them, while Mrs. Davis wished to give birth to them. Judge Young ruled in favor of Mrs. Davis on the ground that, 'From fertilization, the cells of a human embryo are differentiated, unique and specialized to the highest degree of distinction . . . Human life begins at conception.'

"One of the key witnesses in the trial was Dr. Jerome Lejeune, a world famous geneticist from France. In the course of the trial he was asked, 'What ethical considerations do you have about freezing?' He responded, 'I think love is the contrary of chilly. Love is warmth. . .'

"The process being discussed was cryopreservation—the freezing of a living being in order to preserve it. It is a process now being used—as it was in the case of these embryos—to keep embryos alive but arrested at the earliest stage of development, when there have been only a few cell divisions.

"At this earliest stage, the embryo is referred to by some as a 'pre-embryo,' another example of the sanitized language of abortionists and of those who want to feel free to manipulate human life in its earliest stages. As Dr. Lejeune said, this is simply a term invented to give the impression that the first few stages of development are something other than a human being. He described it as a change in words so that you could then justify changing your behavior. In other words, what is being frozen, even at the very first stage of cell division, is a human being—a human person.

"Dr. Lejeune also gave a clear explanation of just how cryopreservation works. *Tempo* and temperature are interrelated. If you gradually lower temperature, you also gradually lower *tempo* of the movement of molecules and atoms. If it is done with sufficient care, the cells will slow down until time almost stands still and they are in a state of suspended animation. Of course, there is the risk that the frozen cells may crystallize, and then the embryo is dead. Gradual raising of temperature should reverse the process, if the freezing has been done successfully. The embryologist who had done the freezing (and who was named appropriately Dr. Shivers) testified that about 30% of the embryos thus frozen are accidentally killed.

"Dr. Lejeune described the process as 'putting inside a very chilly space tiny human beings who are deprived of any liberty, of any movement, even . . . deprived of time.' Time is frozen for them, making them survive, so to speak, in suspended time in a 'concentration can.' This is not the way in which any human being should ever be treated. The intent is to help people to have children. The reality involves manipulation and possible death—things to which no parent would want to subject a child.

"The Instruction on Procreation sums it up: 'The freezing of embryos, even when carried out in order to preserve the life of an embryo—cryopreservation—constitutes an offense against the respect due to human beings by exposing them to grave risks of death or harm to their physical integrity and depriving them, at least temporarily, of maternal shelter and gestation, thus placing them in a situation in which further offenses and manipulation are possible." The warmth of human love demands more than this [Mulligan, 1991].

Cold-climate hibernation has no place in human procreation which is a blessing given to men and women who love each other exclusively, get married for the primary purpose of expressing their love in having children with the assistance of the Divine Creator. A frozen embryo is not the fruit of love. It does not represent the product of mutual self-giving of the spouses, their love, and fidelity. "A medical intervention respects the dignity of persons when it seeks to assist the conjugal act—not to replace it technologically—either in order to facilitate its performance or in order to enable it to achieve its objective once it has been normally performed" [Origins, 1987].

Cryonic Preservation

Popular knowledge of frozen sperm, ova, and embryos inevitably would infiltrate into a novelty of preserving the entire body or parts thereof. With the intention of having the deceased revived and anatomical parts available for transplantation. More of an industry than a scientific project, the real issue is one of business ethics than an infringement on medical probity.

Insurance companies are major participants in these enterprises. They offer to the public what is termed either resurrection coverage or afterlife insurance. These policies are a recent addition to fashionable, financial service which is a modern clamor since America is becoming a service oriented nation.

Several large, financially stable, insurance corporations are involved in cryonic preservation. In 1974 about six cryonic providers offered to preserve clients in liquid nitrogen. At the appropriate time a promise is made to return life to the frozen body when, and if, future biotechnology perfects a technique to accomplish this miracle. Freezing a human body is bioethically neutral. It is construed as a form of burial. To have a business arrangement that considers revitalization of hyperthermic corpses may be a deception. But in the insurance policy issued, the promise made is contingent upon the development of technology to resurrect the dead.

"Afterlife insurance is the newest thing in financial services. As more people request to be cryonically preserved, insurance companies such as New York Life are covering the process.

The concept of reviving a human embedded in ice was first developed as a story line for W. Clark Russell's 1887 yarn 'The Frozen Pirate.' In 1974 the American Cryonics Society began freezing bodies, and now a half-dozen cryonic providers, such as the Scottsdale, Arizona-based Alcor Life Extension Foundation, promise to pickle their clients in liquid nitrogen in the hopes of bringing them back if and when technology allows. The tab? $50,000 for the head, $120,000 for the whole body.

"Mary Naples, a San Francisco insurance broker, has sold more than 200 contracts to people seeking cryonic suspension. It's about 10% of her business. An annual premium for, say, a 40-year-old man could be $2,000, with a death benefit of $192,000 at the age of 65. The kicker is that suspension providers, such as Alcor (it has 35 people in deep freeze; 400 on a waiting list), require clients to designate the provider as the policy's irrevocable beneficiary to cover all freezing costs. That money can not be touched by a family who feels the deceased's investment is misguided. Would-be resurrectionists beware: The insurance money only covers the freezing. Thawing and reviving will, presumably, be COD" [Kellen, 1998].

Chapter 12

Feminist Approaches To Bioethics

Women are so essential to the creation of human life it is inescapable that feminine input would become a specificity in bioethics. So it has come to pass that dialogue commenced in 1999 has continued [Tong, 1999]. Depicted in writing are feminists approaches to ethics generally and bioethics in particular. The core of this discussion is quoted with permission of the author.

"I begin with what she calls 'power-focused feminist approaches.' Simply put, these approaches pay close attention to the experience and interests of women—and to the way those interests may be overlooked or denigrated in the organization and delivery of health care. More stridently put, this approach might focus on ways in which men are privileged and women oppressed in a still too patriarchally ordered world of medicine. And there are legitimate questions to be raised here, some of them noted by Tong (through the prevalence of eating disorders in women may be attributable less to patriarchy than to a world shaped, to some degree, by feminism). Important questions have been raised about, for example, the different levels of participation of men and women in medical experimentation, or about the way new reproductive technologies may alienate women from their bodies, or about the respective rôles in caregiving of nurses and physicians.

"Granting all this, we should still pause to reflect upon the fact that this is an approach to moral reasoning that places at the center the interests of women—that is, one 'special interest' among others. Perhaps one might try to justify this as a temporary measure, necessary in response to a gravely unjust world. But pressing special interests and putting one's ideal of fairness on hold for a time should, at least, be worrisome. This 'power-focused feminist approach' will need to explain how it differs from unjust special preference.

"One way of responding to this concern—the concern that this kind of feminism seeks to justify special preference—is to broaden the range of those whose interests are favored by a feminist ethic. Thus, for example, Tong suggest that power-focused approaches are concerned groups' interests, issues and identities.' They are opposed to a society 'in which sexism, racism, ethnocentrism, classism, and heterosexism thrive.' It's hard to know what to think of this move. On the one hand, large numbers of women believe quite strongly that the heterosexual bond is normative for human life. Evidently the feminism Tong describes (which brings 'heterosexism' into its fold) would have to excommunicate such women—or, perhaps, develop a theory of false consciousness, contending that such women may be oppressed even though they deny it. On the other hand, if we eliminated heterosexism from Tong's list of 'isms,' this broadened feminist concern for vulnerable groups would begin to sound rather like the Roman Catholic emphasis upon preferential option for the poor—making for unusual allies, to say the least.

"In short, these are not promising ways to deal with the charge of unjust special preference. It might be better to turn to what Tong calls 'care-focused feminist approaches,' for they argue that there is more to moral reasoning than considerations of justice alone. There is also care—an emphasis on relationships and fitting action within the bonds that tie us to others. This is, I think, a more promising approach. To be sure, it can be abused, as Tong notes (though I do not myself believe it is possible to 'care too much about others').

"Feminists themselves often disagree about the language of care, however. It might seem to support the notion that the sexual differentiation between male and female is of moral significance, that there are womanly and manly ways of being in the world—suggestions that will make certain feminists edgy. Others might wonder why men may not be as caring, as devoted to special relationships, as women. Tong herself seems disinclined to adopt a care-focused ethic; indeed, whatever havoc this may play with our categories, I suspect that I am more sympathetic to it than she!

"Surely it is best, though, to say that somehow 'care' and 'justice' must be held together within any sound moral perspective. (And this must be part of what Tong means by an 'integrated perspective,' though

I do not think it is adequate to describe care only as a passion or motive that inclines us to be just.)

Joanne Lynn is simply a good physician of the sort to which anyone, male or female, might aspire. I doubt, though, whether her first instinct—to provide the feeding tube—was acting like a 'traditional non-feminist physician.' Rather, it was a quite proper attempt to provide useful care for her patient and to be certain that she did not treat him unjustly by deliberately hastening his death. Likewise, her second thoughts about the feeding tube were not, I think, so much the result of an imaginative breakthrough as they were a realization—perhaps possible only after trying the tube—that for this patient such a treatment was excessively burdensome and, hence, not warranted. It looks less like the insight of a feminist bioethic—or of both feminist approaches integrated in some way—than simply of good moral reasoning that is sensitive to considerations of both care and justice. And, if there is anything at all to the care-focused ethic, it may best be achieved when men listen to women and women, likewise, listen to men" [Meilaender, 1999].

In response to the above quotation, the original author of the Feminist Approach to Bioethics wrote:

"Meilaender's concern about power-focused feminist approaches to bioethics is a reasonable one. However, just because feminists want bioethicists to look intently at women's interests, it does not mean they want bioethics to ignore men's interests. Similarly, just because feminists stress that women's perspectives on moral issues in the realm of health care are insightful, it does not mean feminists believe that women's moral authority is incontestable. Rather, power-focused feminist approaches aim to broaden and deepen traditional ethics (which tended to neglect or trivialize the interests of women and other historically vulnerable groups) with the perspectives of those previously marginalized groups.

"Admittedly, feminist approaches to bioethics are not neutral. They wear their primary interest (women) on their sleeves, opening themselves up for criticism voluntarily. However, just because an approach to bioethics emphasizes gender, it does not mean it is sexist. An approach to bioethics becomes sexist only when it systematically excludes the interests, identities, issues and values of one sex in favor of another.

"That feminists are concerned about vulnerable groups, including gay men and lesbian women, does not mean they disregard the interests of other groups. Most human beings oscillate between rôles of oppressor and oppressed and positions of power and vulnerability. However, some groups of human beings—according to race, gender or class, for example—are oppressed more frequently and severely. The fact that I oppose heterosexism does not mean that I think all heterosexual women (or men, for that matter) should renounce the values they associate with being heterosexual (e.g., beliefs about what constitutes a proper family, a meaningful sexual liaison or marriage). However, it does mean I think it is wrong for heterosexual persons to discriminate against gay men and lesbian women in the public realm (including employment, insurance, housing and so forth).

"I also found Professor Meilaender's comments on Dr. Joanne Lynn's style of practice provocative. When Dr. Lynn prescribed a feeding tube for her patient, she was, by her own admission, doing what the book proclaims as standard operating procedure. Lynn admits she started a treatment that she might never have ordered in the first place had she initially taken the time to listen to her patient's spouse and respond to her and the patient at an emotional level, precisely the level that physicians have traditionally been acculturated and taught to view as dangerous, irrational or unscientific territory. Thus, Lynn's initial actions, like those of some physicians and healthcare practitioners, may be seen as non-feminist because they did not reflect any of the culturally-associated 'feminine' values (such as caring, connection, emotion), but only culturally-associated 'masculine' values (such as justice, independence, reason).

"Feminists who espouse care-focused or power-focused approaches to bioethics are not advocating women's perspectives *über alles*.[1] Far from it. It's just that by focusing on how gender shapes and misshapes one's power to care and be cared for in the world of medicine and sci-

1. The phrase *über alles* is a common component of every day German. The word *alles* means everything, as in *Das ist alles*, that is all, that is everything. Grammatically, *alles* can refer only to a thing, a neuter. If it was intended to signify other countries or people of different nations, it would have to be *alle*. *Das Land* [the land/country] is neuter singular. *Die Länder* [the countries] is pleural. *Alle* is generally followed by a plural noun when it refers to countries, people, animals, clothes, and other specific things. If the sentence is clearly understood then *alle* suffices.

ence, they are identifying ways for everyone to improve bioethical reasoning" [Tong, 1999].

It is a sadness to believe that any intelligent person would apply double standards to bioethics. The ever-growing bioethical codes would be vulnerable to injury like a blossoming rosebud with a deadly worm in its petals if this occurred. If bias exists, it is a grievous fault and grievously should perpetrators answer for it. More worthy is to concentrate on finding moral solutions in response to the multiple bioethical griefs that are rampant. To discourage prejudice between genders is an obligation of those who are learned. Not to do so will divide the art of bioethics leaving it a half-orphan.

Chapter 13

Fetology

Among the rapidly respected disciplines in the specialty of pediatrics is fetology. It has demanded that a fetus be accorded the same careful considerations as any other patient. Astonishingly *in utero* treatment is a major boon in pediatric care. The contribution in biotechnology, the acumen assistance of ultrasound, intra-uterine surgery, ultrasonography, and amniocentesis have become diagnostic tools with accuracy in diagnosis for the detection and prediction of birth defects.

These technical modalities deflate the legal right to abortion for a birth defect. The constitutional permission for a woman to prevent the birth of her child is founded upon a weak explanation. Justification for the reasoning and the constitutional foundation of that decision is very tenuous, specious, and seems fabricated.

Fetology may weaken the Roe vs Wade foundation upon which the Supreme Court established a constitutional right to abortion. A decade after this pioneer decision the highest court reaffirmed the Roe decision in the City of Akron vs Akron Centre for Reproductive Health in 1983. However the presentation before the nine judges demonstrated the weaknesses in the origin of the basis for the decision rendered.

The fallacies of the majority opinion and the Roe decision upon which the Akron verdict was reached were highlighted in the dissenting opinion of Justices O'Connor, White, and Rehnquist. They wrote:

"As the medical risks of various abortion procedures decrease, the point at which the State may regulate for reasons of maternal health is moved further forward to childbirth. As medical science becomes better able to provide for the separate existence of the fetus, the point of viability is moved further back to conception.

"The Roe framework is inherently tied to the state of medical technology that exists whenever particular litigation ensues. Although legislatures are better suited to make the necessary factual judgments in this area, the Court's framework forces legislatures, as a matter of constitutional law, to speculate about what constitutes 'accepted medical practice' at any given time. Without the necessary expertise or ability, courts must then pretend to act as science review boards and examine those legislative judgments" [Akron, 1983].

"The court stated in Roe vs. Wade that 'with respect to the State's important and legitimate interest in potential life, the compelling point is at viability. This is so because the fetus then presumably has the capability of meaningful life outside the mother's womb.' The Court said 'viability is usually placed at seven months (28 weeks) but may occur earlier, even at 24 weeks." Advances in neonatology since 1973 have lowered this to 24 weeks and, in some cases, to 21 or 22 weeks. These advances clearly call into question 'viability' as a standard for existence independent of the womb. At the other end of the viability question, we have seen the necessity of confronting the survival of late-term fetuses. The use of prostaglandins does not guarantee the death of the fetus, and their survival only renews the question of the reality of abortion" [Akron, 1983].

The time during which the unborn child is totally dependent on his or her mother's body is also continually becoming shorter because of advances at the other end of pregnancy. Artificial conception and in vitro fertilization are already realities; many believe that artificial placentas or other forms of extended life support outside the mother's body can not be far behind. Thus the court's use of viability as a standard is becoming irrelevant; it is losing its significance with the advancement and development of support technology [Vanderhoef, 1987].

Ultrasonography has become an especially desirable procedure because it presents no discernable risk to the fetus. By measuring the reflection of transmission of ultrasonic waves, it locates, measures and delineates the deep structures within the uterus, making it possible to visualize the fetus. It assures the accurate determination of gestational age as well as diagnosis, thus becoming an important new non-invasive clinical tool. It is a treasured diagnostic modality that can assist in determining fetal viability.

The abortion-right law is fraught with flawed reasoning. An underlying conflict is present in which the unborn baby's rights are not given the same consideration as the privacy rights of the mother upon which the Roe decision was based. Abortion is not a private matter when every politician, legislature, candidates for public office, hospitals, physicians, clinics, the media, boards of health, TV, Hollywood and many more institutions are not silent on the matter.

"Nowhere is this more dramatically demonstrated than in the new theories of law designated as wrongful birth and wrongful life. The theory of such relief is based upon the legal rights of parents to prevent the birth of a child by holding that a woman has a constitutional right to abortion. Our advances in technology in ultrasound, intra-and extra-uterine surgery, and amniocentesis have enabled us to become increasingly accurate in the detection and prediction of birth defects. Because these changes in our technology, the courts have been called upon with increasing frequency to resolve claims by children with birth defects and by their parents. The parents, under wrongful birth claims, seek damages for the financial and emotional costs of raising an impaired child. A child, under a wrongful life claim, asserts that he or she would have been better off not being born, hence the compensation for birth in an impaired condition.

"The frightening concept that birth can be 'wrongful' is the direct and logical progression of a legal system that authorizes and sanctions the destruction of life through abortion. Wrongful life claims have required the courts to conclude that non-life is preferable to life with defects. Wrongful life has presented us with a frightening example of how the rapid and awesome advances in medical technology have been matched by the rapid and awesome advances in the application of a death ethic by our legal system.

"Nearly all of the medical and legal arguments have been exposed as being insufficient in their foundation as a standard and have now brought us directly to confront the basic issue of the abortion question—abortion is a moral issue.

"Our advances in the biological and medical sciences only increase our responsibility to develop the criteria of respect, deference, and promotion of every human being's primary and fundamental right to life. Our courts and our legislative bodies must accept their responsibility in these moral areas" [Vanderhoef, 1987].

Chapter 14

Fetal Tissue Research

At a well-attended conference on "Fetal Tissue Use: Is it Ethical"? sponsored by the Castello Institute of Stafford, Virginia, the answer was "no". Speakers and audience were physicians, physiologists, surgeons, lawyers, and others. They concluded that there was little reason to support it. Arguments were dismissed that the fetal tissue usage can be separated from abortion because the fetuses used would have died anyway. This statement supports the dictum: "The greatest enemies are ignorance, sin, and death."

The biomedical researchers and clinicians have had no cures from fetal tissue administered for Parkinson's disease and diabetes mellitus. "It is a tragedy and a travesty to argue that we are going to save Americans from all these diseases by this procedure," stated neurological surgeon, Robert White of Cleveland [O'Brien, 1992].

Parkinson's Disease

As to Parkinson's disease the proposed use of fetal tissue in its treatment is superfluous in view of other new therapy. Scientists in Colorado have isolated a natural "nerve growth factor" [a protein] that appears to promote the growth of those nerve cells that are disabled in Parkinsonism.[1] Experiments with rodents give promise of alleviating nerve debilitating symptoms in human beings. Present medications have limited effective-

---

1. It is dubbed glial-derived neurotrophic factor [GDNF].

ness after several years. This includes the new drug called Antril which was developed to treat nosocomial infections [Waldholz, 1993].

Implantation of fetal tissue has occurred at the University of California in Los Angeles. It is reported that seven patients with Parkinsonism received implants of fetal tissue [PDF Newsletter, 1993-94]. The patients had been followed carefully at 3-4 month intervals for at least one year preceding the operation. Levodopa was reduced following surgery in order to prevent possible injury to the fetal tissue implant but was gradually increased to preoperative levels. Patients worsened somewhat following surgery, but by 3 months postoperatively they began to improve.

It seems that the implantation of fetal tissue is helpful to some Parkinson patients. The procedure has been performed at several centers around the world, and scientists are cautiously optimistic. However, they are still not sure which patients will improve, nor how long the improvement will continue, or if the improvement will be maintained. To date there has been no double-blind study (in which neither the patients nor the treating physicians know which patients received the tissue). Some will be conducted by scientists at Columbia-Presbyterian Medical Centre in collaboration with others at North Shore Hospital-Cornell University on Long Island. Proponents of using fetal anatomy parts have overstated the alleged improvements attributed to fetal tissue. Alternative therapy has more promise of ameliorating Parkinsonism than questionable unproven benefits from fetal tissue.

For example, "preliminary investigations in animals indicate that several other tissues, besides fetal mesencephalon from aborted babies, may prove appropriate for grafting. Ultimately, advances in molecular biology may allow either transplantation of genetically engineered cells or direct modification of existing brain cells by transfection [transference] with viral vectors.[2] The favorable preliminary experience with cerebral transplantation in patients with Parkinson's disease has resulted in the consideration of this strategy for other neurologic disorders" [Mayo Clinic Proceedings, 1993].

Parkinsonism is a physiopathologic entity that lends itself to treatment by transplantation. The motor function deficits are related prima-

---

2. In pathology a vector is an organism that carries pathogens from one host to another.

rily to the loss of a single group of cells within the brain named the *substantia nigra*. This disease is treated currently with levodopa which supplies and replenishes the brain with dopamine. The absence of which results in the clinical picture of the disease, i.e., slowness of movements, peculiar gait, muscular tremor, partial facial paralysis, and salivation. This illness is called *paralysis agitans* and sometimes referred to as shaking palsy.

Fetus-to-Fetus Transplant

Due to genetic defects there are many diseases which researchers are attempting to correct by transferring specific aborted fetal tissue to another defective living fetus. In theory many genetic disorders, including sickle cell anemia and Hurler's syndrome,[3] would be potential candidates for cure by tissue taken from an aborted fetus.

Specialized experimental researchers took precursors of blood cells [stem cells] from the liver tissue of a fetus that had been aborted due to a tubal pregnancy. These cells were injected through the pregnant woman's uterine wall into the chest cavity of her fetus. The cells settled in the fetus's liver and from there migrated to bone marrow, where they gave rise to cells that circulated elsewhere in the body, where they formed the needed enzyme [Slotnick, Zanyani, 1993]. Further details were not disclosed. But it is known that the amount of enzyme being produced by this hepatic tissue method is about 85 units per deciliter of blood, a minimum of 80 units per deciliter is needed to prevent symptoms of the disease. A normal range is 80 to 700 units per deciliter [Hilts, 1994].

Fetal Ovary Transplantation

Adventuresome experimentation by an Edinburgh scientist suggests the feasibility of transplanting ovaries from aborted fetuses into infertile women who do not produce viable ova on their own. The procedure is

---

3. Hurler's syndrome is an inherited disease in which cells do not produce an enzyme crucial to breaking down sugars in some cells. As a result sugar molecules accumulate and ultimately cause these cells to break down. Children with Hurler's syndrome usually die in the early years of life.

reported as a success in mice. This accomplishment was taking ovaries from mouse fetuses and transplanting them into adult mice. The transposed ovaries produced eggs that could be fertilized and developed into normal mice. The researcher stated that it might be possible to do the same procedure in human beings [Gosden, 1994].

"In Britain, the Health Secretary, said the Government's national health program would not pay for that effort. The ethics committee of the British Medical Association is preparing a report on the doctor's proposal for ovary transplants. Some ethicists say reproductive technology may finally have gone too far. The idea of implanting an ovary from an aborted fetus, whether it proves feasible in human beings or not, raises questions about the extent to which science should intervene to help infertile couples" [Kolata, 1994]. Sinister mutations in bioethics are becoming more evident as bioscientists are motivated to do good by means of questionable morality.

Does fetal ovary transplantation reduce reproduction from a biological function to a commodity? Moreover, "a long-standing principle in ethics forbade the use of a vulnerable population merely for convenience. Thus it is no longer considered ethical to do research on prisoners or retarded children if the same studies could just as easily be done with people who were free to volunteer. In this case, human eggs can be obtained from adult women who volunteer to donate. So that raises the question: Are fetuses a vulnerable population? [Levine, 1994]. Manmade moral diversity has no restraint.

Public, private, and professional debates, discussions, disagreements, and disenchantment over the emerging reproductive technologies in some ways have become illogical due either to emotionalism or passionate devotion to a cause. However startling the promise of these amazing technologies, there remains the ethical and legal challenges posed to science and society. It is unclear how many of these indicate future success. If bioscientific hopes are fulfilled by preliminary, positive, clinically confirmed results, ethical and legal problems surely will follow.

Among the most flagrant of which is the subterranean trade in fetuses. In 1980 it was estimated that ten thousand fetuses per year are sent to biology and pharmacology research laboratories. This was before the breakthrough in fetal cell transplantations which have increased the demand for aborted babies. Even before the beginning of fetal tissue use allegations of abuse were heard [Hillebrecht, 1989].

Some hospitals were stained by serious scandal. In 1976 newspapers revealed that $68,000 from the sale of aborted fetuses had found its way into the pockets of a pathology department's administration. Also it was disclosed that doctors at the hospital may have encouraged unneeded abortions on welfare patients as a way of adding volume to the fetus trade. In the wake of the resulting bad publicity, fetus-procuring agents went off-shore. For a time, South Korea, Argentina, Brazil, and Haiti became the major suppliers. Potentially there is a great deal of money to be made in this international capital-investment chicanery. How easy it is for those without scruples who are spiritually weak to be induced into the *imbroglio* of an immoral enterprise that dethrones bioethics.

Opposition To Fetal Tissue Research

Removing tissue from aborted fetuses shows a disrespect for human remains. Legal abortion is the culprit that has masterminded distorted judgment in the bioscientific community on medicomoral principles. Forgetting that medicine/surgery are studied in order to preserve human life not to destroy it. Scientists of merit "are not divided about the beginning of life.[4] They are divided on the subject of respecting life" [Lejeune, 1993]. Nature knows more than it discloses. No scientist has discovered the mysterious secret of nature's physiology, its orderliness, and immutability. Its consistency secures moral integrity which is not inimicable to any science.

Researchers sometimes forget that people are real persons and not animals or inanimate objects. Medical science by clear observation and appreciation of what it knows must come to reëvaluate human personhood. Researchers and bioexperimenters must not forget that no matter how small or old, human life is not an object. In an experiment on a material object like stress tests on steel for building a bridge or constructing a skyscraper, it may be cracked, broken, even destroyed in the testing

---

4. Major textbooks written by highly respected embryologists agree that life begins at the moment that all genetic information necessary for development is gathered inside the living system initially. That occurs in human beings when the male sperm fertilizes the female ovum. At conception the new entity identified as a fertilized ovum becomes a member of the human species and a kinsman.

process. An animal experiment may result in severe injury or cause its death. In terms of benefit to humanity the loss of an animal is warranted [Mulligan, 1990].

This notion does not prevail when human beings are studied. They should not be broken, injured, destroyed, and subjected to anything inhuman. Moral theology has precise norms in this regard which require a differentiation between research and experimentation. Both words are used incorrectly as synonyms which they are not. Research is a process of systematic observation that is primarily looking, recording what is seen, and learning from the gathered information. In the usual course of events research would not be hurtful, harmful, fatal, and no moral objection to it would be entertained. Of a certainty, there are moral restrictions placed on the means of observation.

Examining brain function by CAT scan, electroencephalography, physical examination, and xray study of the skull is far different from doing ventrilography, burr holes, and craniotomy. Xray observation of an embryo could cause a defect or congenital anomaly. Sonography seems to be innocuous. Therefore there is moral responsibility in research not to use a method that can cause injury, complications, or mortality. Bioethical research requires concern for the persons well-being at all times.

"Experimentation is more than observation. It involves not only research (looking) but active intervention (doing something). Experimentation on a human being (at any stage of life from zygote to adult) involves doing something to that person. In medicine this could involve the performance of surgical procedures or the use of drugs or new technologies. The purpose is to verify some result or effect that which is not yet known or not yet understood. It is clear that the unborn must be especially protected, since they have no way of knowing what is to be done, or of choosing or giving consent. Both research and experimentation are performed with the goal of knowledge. Work with human beings, at any stage of life, is work with persons. The researcher or experimenter would do well to keep in mind that he is not simply "getting to know it." He is "getting to know you" [Mulligan, 1990].

"The simplistic assumption that one life can be 'harvested' to benefit another would appear to undercut a basic criterion of justice which has prevailed in all civilized societies. An alternative is to acknowledge the wisdom and inevitability of our shared vulnerability and calculate the moral cost of a frantic search to avoid the consequences of human fragility. Such options are bitter and unpopular medicine for those raised in a society preoccupied with bodily perfection of youth. . . .

"Yet we flee from recognition of our own interdependency, vulnerability and decline. We are outraged that we grow older and more limited each day. Life takes those little nibbles at our physical being but doesn't destroy our souls. It is we, individually or as a society, who allow that important aspect of human life to shrivel and wither. Within this context, our frantic rush toward fetal tissue transplants would appear to sprout from the same seeds which yield a caustic crop of social alienation and disharmony. If we care only for ourselves, our children will not value themselves and will find their own destruction in our streets. If we care not enough to find the resources to enable our weakest members to find ways to live productively, we face our own dependent stagnation or death when we fail to fit the utilitarian standards we have embraced.

"When our desire to postpone or avoid sickness, disabilities or discomforts outweighs all lingering concerns about preserving an essential recognition that all human life merits respect, we are lost as moral people. The point where human life ceases to be valued and becomes a 'thing' to be harvested and used by others more 'worthy' is of deep concern to all those who recognize the potential of life in spite of imperfections. . .

"When medical science or political systems encourage 'cannibalism' of one life to nurture another, we will have lost the sense of our unique dignity and value. We will have sacrificed the health of our society for the temporary well-being of a few. And we will have fostered the alienation which stalks our society" [Owens, 1992].

Recital Of Objections

1. Enthusiasm for medicosurgical research on and experimentation with fetal tissues that accentuate promised benefits places a mask on the unethical, abominable practice—a dogooders feeble excuse for being pro-abortion.
2. It encourages a dependency on fetal anatomy which emboldens those who perform abortions.
3. Search and destroy methods seeking new discoveries do not validate taking fetal tissue from aborted babies.

4. Unwarranted is the premise that fetal tissue transplants are promising in the treatment of Parkinsonism and diabetes mellitus.
5. Experiments on human beings at any stage of life from zygote to senescence involve active doings which may institute morbidity and/or mortality.
6. Women are exposed to greater risks to their persons as unscrupulous physicians perform dangerous pre-birth abortions to obtain aborted babies for sale.
7. Exploitation of poor women persuaded into pregnancy and abortion for economic security.
8. Cash commerce in fetuses is not stoppable as long as tissue transplantation persists.
9. As a composite, all-inclusive term, "fetus-farming" for financial funds, even for an intended family good such as a loved-one needing fetal tissue to combat disease, is misplaced loyalty.
10. Harvesting abortees, like an agricultural crop to be sold, is a debased occupation of unprecedented malice.

In 1992 a strong campaign to support *via* letters to congressmen the continuance of the ban on fetal tissue use was made by energetic physicians. The major contents of the formal letter, dated March 24, 1992 is reproduced partly as follows.

"We are writing in support of the current moratorium on federally funded human transplants using tissue from induced abortions. In our opinion the effort to overturn this moratorium through H.R. 2507, the National Institutes of Health reauthorization bill, is ill-advised for several reasons:

1. *The Administration's concern that such federally subsidized programs could become an added inducement to abortion has not been rebutted.* In one recent study, a significant number of college students showed a willingness to induce abortion for the express purpose of providing fetal tissue (*Lancet* 335: 1594 [1990]). Clearly, some women could be swayed in their decision to abort by the perceived medical value of aborted fetal tissue.

2. *The therapeutic value of tissue from induced abortions has been greatly exaggerated by some involved in the political debate.* Some experiments hailed as examples of therapeutic success actually used tissue from ectopic pregnancies (the Walden case in Texas) or from spontaneous abortions (Dr. Madrazo's research in Mexico)—and thus would be eligible for federal funding even under the current moratorium. In one much-reported experiment, Swedish researchers obtained fetal brain tissue for treatment of Parkinson's disease by aspirating the brain out of the fetal skull *before* terminating the pregnancy; yet despite this unrestricted zeal for 'fresh' brain tissue, the researchers admitted that "no major graft-induced improvements of therapeutic value to the patients have been observed up to 6 months postoperatively and concluded that this is 'an experimental approach and not a therapeutic alternative' for Parkinson's disease (*Arch. Neurol.* 46: 627 and 630 [June 1989]).

3. *Alternative sources of tissue as well as alternative therapeutic approaches are available for many of the ailments in question, and have not been fully explored.* Diverting federal funds to research that depends on the continued availability of tissue from induced abortions will detract from these alternative approaches, and make federal research on such ailments dependent on the continued legality of abortion. Once such a policy decision is made, federal or state changes in the legal status of abortion will correspondingly jeopardize the therapeutic practices that depend on this status. No such problems would be created by alternative approaches, such as the development of a tissue bank using tissue from ectopic pregnancies or spontaneous abortions."

Chapter 15

Ethical Challenges In Genetics

Younger generations want to subvert basic, time-tested rules that stood firm throughout past moral storms, ethical conflicts, and pseudo-philosophical destructive criticisms. Modern, negative sounds are familiar. Same words not stiff *staccato*, sounds much louder, and more off-balance. Trying to be persuasive in defense, wrong words are spoken cringingly that do not express well what was thought to be convincingly changeable to any opposition. Criticism comes easily. Too often speaking shows ignorance. Silence hides the inferior intellect. But evil will out no matter how clever it is hidden and the excuses made for its existence and the supposed good intended.

"In 1952 the German Supreme Court passed judgement on some doctors who had participated in the selection of mentally handicapped people for euthanasia during the Nazi regime. The doctors claimed in their own defense that they had saved the lives of countless sick people by forcing them into religious houses. These sick people would have died had the accused given up their activity and yielded their jobs to 'harsher' colleagues. The court rejected this line of defense. Appealing to the general Christian and European moral view, it declared that 'the prevention of a greater evil' could not justify the deliberate taking of innocent human life. Such manslaughter is always a crime. Even the best of intentions does not justify the means" [Spaemann, 1993].

This was a shameful reason which is an expression of contemporary morality that has eliminated the idea of shame. The guilt of shame and betrayal of fear as lack of courage were intricately woven into the architecture of ancient ethics. Not surprisingly atheism is protagonistic to an ethical culture that does accept trust, while seeking to remove the concept of shame in its teaching even when it does not fortify moral life. "Atheism involves a number of trends which can be recognized under the headings: utilitarianism, consequentialism, proportionalism or teleological ethics[1]" [Spaemann, 1993]. All these -isms singularly and collectively do not include God as the hub of their isms existence. Hence God's Commandments are a fantasy, whose consequential restitution for disobedience is a myth.

Human beings including bioscientists are never forced to do evil. To do so would be contrary to the teaching regarding the correct human, worthy way of living morally. Guardians of human identity and freedom of conscience defend the conviction that there are types of behavior that are not expected of any human being. Reference is to those actualities done that are contrary to given nature which is not subjected to the weighing of *pros* or *cons* as to performance. By this is meant no discussion is valid that maintains a person is forced to do evil.

There are types and kinds of behavior which can never be proper no matter the coercive force and situation encountered. To do otherwise would not be in conformity with the pristine dignity of the person made to the image and likeness of God. "Finally, it is always possible that man, as the result of coercion, or other circumstances, can be hindered from doing certain good actions, but he can never be hindered from not doing certain actions, especially if he is prepared to die rather than to do evil"[2] [Pope John Paul II's encyclical *Veritatis splendor*]. Once a person abandons his/her created nature and does what is not in accordance with it, everything becomes unbearable as morality deliquesces. This is not a

---

1. Teleology is the theory of purpose, ends, goals, final causes, and values. As opposed to mechanism, which explains the present and future in terms of the past, teleology explains the past and the present in terms of the future. Teleology as such does not imply personal consciousness, volition, or intended purpose.

2. "Better to die than to do evil." Recent works of moral theology have criticized the martyrs' refusal to do anything, under any circumstance whatsoever, that could be interpreted as emperor worship. However the Church of Christ is the Church of the martyrs, the witnesses to the faith, and is not the Church of scholars, even though the scholars have an important rôle in the service of this witness. As servants of God human beings who believe in Him are the highest witness believers in the Resurrection.

sentiment recollection. But ethical tenets that are imposed upon geneticists as bioscientists whose memorable work is under microscopic scrutiny world-wide.

Genetic Advances And Ethical Risks

Human genome is the complete set of instructions for making a human being. The long-term effort to map out and discover the sequence of events in human genes is called the Human Genome Project. Laboratory methods are able at this time of bioscientific acumen to discern the function of the genes in the human body. Each day scientists find more and more information that accumulates a wealth of knowledge on genetics.

An example is the experience of "A graduate student at Johns Hopkins who sequenced 8 million chemical components of genetic material in a single year, all of them located on chromosome 21, the smallest of the 46 human chromosomes. Eight million is small potatoes in genome work; the human body has more than 3 billion such units. But the interesting news is that the student worked 10 times faster than was possible only a few years ago. More-powerful computers are speeding up the task every year, bringing us every closer to conquering most diseases" [Leo, 1989].

"Annas fears that the mapping of the human genome may lead to a very narrow notion of what a physically normal person is. This, in turn, could promote an increase in the number of abortions, or even create a market in prescreened high-grade embryos guaranteed" to look like a movie star or an Olympic athlete" [Leo, 1989]. Fictional as it may appear the eugenic thought may be promoted to weed out the less than perfect. Premarital inquiry of the genetic history of a future spouse is a probability.

Apparently there is more to human genome research than finding cures for diseases. People modification is a popular theme witnessed by the rise in cosmetic surgical procedures. It is not a fantasy to think that people are adverse to taking charge of their physical appearance and alter their own biology. Human beings have fewer genes than was estimated. A lesser number means a greater effort to influence them. Hence scientists opine it will be easier to create genetically modified people with safety plus reasonable degree of success by germ line gene therapy.

Ethical issues are unavoidable in the genome project. At present the relationship of the bioethicist to the bioscientific researcher is not very strong. No starting point exists between them that mutually accepts the fact of the recognition of the dangers as well as the benefits with genetic advancement. A now hypothetical supposition may become perilous if based upon genetic findings. An excuse may be found to divide populations into superior and inferior groups by value judgments. This would be a pursuit of Hitler's dream of a master race. What if a genetic defect is found in the majority of the population and abortion is the therapy for the prevention of physical deformity, congenital, and hereditary diseases? Does wholesale abortion take the place of gas-chambers and cremation ovens? Does spiritual beauty go unrecognized? No beauty is to be ignored even in human beings with physical imperfections.

Genetic research can lead to ethical abuses. A profound interest is apparent in biological and genetic manipulation. There is an enormous curiosity in the recombinant DNA [deoxyribonucleic acid]. Found in the nucleus of cells it is responsible for the transfer of genetic characteristics from one generation to the next. The restructuring of inherited characteristics by manipulation of DNA has been done in lower forms of life. Scientists have been able to change on-cell organisms in such a way as to give them new characteristics which is tantamount to a new life-form.

Other indications of the rising ethical upheavals that are to be expected occurred in 1990. A National Institute of Health panel approved the insertion of new genes into the blood cells of children suffering from a genetic disorder that destroys the immune system [Mulligan, 1991]. In China a plan was presented by a lecturer in which experiments were to be done on human and chimpanzee cells.[3] The object to be obtained was a new, strong, docile, not-too-intelligent hybrid species of agricultural workers. Another fantastic suggestion is cross-fertilization of human and animal gametes and the gestation of a human being in the uterus of an animal [Mulligan, 1991]. Moral objections would be many as the ethics of these proposals are morally distressful.

An evil-eye is cast upon geneticists who are consulted by would-be parents who wish to select the gender of their baby. A genetic institute is available for this purpose. "The institute's latest product is MicroSort, a machine that sifts through sperm and separates the X's from the Y's, allowing customers to choose whether to have a boy or a girl. The process is not quite foolproof—in trials thus far, 93 percent of couples who

---

3. Arthur Clarke, author of 2001, quoted by Msgr. James J. Mulligan 1991

wanted a girl have gotten their wish and 73 percent of couples seeking a boy got one—but it's convincingly better than God's even odds. Price: $2,500 per menstrual cycle (on average, it takes four cycles to achieve pregnancy).

Nature's way isn't faring too well in reproduction these days. Science is gaining in many ways. In the past decade, the proportion of women who pick their delivery date by having their doctors induce labor has doubled to 18 percent. Geneticists can screen fetuses for dozens of diseases, allowing parents to decide whether to let nature take its course or halt the process and try again. The infertility industry has become a robust profit center in medicine, extending women's childbearing years almost unimaginably. But gender selection is a big step. It's the closest we've come so far to designer babies.

The American Society for Reproductive Medicine frowns on using gender selection for "family balancing," and the American Medical Association's president is even blunter. "We have to draw a line in the sand," she thunders. But if we have learned anything about technological advances in this century, it's that there's no stopping them, no matter their ethical or moral implications" [Fisher, 1999].

"Biologists have for the first time deciphered the full genetic programming of an animal, a landmark achievement both in its own right and as a milestone toward understanding the human genome.

"The animal is a microscopic roundworm known as *Caenorhabditis elegans* and used in laboratories throughout the world as a means to explore biology at the genetic level. Its genome, or full DNA, has now been found to consist of 97 million chemical units and is expected to contain 19,099 genes. If printed in ordinary type, the DNA sequence would take up 2,748 pages of a newspaper.

"The genome, deciphered by two teams of biologists, gives biologists their first sight of the information needed to develop, operate and maintain a multicellular animal.

"The worm genome has paved the way technically for decoding the human genome and will also help to interpret it. Understanding the human genome is expected to lead to profound changes in treating the many diseases that have a genetic basis.

"The only genomes sequenced up until now have belonged to single-celled organisms like bacteria and yeast. Worms and humans have turned out to have many genes in common. The worm genome is regarded by biologists as an essential basis for understanding how the human genome works" [Wade, 1998].

This is an example of the benefits to be derived from genetic research without any fear of bioethical violations. Another benefit is the good example of an occasion in which genetic screening serves a good purpose. In this way genetics is helpful and has no negative implications. An example is the subject phenylketonuria.

This is an inherited disease transferred genetically as a defect in metabolism. Causing mental retardation it can be diagnosed soon after birth by a blood test. No contrary moral implications of screening for phenylketonuria [PKU] is appended to the laboratory test.

"First of all, the method of diagnosis by blood test of the already born child does not involve the serious risks that are always present when amniocentesis is performed on the unborn child. Furthermore, a positive finding in the diagnosis is not going to result in the imposition of a death sentence on the child.

"The treatment which is offered does not change the genetic facts. In other words, this is not a case of genetic engineering. The patient has PKU both before and after the test. But the treatment does take care of the undesirable effects of the PKU. All the indications are that both the test and the treatment are morally acceptable" [Mulligan, 1991].

Genetic Engineering

Genetic screening is a search procedure which involves the diagnosis of some genetic diseases. The exploration does nothing to either modify or alter genes. The process of attempting alterations is genetic engineering. The former [screening] is innocuous bioethically, the latter [engineering] is not always innocent.

Engineering is more complex, may be dangerous in its own specific fashion, and bring about alterations that can be transmitted to subsequent generations. This moral burden is a risk to this genetic enterprise which involves causing most serious physical effects on humanity. Such activity raises profound moral questions.

To employ genetic engineering to inhibit transfer of diseases from parent to child is a laudable enterprise. Such diseases as neurofibromatosis may be controllable. It is a genetic disease that produces flat, brown areas on the skin, plus nodules along the course of nerves. Not always hereditary, it is caused by spontaneous genetic mutation at conception according to geneticists.

Using sophisticated genetic engineering, agricultural biotechnology aims to improve wheat and corn crops. In another project animals are to be used for growing human disease for the development of prophylactic vaccines, containing antibodies. Cows will produce more milk by feeding them recombinant growth hormone. Life sciences companies will combine their biotechnical talents in pharmacy and chemistry to form new industries which should not dethrone bioethical norms.

Many recurrent classical problems of laboratory safety have become less worrisome because of genetic engineering techniques. The basis for which is the progress in molecular biology that has successfully decreased rather than increased laboratory "hazards by allowing study on smaller amounts of material and providing gentler reagents" [Davis, 1987]. This is a plus for genetic engineering without any bioethical infringement. Genetic engineering is growing rapidly as simultaneously it challenges basic assumptions in molecular biology [Makulowich, 1987].

Another good side of genetic engineering is in the fight against neoplasms. A report in the science journal "Nature" indicates that scientists have transmuted a normal cell into a cancer cell by genetically altering it in the laboratory [Weinberg, 1999]. The importance of this ability is its possible application toward the development of medication to combat tumors. Research bioscientists are aware that cancer is caused by genes that have changed for the worse. Genetic engineering may assist in preventing the flaws.

Genetic Enhancement

Like all scientists, the aim of geneticists is to be constructive and not destructive to humanity's well-being. All those participating in genetic enhancement endeavors through gene transfer have the ethical burden not to collude with any decision whose purpose is immoral, illegitimate, and/or abnormal.

Vanity has prompted dissatisfaction with the faltered appearance of the visible anatomy in some people. They are not content with themselves as partners conforming to conceptual creation. Hence plastic surgery became a distinct specialty unto itself. Recently it has redefined itself and has refined its name into cosmetic surgery. Now research scientists have entered the beautifying scene with genetic alterations to improve the human body. Conceitedly this is an attempt to better God's handiwork. Genetic enhancement has instigated a conceptual and ethical challenge for gene therapy regulation.

"One of the fruits of the 'genetic revolution' in biomedicine has been the ability to splice functional genes into the DNA of human cells to produce stable changes in the bodies of patients. The use of these 'human gene transfer' techniques to treat genetic disease has been widely endorsed, as long as two lines are not crossed: no changes are made that would be passed on to the patient's children; and no attempts are made to exceed restoration of the normal, that is, to 'genetically enhance' human traits like stamina, strength, beauty, memory or intelligence. This second boundary is particularly interesting, because it captures an important moral intuition and, at the same time, is at constant risk of collapsing under the weight of basic conceptual arguments. If the boundary between gene therapy and genetic enhancement is to serve as a useful line for policy, we should be clear about what it is demarcating" [Juengst, 1999].

"The treatment-enhancement distinction is often employed to argue that therapeutic uses of genetic engineering fall within the boundaries of medicine's traditional domain, while enhancement uses do not, and therefore are more problematic" [Anderson, 1989]. There are several rejoinders to this argument. Some argue that medicine has no essential domain of practice, so that a coherent distinction between medical and non-medical services never can be drawn in the first place. Others accept the distinction between treating and enhancing, but challenge the traditional values of medicine by arguing that privileging treatment over enhancement is itself wrong. Others argue that, in any case, for psychological and economic reasons, the line between treatment and enhancement will be impossible to hold in practice [Parens, 1998].

"There is another response to the distinction between treatment and enhancement, however, that is particularly relevant to gene transfer research. This response criticizes the distinction by showing how it dissolves in the use of human gene transfer techniques to prevent disease when such interventions involve the enhancement of the body's health maintenance capacities. For example, many new cancer protocols involve transferring genes that improve the ability of the human immune system to detect cancer cells, while other gene therapies already give their recipients better than normal abilities to lower cholesterol levels.

To the extent that disease prevention is a proper goal of medicine, the use of gene transfer techniques to enhance human health maintenance capacities will help achieve that goal.

"There have been a number of attempts to explain how the concept of enhancement can function as a boundary for medical practice and still include legitimate forms of preventive medicine. Some argue that any intervention designed to restore or preserve a species typical level of functioning should count as treatment, leaving only interventions that would create capabilities beyond the range of normal human variation to count as enhancement. Others attempt to draw the line between interventions for diagnosable pathologies and those aimed at improvements unrelated to the individual's health" [Juengst, 1997].

Genomic medicine has not shown what it can do. Only the surface is seen. Beneath it may be found potential means of therapy that can assist in neurological improvements in the disabled. Perhaps discoveries will diminish the aging process and block the progress of Alzheimer's disease. Improvements such as these are credits to the tuned talent of geneticists.

Much of genetic enhancement is envisioned in the future. Many of the theories advanced may remain simply anticipations. Technical impossibility may be a berm that is impossible to scale. Many complex human traits that would be chosen for augmentation, like intelligence and memory retention, are influenced remotely by genes.

Ethics Of Genetic Counseling

Pride in genetic technology is demonstrated by obstetricians who have assisted their patients in many ways. Especially in detecting inherited defects before birth. Attached to which are bioethical dilemmas. Genetic probing and ultra-modern techniques allow these discernments to be accomplished during the first few months of pregnancy. Identification of such diseases as cystic fibrosis, hemophilia, Huntington's chorea, muscular dystrophy, and other genetic disorders are diagnosed while the baby is in the uterus.

Prospective parents can be informed as to the health status of their unborn child. The ethical burden is very critical when a negative diagnosis is made. Abortion enters the parental minds. No statistics are available that count exactly the number of abortions performed because of genetic defects. Sociologists attach to this situation the term "tentative pregnancy" the time when the decision for or against abortion remains undecided [Rothman, 1986].

Genetic testing has a brighter, better side in the same situation. This test allows persons who are at risk of an inherited disorder not to be intimidated and decide to have a baby. Whereas in the absence of the test, they might have decided not to have any children. The explosive growth of genetic research with its diagnostic answers has appended to it ethical questions that require answers.

There is much distance between diagnosis and treatment. Bioethical decisions must be made after the diagnosis and not delayed by unavailed therapy. The ethical dilemmas will intensify as recombinant DNA technology will develop eventually tests for more and more genetic diseases. "Studies show that when prenatal testing is readily available, 60 to 80 percent of women 35 and older will accept the test and virtually all will have an abortion if the fetus is affected" [Squires, 1986].

Who are candidates for genetic counseling? They are those who either had a child with a genetic disorder or who are at risk for a genetic problem themselves. Because of age-related risk women 33-35 years of age who expect to be mothers seek guidance. By age 40 the risk of having a baby with a chromosome abnormality is one in 100, or approximately one percent [National Centre for Education etc, 1999].

"A typical session would involve getting a little information about the current pregnancy: How have things gone? Have there been any problems? Was it a planned pregnancy? Had the couple been trying for a long time to conceive? Typically taken is a family history to see if there is any other disease or medical problem of concern in the family aside from the reason the patient came. If a woman comes to talk about amniocentesis, then we talk about where the chromosomes are. Everybody seems to know about Down's syndrome [a chromosomal abnormality that causes mental retardation], but trisomy 13 and trisomy 18 are two other chromosome problems [associated with the mother's age] that are usually lethal for newborns. Then we talk about what their risk is at their particular age.

"Next we talk about the actual testing, about what happens, what the sonogram [a test using sound waves that helps physicians 'see' the fetus] is. We talk about the risks—which are primarily miscarriage—of amniocentesis. We discuss what we do when we get the fluid, what we analyze, and how we communicate the results. We talk about what happens if there is an abnormality.

"Many patients already know that they want to do the testing. Other patients are very ambivalent and do have a very hard time making a decision. We do not make those decisions for them, although we try to help them look at the decision, the possible outcomes, the possible risks, so that they can feel comfortable whichever way they go. They must take some risks. Either they have the test and take a risk of miscarriage—which we believe is small but still may be unacceptable to some people—or they don't take the testing and risk having a genetic problem.

"Do you ever have couples who come to genetic counseling solely to determine the sex of their child? It's not been a major problem. Over the years, it has happened less than once a year, more like once every two years. It's certainly a controversial issue. We are in the healthy baby business, and so aborting a healthy baby as we know for the wrong sex is very difficult for us to consider. We certainly will not withhold the sex, and if they've got a good reason to have the amniocentesis, we wouldn't consider denying the procedure either" [Corson, 1986].

The above paragraphs by Corson are an interview partial protocol that is followed by the interviewer of a patient who seeks genetic counseling. As practical clinical examples they are testimony to the real life scenes in which ethical questions must be answered. These inquiries concern average people who are not bioscientists, do not know the mysteries of genetics, and the bioethical conflicts they engender.

Modern biological thinking is compelled to focus on the unification of facts pertaining to all aspects of genetics. This includes more than Mendel's principles, but also the intrinsic nature of genes, their transformations, and the exact reading of genetic texts of living things. All these endeavors by inquiry lead to an enlightenment that unfolds the secrets hidden in genes. Pursuits in human genome studies include manufacture of monoclonal antibodies and the production of human therapeutic proteins in bacteria and yeast. Hopefully none of these expected benefits will not conflict with bioethical standards.

Like any other great discovery, the announcement in February 2001 on the entire genome sequence alerted the staunchest supporters of the project who were stunned. Some of their assumptions have been proven to be delusional. Uneasiness ranges from trivial to the profound at a most glorious shining moment in bioscientific research. Startling was the revelation that human beings have only three times as many genes as a fruit fly and perhaps only a few hundred more than a lemming. This knowledge is a lesson that argues for the remembrance of humility. With this unveiling comes the suspicion of future ethical missteps [Keller, 2000].

Chapter 16

Embryo Stem Cell Research

The world of bioscience holds so many magical secrets that it astonishes even the master researchers. Danger is appended to revelations when experiments are chosen that have a myriad of moral transgressions attached to them. Many of which culminate in ethical perils easily comprehended. Aspirations for desired accomplishments are not to be satisfied by using science immorally.

Audacity of biological research scientists minimize actual and constructive bioethics as science is glorified. Undaunted in violation of ethical standards, most bioscientists believe unorthodox experiments do no harm as they curve around their activities that stretch the conscience to conform to intended conclusions which violate ethical acceptances.

New bioscientific technology does not and is unable to supply its own moral values because it is prejudiced to succeed at all costs. Moreover most laboratory scientists engaged in specific forms of research believe they have no duty to follow ethical codes that are restrictive. Also as they deny selfishness and greed they vaunt their altruism as a dedicated service to the needs of humanity.

Above all as an author suggests scientists should stop playing God. Implying all scientists and explicitly biotechnology are mentioned. By their ideas, intentions, and accomplishments these "technoutopians" desire to do no less than to remake other human beings and to redesign human nature [D'Souza, 2000].

This techno-affluence usurps God's divine prerogative which is common in modern scientists and current biotechnological entrepreneurs. Therefore not a solitary thought is given to bioethics, matters of faith, and religion. All of which generally have no appeal to scientists.

No ample reason, no initiative, and no visible sign allow belief that either religion or civil society exert any influence on current scientists. In the realm of research bioscientists, bioethics has not found a home. Scientific enthusiasts and biotechnical investors are doing much to usher in a new era of bioscientific and intellectual prosperity. Hopefully they will reawaken the value of bringing into their laboratories a vibrant sense of virtue. With energetic moral strength they can accomplish a great deal more while knowing science and ethics are easy to manipulate.

A discovery in November 1980 brought attention to research that focused on human embryonic stem cells. As primordial cells they can give rise to differentiated human tissues. These cells have the potential use to repair anatomical structures in disrepair because of illness, injury, and senescence. To obtain these precious stem cells, human embryos are needed as the supply source. The two major places from which embryonic stem cells would come are extra embryos from fertility clinics and aborted babies [Wade, 1999].

To destroy a human being for a potential benefit presents an ethical quandary. Human destruction no matter the stage of development from the most minimal to the fullest maximum is not morally defensible. This prevails no matter the intended good—even one of majestic magnitude.

For thousands of years medicine has been allied with God in a beautiful tradition that recognized physicians as God's intermediary. Together they acted in an ongoing service to the sick. Disagreement with the intellectual concept of stem cells usage can bring about an alienation of affection between laboratory medicine and the divine First Physician. As an entity in His creation physicians, like all human beings, have been given an intellect and free-will. The keener these attributes the greater obligation to use them well. Encumbent upon physicians is to realize, accept, and adhere to the moral duty which dictates that the greater the intelligence the greater the ethical care to use this gift wisely, justly, and morally.

Embryo stem cell research has a clash of values. Unfortunately added to it is that many challenges accepted and undertaken are easier made than met successfully. Many remain speculative. With eternal hope solutions may be found due to the multiplicity of researchers. Many approaches are plausible they are as numerous as there are investigators. Discovery remains the persistent *texte de base*.

Much-heralded as it is, stem cell research has not heeded the impending moral consequences of the application of this potential power.

Lesser ethical minds opt to be scientifically fashion-conscious, servant-models of relativism, lip-service sycophants to moral indifference. This stance gives an ethical impoverishment to the biosciences. Many cellular researchers are unwilling to be initiated into clarification by bioethics which to them is a mysterious phantom. Many cell-biologists are unable to understand that the image of science should be intimately united with ethics. This unity not divergence makes a moral icon of medicine that highlights classical, well-established professional conduct which simultaneously is ever ancient, yet ever new.

Ethical questions abound which do not diminish the enthusiasm for stem cell research. The voices of those debating the justification for this form of research are not silent. Doctrinal positions have been expressed by many theologians. However advantageous it may be to ailing bodies, the ethical disadvantage is the origin of the tissues that has caused dissonance. To destroy and manipulate human embryos under the guise of medical science progress is a threat to humanity. An embryo is destroyed to gather generating stem cells. "As long as embryos are destroyed as part of the research enterprise, researchers using embryonic cells [and those who fund them] will generally be directly or indirectly complicit in the demise of embryos" [National Bioethics Advisory Commission, 1999].

"The availability of the embryos does not justify their use. Here is one of us, however primitive, and the question is whether members of the human species should be treated as other than ends in themselves" [Cameron, 1999]. Advocates of abortion, plus those who advocate stem cell research, tissue for which is taken from aborted fetuses, present justifications in a style that appeals to a wide audience as a valuable addition to human improvement and longevity.

If humanity resided in a moral utopia there would be no improprieties and no discussion necessary on situational ethics. Presidential advisers are forceful advocates of embryo research. The theme-song is "the research's promise for the betterment of mankind merits the recommendations" [Associated Press, 1999]. A draft report of the National Bioethics Advisory Commission states, "This research is allied with a noble cause, and any taint that might attach from the source of the stem cells diminishes in proportion to the potential good which the research may yield."

Janet Parshall, chief spokeswoman for the Family Research Council, criticized the recommendation as "a classic example of situational ethics."

"I think it's the worst kind of utilitarianism . . . to say we will destroy these so those can live," she said. "One would only hope that common sense and compassion would rule the day rather than scientific advancement."

Judy Brown, president of the American Life League, also attacked the commission conclusion.

"There are not two classes of human beings," she said. "The embryo baby is no different than any other human being and should never be subjected to destructive research" [Wade, 1999]. Research on aborted babies is not appropriate for biomedicine whose sword of justice should remain sheathed when there is slaughter of the innocent.

Revolutionary prospects for stem cell research is bogged down in bitter bioethical controversy. Mired down with doubt is the revelation that "genetic factors may play a much smaller rôle than was previously thought, for example, in the causation of Parkinson's disease." Stem cell researchers had a great assurance that their work would be most applicable in alleviating diabetes mellitus and Parkinsonism [PDF News, 1999]. The great expectation did not materialize.

"Ethical relativism does not stop even at the threshold of the identity and dignity belonging to every human life and leads to illicit and disturbing experimentation. The universal conscience rightly reacts. How can one not be deeply troubled? In fact, once even this limit has been crossed, one senses that nothing else will safeguard man from illusory manipulations or from the temptations of a self-destructive madness, which can easily be imposed also by various courts of law or parliaments, as we know from the history of this century. We know this well. I do not have to cite examples.

"Respect for human beings from the moment of conception, as I recalled in the Encyclical *Veritatis splendor*, is one of the basic and inexorable demands of the moral law.

"So many things change in and about man. There is, however, something that does not change: it is his 'nature', as seen in the light of reason and, in turn, as confirmed and enhanced by divine Revelation.

"It is on this eternal law that the universal and unchangeable nature of the moral law is based, a law which shows us the boundless horizon of the good and indicates the limit not to be transgressed of those intrinsically evil acts, that no circumstance or intention can make acceptable and good (cf. *Veritatis splendor*, nn. 80-81)" [Pope John Paul II].

The spiritual nature of human beings has a transcendent vocation that implies a primordial solidarity among all individuals composing humanity. Because of which we are all responsible for each other. Respect for natural law, the correct, and proper use of what has been given to us—especially life—is an individual's moral obligation toward each other, and all others.

To mollify debate and avoid bioethical conflict, all that is required is to gather stem-cells from other available sources. A rich supply is available from umbilical cord blood, umbilical cord tissue, placenta, fat removed by liposuction, margins of skin from operative incisions, and any tissue removed at the time of either intra-uterine or extra-uterine fetal surgery.

Chapter 17

Cloning

Scientific freedom does not mean escape from the moral law. Science and morality are not opponents. Both entail a duty that should be homogeneous since each finds a common basis for their actions, namely, love and life. As a precept it may be beyond mortal means of expression, definition, and description. In its own way each tries to heal, restore, and transform humanity for the better. The crisis in morality afflicting the bioscientific community from within calls attention to the lack of harmony in bioethics on recent experiments that have caused consternation.

The loss of unity between bioethics and bioscience is caused by the inability to recognize universal, concrete, ethical norms. Many scientists have the explicit conviction that science and ethics are heterogenous: reciprocally antagonistic. This leads to the conclusion that laws of ethics are an impediment to biomedical progress. Categorically some bioscientists deny that particular norms are not universal and necessary. Hence a danger is imminent that elaborates on the glory of certain experiments without any ethical consideration of what is done, and will be done.

Such is the new sociology of bioscience indicating each scientist is his/her own bioethicist. Even if the experiments are or become a colossal nuisance. Before undertaking questionable, highly-sensitive experiments, the researcher should renegotiate the scientific production with morally sustained bioethics. This reflection is poignantly appropriate to cloning as a consoling certainty in which a scientist's identity may shine brilliantly in ethical splendor or paint himself/herself as a moral dullard.

Good militant scientists are not oblivious to the consequences of their professionalism.

Biotechnical entrepreneurs without virtual reality checking are advancing stratospheric scientific accomplishments that are startling. Their perceptions may be bizarre but they are coming closer and closer to actual production. Many attitudes augur for triumph of mechanical bioengineering over bioethics. In the guise of research progress and advancement they mutter encouragements to themselves until they conquer the impenetrable. Shaving of moral platitudes and ignoring unpleasantries such as ethical restrictions give occasion to construct an *ersatz* protectivism that annihilates the ethical standards past generations knew and upheld.

Surges of pride stimulate uncovering other surprising developments that are equally and/or greatly more deviating from ordinary, basic, natural bioethics. Myriad scientific breakthroughs are anticipated during this new millennium of admirable research. Remarkable as they will be, one major item will be missing. Which is the failure of faith, reason, and research to unite. No spiritual inclination will be visible that sustains metaphysical truth within the boundaries of bioethics. There can be no merit to bioscientists' argument that ethics has no place in research because it hinders free-expression, freedom to act autonomously, and retards liberty in completion of scientific transactions.

Since 1997 the world was startled with the birth and survival of Dolly, a sheep that is genetically identical to a six year old one. With this accolade to husbandry the immediate thought was to apply this strategem to human beings. The mere thought of it transformed science fiction to possibility. Many ethical and legal issues surround the potential cloning of human beings. Basic ethical principles prohibit human cloning.

An objection to cloning is that "severing of procreation from love and intimacy is inherently dehumanizing, no matter how good the product" [Kass, 1997]. "Arguments in support of human cloning have been made on the basis of procreative autonomy, freedom of scientific inquiry, and the potential benefits of cloning. It has been argued that the decision of human cloning is one that each individual should make for himself/herself because of personal autonomy" [Nangia, 2001]. An author outlined an argument that individuals have a right to procreative autonomy" which he defined as a "right to control their own rôle in procreation unless the state has a compelling reason for denying them that control" [Dworkin, 1997].

At this point in time, 2001, many ethical issues surround human cloning by somatic cell nuclear transfer [SCNT]. Right reason dictates that constraints should be placed on human cloning. "An excessive focus on [autonomy] can prevent us from seeing why other values as well are socially important and protectable and why certain freely chosen practices can still be wrong even if they do not result in immediate or quantifiable harm or direct infringement on the options of other free agents" [Cahill, 1997]. Decisions on human cloning are not to be on emotion, risky thinking, and desire for fame. Many ethical, moral, legal, and scientific arguments have been made against human cloning. Well-intended research may have side-effects that border on the macabre.

The advocacy of human cloning may be a triumph of hopeful expectations over research experience. Non-speculative fiction is applicable to cloning technology as a device without consequences. Shocking aspects of which are not publicized. They are not recorded in scientific journals and may be hidden in laboratory vaults. Such knowledge could sober enthusiasm for this identical, twin reproduction which is a scientific revolution against natural reproduction. Well-crafted expositions on the intellectual propulsion of cloning are tainted with subtle socialistic goals. State interference and control of human cloning is an aspect of creeping socialism. Which when enforced vigorously leads to political despotism over medicine. Also dominating scientists have influenced national rulers as is recorded in the annals of biography and past historical events.

Fabrication of human beings by interference with nature changes the biological order which distorts the normalcy of life as it was ordained. Collective similarities are not automatically a gift of health and happiness. Searching for that which is already known is neither a labor of love nor a happy holiday. Hiding defects of any kind is intellectual dishonesty. A hazard that corrupts the mind to claim an imperfection as perfect. Then excessive violations of bioethics proliferate and prosper. Many research bioscientists have the intellectual capacity to do what is morally correct. However they discard bioethical propriety for gain, greed, and the taste of immortality.

Is cloning to lead to the indeterminate question? Is it a wolf in sheep's clothing or a cow in people's clothing? This *divertissement* is the probable product of those with mystical minds and creative hands. United together they concoct and mold curious creatures which they sculpture figuratively by microscopic cellular enucleation. Is this a skill that brings forth questionable problems?

To some bioscientists cloning is the starburst breakthrough in the panorama of 20th century science. With spontaneity and vitality it has opened the shutters of imagination that lights the mind to explore the unknown. Appreciated, but not sanctioned is the self-boosting urge to have a jumpstart on cloning a human being. A challenge that will have performance under high-pressured stress. Care must be given to a decision that may display an epitome of conceit with flawed bioethics.

Ignored may be the demands of precise, effective research, and clinical studies to discern no violation of ethical priorities. Zeal is willing but the accomplishment may not be good. Bioscientists can not afford to be unethical black-guards. Fault may be found in the bioscientist who did not give an honest heart to the research project. Which is the time-honored requisite for obtaining merited glory.

> Give therefore thy servant an understanding heart to judge thy people, that I may discern between good and bad. For who is able to judge this thy so great a people?
>
> 1 Kings 3:9

Animal Clone *In Actu*

When Ian Wilmut cloned Dolly in 1996, the eyes of the scientific world were upon him. Duplication of the feat has not been acclaimed. Born without complications, it seems Dolly's cells are older than her birthdate. This is an example of the difference between being able to affect an outcome with technological interference with a normal physiological function, and knowing the entire future outcome from what was instigated.

De facto a cloned mammal begins life with the same degree of cellular deterioration that is present in the donor cell. Dolly's original cell came from a 6-year-old sheep. Therefore at the time of birth she was already six.

"Cloning is a popular name given for somatic cell nuclear transfer, a process in which the nucleus containing the genetic blueprint of an animal is removed from a non-reproductive or 'somatic' cell—an udder cell in Dolly's case—and put in place of the nucleus of an egg cell or ovum" [Beresford, 1999].

From cloning an animal to cloning a human being is a giant step morally. Even if the bioscientists intending to do it speak in terms of improving the quality and length of life.

"Lee M. Silver, a professor of molecular biology at Princeton University and author of the book *Remaking Eden: How Genetic Engineering and Cloning Will Transform the American Family*, is a vocal advocate for human cloning.

Asked about the threat to human dignity that cloning poses, Silver answered that "Somatic cell nuclear transfer—what people refer to as cloning—in vitro fertilization, and sexual intercourse, are all methods of creating a baby. When done intentionally, the purpose is always to have a baby to love. If cloning is considered to be treating human beings as a means rather than an end, then so is sexual intercourse with the intention of getting pregnant and having a baby. I don't see the difference because cloning will never create a particular human being. All it will do is allow the birth of an unpredictable boy or girl, who will happen to look like a parent looked a long time ago'" [Beresford, 1999].

The National Institutes of Health, the principal distributor of tax dollars in the U.S. for scientific and medical research, is pushing for stem cell research [cells obtained from human embryos] through somatic cell nuclear transfer in order to produce stem cells that will not be rejected by a patient's body.

"A fact sheet issued Jan. 28, 1999 by the health agency maintains that the federal ban on funding research using human embryos does not apply to research using human clones. It states: 'The use of somatic cell nuclear transfer would be another way to get around the problem of tissue incompatibility for some patients'" [Beresford, 1999].

Human Clones *In Potentia*

Many prospects of producing human clones have surfaced from different geographically dispersed research centres. Contemplated is the use of the same method that gave husbandry the notorious Dolly. Human cloning is perceived as a perverse technique which could destroy the fabric that makes a human being. Moralists declare human cloning is an insult to the uniqueness of the human person as to identity, individuality, and freedom to become an *ens a se*.[1]

Bioethicists of distinction have written on the subject of why human cloning should be banned [Annas, 1998]. The news that scientists in

1. Being standing by itself as a totally complete entity.

Worcester, Massachusetts used a cloning technique to create a human embryo by placing DNA from a scientist's leg cells into a donor cow leg was greeted with horror and repulsion [McKling, 1998].

Moral Offense

"A real horror story", a 'tunnel of madness': these are the reactions, respectively, of George Annas, an expert in medical ethics and legislation at Boston University, and of Gianluigi Capitanio, chairman of reproductive physiopathology at the University of Genoa, to the news that Robert Stillman, an expert in the Fertility Center of George Washington University had 'cloned' or reproduced a human embryo in the laboratory.

"Cloning, or making a reproductive 'photocopy', has already been performed in the vegetable kingdom and the animal world. However, no one—although the procedure is not difficult to carry out—dared to try it on a human being. Robert Stillman has done so for the first time (as far as is publicly known), challenging every sort of legal obstruction and clearly violating the code of medical ethics regulating experimentation.

"The reasons why he ventured into this disturbing and alarming experiment do not justify an intrinsically perverse decision. Providing children for couples who are naturally unable to have any is not enough to justify starting a process that the common conscience rejects as contrary to the dignity of the human person. And what is to be said of the prospect of using cloned embryos for organ transplants, a most detestable procedure, or of 'programming' children by selecting them from frozen embryo banks, using as models those children already born, whose psychological and physical features are verifiable and controllable?

"It has always and everywhere been held that a good end or the attainment of useful goals can not alone be the criterion for human moral conduct in any area whatever, including that of medicine. Genetic engineering is doubtless a science that offers advantages to humanity and to the reproduction of the species. However, in order for it to be 'human', i.e., corresponding to the values of the dignity of the person and of his rights, it must always serve him by improving the quality of his life through the elimination of hereditary defects or other possible disorders.

"When genetic engineering goes beyond these rigorous limits, when it places itself above or beyond ethical and legal norms based on the primacy and dignity of the person, when, in short, it violates the rights of even one human being, it becomes a perverse tool that can be neither accepted nor permitted. In this regard, lawmakers, i.e., States, have the duty to lay down precise norms within their own legal framework, not to halt scientific research, but to discourage the unscrupulous from venturing into a 'mad tunnel' or from wanting to write a 'horror story' by humiliating and offending all of humanity" [Concetti, 1993].

"In Strasbourg on October 28, 1993 the European Parliament issued a strong condemnation of the cloning of a human cell announced several days earlier by an American researcher and requested the banning of this method of genetic engineering. In an emergency resolution, the Europarliament also called for a world conference regarding a total ban of cloning and asked the European Commission to guarantee that this type of manipulation not occur in the European Community" [News Briefs, 1993].

"A renowned geneticist, Dr. Jerome Lejeune,[2] strongly criticized the reported cloning of human embryo cells . . . that the case was 'not a breakthrough in science; it is a breakdown of common sense.' The reported cloning of human embryo cells at George Washington University Medical Centre was widely reported . . . Lejeune said the case did not even involve cloning. 'What they did was splitting of the embryo which is twinning . . . such artificial twinning has been done for years with goats, sheep, and cattle. Cloning, he said, occurs when you get new individuals out of tissues not obtained by sexual reproduction. We should respect the embryo because it is a member of the human species. . . The only thing new [in the GWU case] is playing with human beings as if they were animals. . . [T]he spark of intelligent love—in—primitive man often depicted love with the image of a child, but today the ancient Hippocratic Oath has been revised to remove provisions against abortion. . . He compared the use of fetal tissue in research as 'cannibalization' because brain cells are removed from living fetuses to be used in the bodies of elderly victims of Parkinson's disease. The test results [in which] are very poor. . . The science of genetics has much to offer humanity, as long as it is used to protect and not to end life. . . Genetic

---

2. French geneticist, professor at the University of Paris, author of the book, *The Concentration Can*, published by Ignatius Press, 1992, discoverer of the chromosomal abnormality that causes Down's syndrome: Well-known lecturer in USA, expert witness in American courts, and testifier before Senate subcommittee on origin of human life.

engineering can also be used for the service of humanity—pointing to the example of genetic manipulating of bacteria that has proven to lessen bleeding in hemophiliacs" [Zimmermann, 1993].

Although spectacular advances have been made since the first child was born from in vitro fertilization more than two decades ago, no national board has either discussed or debated [in a designated plenary session] the serious ethical issues surrounding this embryological research. Cloning brings to the forefront the profound lack of national scrutiny in this matter of grave importance to ethical integrity and the status of our nation as a moral state. An ethicist at the University of Virginia said, "Our policy on embryo research is in total disarray" [John Fletcher, 1993].

Cloning For Therapy

"After the cloning of the sheep Dolly had been announced in the early months of 1997 (it will be recalled, it was precisely a question of the cloning by fusion of an enucleated egg cell with a somatic cell taken from the udder of a six-year-old adult ewe and cultivated in the laboratory), the alarm immediately focused on the possibility of transferring this procedure to human beings. There were numerous moral condemnations of this possibility: many sides, while deferring judgement on the use of this procedure with animals to a prudent, qualified evaluation, called for clear, definitive legal norms on human cloning. . .

"In this regard, hypotheses and comments were widely publicized, describing particular procedures for producing cells and tissue for subsequent use in experimental and clinical medicine, especially in the area of therapeutic transplants. Mention was made of the production of multipotent cell lines from embryonic stem cells (to be precise, cells from the internal cellular mass of blastocysts), derived from human embryos produced by cloning. . .

"It was announced that the same centre in Scotland which had cloned Dolly was willing to collaborate with a U.S. firm to produce human cells and tissue through cloning procedures and to establish banks of this precious human material . . . An opinion was requested from the Licensing Authority of the United Kingdom, which answered positively in early December 1998, giving the go-ahead for this procedure, that is, it was favourable to cloning for therapeutic purposes, considered as a sort of fruit of biotechnology 'with a human face'.

"Thus a dilemma was created, as often happens in these situations: either give the go-ahead for this 'beneficial' production, or prevent science from marching to victory over degenerative diseases (such as Parkinson's), metabolic diseases (such as insulin-dependent diabetes mellitus), as a means of overcoming sterility, or oncological diseases (such as leukaemia). . .

"What the biotechnical industry intends to achieve with this type of therapeutically-oriented technology seems to be the true and proper cloning of human individuals. It is not a question of reproducing identical cells from one parent cell as currently happens in the area of cell culture, nor is it simply a matter of using the technique of cell proliferation in vitro to produce tissue intended for implantation (for example, skin, bone or cartilage tissue) according to 'tissue engineering' procedures. This technique uses cells taken from a human or animal body, which can then multiply and generate tissue in the laboratory, to replace the impaired tissue in a patient's body, for example, in the case of serious burns. If it were in fact a question of cell reproduction or interventions of tissue engineering, there would be no ethical problem in admitting the lawfulness of these procedures.

"Instead, it is a question—and researchers know this very well—of producing cells and tissue from cloned human embryos, that is, from human beings the interruption of whose growth is planned so that they can be used as a source of 'valuable' biological material to 'repair' the deteriorated tissue or organs of an adult.

"Indeed, we know that the embryo's cells before implantation in the uterus and the pluripotent stem cells found in the human organism even in its later phases of growth have an extensive capacity for self-renewal and differentiation. The desire is to exploit this potential for the variety of therapeutic purposes mentioned above" [Catholic U, 1999].

Among other places stem cells are present are in the yolk sac, liver and bone marrow of the fetus, as well as in the blood of the umbilical cord at the moment of birth. When stem cells are taken from spontaneously aborted embryos or fetuses or from the umbilical cord during birth, there are no particular ethical problems. However, these cells would not lead to that variety of cellular differentiations which can be had from stem cells taken from embryos and so do not seem to satisfy the requirements of the biotechnologist who is looking for numerous and vital cells selected according to clinical requirements. This is why the production through cloning of a human organism at the embryonic stage of development is considered a preferable source and supply for future use through the freezing of the embryo itself. Moreover, the tissue thus obtained would be compatible with that of the nucleus' donor, the patient himself. This would make it possible to overcome the problem of the rejection of transplants made with tissue "foreign" to the patient.

This use of cloning would thus make it possible to have a specific and "abundant" product, to fuel the hopes of a flourishing bioindustrial business. Furthermore, it only takes a moment's reflection to realize that, in effect, the pressure for research in "therapeutic cloning" comes precisely from the biotechnical industry. "The U.S. firm itself, for example, has shown great interest—announcing it on the Internet—in the possibility of patenting products for the treatment of degenerative diseases associated with ageing, for which it had said it is willing to fund research which will lead to the production of stem cells as well as to the identification of the factors of cellular differentiation for the purpose of genetic engineering or for use in transplants" [Catholic U, 1999].

"The bioethical repercussions of these procedures, despite the 'humanistic' intentions of those who predict resounding cures from the cloning industry, are so momentous as to require a calm but firm evaluation which shows the serious moral implications of this project and justifies its unequivocal condemnation. It should first be said that the humanistic goal is not morally consistent with the means used: the manipulation of a human being in his first stages of life in order to take from him the biological material needed for experimentation with new treatments, thus killing this same human being, obviously contradicts the value connected with saving the lives (or treating the illnesses) of other human beings. The value of human life, a source of equality among human beings, forbids any purely instrumental use of the life of a fellow creature who is brought into being only to be used as biological material. Secondly, this practice distorts the human meaning of procreation, which is no longer considered or practised for reproductive reasons but programmed for medical and experimental (and therefore commercial) purposes.

"This project is encouraged by the progressive depersonalization of the generative act (introduced by the practice of extracorporeal fertilization), which becomes a technological process making the human being an object to be used by anyone who can reproduce him in the laboratory. In human cloning for therapeutic or commercial purposes, the rôle of the 'parent' is distorted, reduced to that of a donor of biological material for producing a child/twin intended to be used as a source of spare organs and tissues.

"This practice is also contrary to the European Convention on 'Human Rights and Biomedicine', which, although permitting the use of surplus embryos obtained through artificial fertilization procedures—a decision we consider disgraceful and morally impermissible—nevertheless prohibits their production for experimental purposes (Art. 18b). The fact that the United Kingdom has not yet signed this convention is not a sufficient reason for minimizing the principle expressed in the European Convention, which confirms every human being's right not to be begotten for purposes other than reproduction itself.

"However, such a practice is in obvious contrast with human rights, since it would allow a living human being to be used as a source of cells or tissue, although for the well-being of another individual, even when this means the death of the human being used" [Catholic U, 1999].

The principle actually being introduced in the name of health and well-being sanctions a true and proper discrimination according to the extent of development (thus an embryo is worth less than a fetus, a fetus less than a child, a child less than an adult), reversing the moral imperative which imposes instead the greatest protection and respect for those who are not in a condition to defend or express their intrinsic dignity.

Western civilization, which has emancipated itself from racial discrimination and has confirmed the right of every human being to be treated as a member of the human family, regardless of his health, age or social status, now is in danger of ushering in a new barbarism with the help of technology. The project of human cloning for therapeutic/commercial purposes represents the return of the social Darwinism which was at the root of the pseudoscientific racism of the late 19th century" [Catholic U, 1999].

Redundant as it may be, an embryo is not an ordinary cell, not amorphous genetic material, but a human being who is beginning life's journey. Therapeutic purposes never justify any intended welfare that interrupts the serial production continuance of an altricial embryo. Altruism is the screen behind which the biotechnical marketplace hides and the therapy mirage has no relationship with the cognitive status of science. Calling the embryo an "embryoid body" does not change anything. All these immoralities exploded when artificial procreation dismissed the human presence, separating the personal element from conjugal love. Without parental affection, concern, and supervision the embryo is exposed to biotechnical and commercial exploitation.

Producing a human being without sexuality by twin fission, cloning, parthenogesis or any undiscovered future technique are contrary to the moral law and *ipso facto* are unethical. Cloning human beings ignores the worth of dignity that destroys identity. Cloning for therapeutic benefits is reprehensible as it involves experimentation on embryos and fetuses requiring their suppression before birth. Nothing in biotechnical and medical science however remarkable can usurp human life. Science is to serve humanity. This service does not condone any interference with the life principle. Even when the intention is to alleviate the illness of another person. To bring a human being to the banquet feast of life and put him/her to death before they have tasted the food is a barbaric cruelty that undermines all that is good in a worthy civilization.

A laudable use of cloning for therapy has been promulgated. It concerns "the identification, purification, and cloning of neurotrophic factors [which] have bolstered the hope that [either] administering these factors or activating their endogenous synthesis might delay the devastating brain damage characteristic of chronic neurodegenerative disorders" [Bradley, Vicino, Carmingnoto, 1993]. The anticipated method is slowing down the progressive loss of neuronal populations in diseases such as Alzheimer's, Parkinson's, and amyotrophic lateral sclerosis.

Need is required for cloning popularizers to give their lead endeavor a respite. Their appeal rested on the logo "to do good." This bit of sophism spells trouble no matter how elaborately presented. There were not sufficient followers of those who tried to spread the flawed legacy that morality was of religious origin. And that religion was the traditional enemy of science. Science and religion can flourish side-by-side under one roof like the early astronomers made cathedrals into solar observatories.[3] Reconciliation is in order that puts an end to either any moral paradox or ethical anomaly in bioscience.

---

3. Astronomers "thereby disapproved the very geocentric dogma they were supposed to uphold" [Heilbron, 1999]. This was true until the contretemps between Pope Urban VIII and Galileo Galilei which made Copernician astronomy a forbidden topic for two centuries. Prior to this intransigency, "the Roman Catholic Church gave more financial support to the study of astronomy—Copernician and otherwise—than did any other institution" [Heilbron, 1999]. Cathedrals with apertures in their roofs were used to study the stars: Basilicas of San Petronio, Bologna; Santa Maria del Fiori, Florence; Santa Maria degli Angeli, Rome.

Futurology, hopefully, will broaden the moral horizon of the scientific spirit as an abundant good science is the quest. Among the new millennium's projections is the technology road map that leads to greater deeds that will succeed. The only barrier is not to throw down and overcome immovable bioethics.

Bioscientists of merit honor moral truth that fortifies faith in God and guides all scholars into channels that are mutually supportive. An amalgamation of thought on the continuity of science and ethics leads to the truism that people are neither things nor animals. Likewise, as do all scientists, they realize or should realize that particular competence in special talents should not be self-mesmerizing. Peer popularity with public acclaim may disarrange judicious thinking and prudent decisions with a concomitant loss of intellectual balance. This distortion can disproportion the priority of technology over ethical conduct. No bioscientific researcher should set aside the primacy of persons over things and the superiority of spirit over matter.

Chapter 18

Experiments On Human Beings

Ethical considerations of research on living persons sponsored by academia, federal government, industry, eleemosynary social groups, and tax-free foundations are not to be minimized. Research requirements are necessary especially since some persons subjected to study are ignorant of what is taking place. Informed consent must be obtained and any harm from the experiment must be disclosed with sufficient time and diligence given to the explanation that it is fully understood and consented to without reservation. What is not included in the agreement is automatically excluded. Human experimentation is not without moral, ethical, and legal hazards. Caution is a warning to be taken seriously. In addition to which human research assumes great importance in any scientific enterprise. Special consideration should be given to any financial arrangements, the sponsorship, and capitated remuneration. Each aspect of human experimentation comes under the purview of contemporary bioethics.

Federally funded research does stipulate rules and guide-lines that govern human experiments. These are regarded generally as ethical standards in non-governmental sectors doing this form of research. Included are private foundations, industry, and similar institutions. Weakness resides in private research that is beyond scrutiny since much of it is unknown publicly. Vigilance is not tested by any critic. Therefore, no observer checks either the remote or obvious appearance of ethical lapses.

Many ethical issues in research do not touch on the subject of human beings as objects for experimentation. In old-time England medical ethics, presented as a code of precepts, was available to physicians and surgeons. These were adopted as the proper professional conduct by medical practitioners in 1803.

Précis On Human Research History

Social enlightenment at the beginning of the nineteenth century illuminated the minds of men to take notice of the ethical nescience that prevailed in experimentation. Moral-conscious men took proper measures to correct this deficiency. Among the most prominent was Thomas Percival in England who wrote about consultations with fellow physicians prior to prescribing innovative therapy [Percival, 1803].

In America the startling report of the Army surgeon, William Beaumont in 1822 was a classical human experiment. He treated Alexis St. Martin following a gunshot wound to the stomach. A permanent gastric fistula remained. *Via* this fistula Beaumont demonstrated the physiology of gastric secretion and motility, the presence of hydrochloric acid, and an active substance identified in 1846 was pepsin [Castiglioni, 1941]. With this landmark human experiment arose bioethical questions which Beaumont expressed eleven years later. Namely that voluntary consent was necessary from the person subjected to experimentation and the person must be able to leave the experiment at any time [Myer, 1981].

Claude Bernard, the French master of experimental medicine during the nineteenth century, with cautious optimism postulated that physicians have an obligation to expand medical knowledge by conducting research with human beings. But the subject's welfare must be paramount [Bernard, 1957]. Claude Bernard sacrificed his home and family on the altar of his laboratory. His wife demonstrated an undisguised indignation as Bernard chose science over his spouse which perhaps was a difficult moral decision to make [Robinson, 1943].

"The first national government to promulgate ethical requirements for human experiments was Prussia in 1900, which limited them to investigations with competent and consenting adults" [Moreno, 1996]. In 1931 the Interior Ministry of Weimar Germany issued a set of regulations that included protective restrictions on children experiments. Prior to using human experimentation previous similar animal experiments were mandated" [Sass, 1983].

Post World War II the Nuremberg Code was written by the same judges who presided at the medical war crimes trial. An absolute, procrustean dictum of which was the emphasis on voluntary consent that ruled out research on children and others who were not able to give personal consent [US vs Brandt, 1947].

"An experience with pediatric research is mixed, as the trials with polio vaccine attests. In the 1930s early efforts to develop a polio vaccine using institutionalized children as subjects met with severe public criticism" [Moreno, 1996]. Doubts about the validity of "voluntary" participation discontinued the administration of the vaccine. . . "The successful vaccine development program [1950] avoided institutionalized persons . . . vigorous public education [enabled] parents to understand the nature of the research" [Moreno, 1996].

During the 1960s and 1970s studies on syphilis in Tuskegee, and hepatitis research at the Willowbrook State School caused a furor in the United States as a bioethical outrage. These occurrences resulted in the codification of specific rules of conduct on policies and procedures involving human beings. In 1978 a commission recommended "that the use of human subjects be guided by the principles of respect for persons, beneficence—and justice" [National Commission, 1978]. In 1991 the "Code of Federal Regulations that govern federally sponsored human subjects research were extended to cover all agencies. These regulations are referred to as the 'Common Rule'" [Federal Policies, 1991].

"Ethically, consent requirements are more stringent in human research than they are in routine clinical medical practice; potential conflicts are more than theoretical" [Moreno, 1996]. The defense of the human person from physical harm and spiritual degradation has many supporting groups listed as Bioethical Centres. Separate departments at colleges and universities have highly qualified bioethicists in command positions. Especially is this noticeable at those universities with schools of medicine. Some of these universities offer a doctoral degree in bioethics. The Roman Catholic Church has research centres in the United States and Europe which have a fine international reputation in the field of bioethics. They are defenders of human life, protect it as far as possible. These Centres are never silent in protest against the degradation of humanity at any stage of its existence from womb to tomb.

Examples Of Unethical Research

Analecta gleanings verify that perceptive wisdom with quiet dignity support the concept of ancestral roots' demonstration that humanity cherishes the priceless legacy established by the bioscientific community. This scientific jewel is appreciated by the laity who have thoughts on medicine better than they have expressed in words. Even those silenced by death resting in their *cubilia*[1] will agree.

Necessary currently is a renewed sense of this bioethical nostalgia to be moved into the mainstream of bioscience for its restoration without renovation. Bioethics is threatened to fall apart when staggering ramifications for financial relationships with commercial enterprises determines selection. Then the difference between ethical facts and customized decision-making is submerged by the requisite strategy that is extremely persuasive in the marketplace.

Looking around the biomedical scene it is discovered within the global maelstrom of moral weaknesses a swirling mass of unethical conduct converging on laboratory activities. Here critical medical technologies and profitable business opportunities have joined energetically in questionable biocommercial ventures. Unethical risks are discounted and/or discarded when financial rewards are high.

The promise of new innovative entrepreneurial enterprises has brought profitability into the growing economy. This has made the biosciences suitable allies for the value-oriented profit-destined propositions considered. Sometimes the wisest choice may not be the ethical one. Especially when a business motto does not coincide with the ethical code which becomes insignificant and is not allowed to get in the way of a profitable business deal. Bioscientists should be moral people who remember there is no mortality when good things done rightly are recalled in the human minds of successive generations.

Medical history verifies that in previous years medical researchers used themselves as subjects for experimentation. Some became ill, others had complications like drug addiction. How many died is not recorded. Courageous in their determinations they subjected their own bodies to harm rather than to use another human being as a testing tool. When those in the academic world are not hero-conscious, are afraid to use their own bodies as repositories for science, they turn to other human beings for laboratory study. To do this surreptitiously is unacceptable and ethically repulsive.

---

1. Cubilium [cubilia is pleural] is a burial crypt.

Failure To Meet Standards

"Dozens of human experiments at Duke University came to a halt Wednesday, May 12, 1999 to the surprise of many members of the medical staff as they arrived on a warm and flowering spring morning at the huge medical centre.

"The day before, Duke became the third major research institution in six months to have its research halted because of failure to meet federal ethical rules. The next day, the Office for Protection from Research Risks, the agency that suspended the research, expressed concern about another experiment last summer in which a volunteer was injured. In that experiment, a volunteer briefly lost consciousness during a space-walk simulation at the university, prompting NASA, which paid for the research, to suspend the study for several months.

"A subsequent ethics review, a copy of which was provided to The New York times by NASA, raised serious questions about whether the study subjects were adequately informed of the risks. 'We investigated the protocols, procedures and we took corrective actions,' said NASA's associated administrator in charge of life-sciences research.

"But the agency's director said that reporting is required and described the omission as a serious breach. This sort of revelation is consistent with the picture of human subjects protection at Duke University Medical Center that OPRR has pieced together through the past five months.

"His office's decision to suspend Duke's federal license to conduct medical research is only the fourth such move by the government in nearly a decade. While cited as a wide variety of oversight lapses in experiments on human subjects, Duke officials have characterized the problems as mostly administrative" [Hilts, Stolberg, 1999].

Growth Study Parameters

Lesser known is that children's growth parameters vary according to the type of fruit juice consumed. Without satisfactory disclosure and parental consent it is unethical to conduct fruit juice experiments on children. The relationship of children's fruit juice intakes with short stature and obesity have been observed.

"Decreased child height or length has been reported previously with high intakes of fruit juice. Consumption of excessive fruit juice (more than 12 oz/day of 'primary apple juice') was a contributing factor in eight children with non-organic failure to thrive" [Smith et al, 1994]. Five of the children (63%) had a length <5th percentile for age and gender, and two (25%) had a length of equal to the 5th percentile. In previous children who consumed >12 oz/day of fruit juice, were significantly shorter after adjustment for maternal height, child age, child gender and child age-gender interaction" [Dennison et al, 1990].

"Based on fourteen days of dietary data and analysis by type of fruit juice consumed, the relationships between fruit juice intake and adiposity (BMI and ponderal index) persisted for apple juice only. Apple juice was also the most commonly consumed fruit juice by this study population.

"The relationship of children's fruit juice intakes with short stature and obesity observed with seven days of dietary data persisted after analyzing 14 days of dietary data. These relationships, however, varied with the type of fruit juice consumed. Intakes of orange juice or "other" fruit juice were not related to either child height or obesity. Apple juice intakes were significantly correlated with both child adiposity indices and were negatively correlated with child height. Grape juice intakes were also negatively correlated with child height" [Dennison et al, 1997].

"While signs of malabsorption commonly appear after ingestion of apple juice, they are less frequently present after ingestion of white grape juice (54% vs. 19%) [6]. Almost none of the grape juice consumed in this study was white grape juice, and only a quarter of the NDS-classified grape juice was actually plain grape juice. Almost half (46%) of the mixed fruit juices (39% of total fruit juices) were classified by the NDS system as grape juice. As a result, 72% of the NDS-classified 'grape juice' was really a grape juice mixture. Thus, one needs to be very cautious in interpreting the findings associated with grape juice intake" [Dennison et al, 1999]. Physicians have an ethical duty to inform parents and child caretakers to moderate prudently young children's consumption as to type of fruit juice.

Human experimentation is not a fiction. No world surveillance is functioning to ferret out where this may be a frequent occurrence. As a prophylaxis against it investigations involving human subjects must be so categorized. Medicosurgical literary editors are aware of the medicomoral implications of such research. As an illustration, in the instructions to authors, the American Journal of Gastroenterology emphasizes that, "All clinical research papers submitted from the United States of America, which involve human subjects, must be accompanied by evidence of peer review. The date the project was approved, when available, should be included."

Legal Liability

Arising from the use of experimental treatment there is the threat of legal culpability. A lawsuit was started against a hospital and an attending physician when a female patient was treated by an experimental technique. The defense was that the therapeutic modality was used in the patient's best interest. Therefore neither the staff physician nor the hospital should be liable. This understanding is incorrect.

Even when treatment is rendered in good faith, liability can result. This can occur when the nature, potential benefits, and foreseeable risks of the experiemental treatment are not specifically, accurately, and adequately explained. Added to this *caveat* is the discussion with the patient of the option of foregoing treatment. In this circumstance of neglected information giving, the patient's informed consent is neither fully nor legally obtained. As a result, the hospital can be vicariously liable for any harm caused by the physician.

An example of this lesson in experimental liability occurred in New England. The estate of a prominent man sued a famous surgeon and a hospital. In 1960, the surgeon, after discussing his intention with hospital personnel, treated his male patient according to an experimental protocol. The plan consisted of radiation treatment for a brain tumor during open craniotomy. This was direct radiation of the tumor site. The neurological surgeon believed this form of treatment would increase the chance of the patient's survival.

The patient died. In 1995 additional information was brought forth regarding this method of therapy. The President's Advisory Committee on Human Radiation Experiments uncovered and publicly documented details of these experiments. The family of the deceased sued the surgeon and the hospital based upon disclosures read in the committee's report.

Under the state law the statute of limitations was tolled. Because of the failure to give the deceased adequate information, the estate of the patient brought a lawsuit against the surgeon and hospital based on fraudulent concealment. Moreover the court allowed an additional cause of action against the surgeon directly for negligent treatment. Further legal allegations were valid against the hospital for failure to exercise control and direction over the radiation experiments since the hospital had actual knowledge of the occurrence [Heinrich V Sweet, 62 F Supp 2d 282, D Mass. 1999].

Both physician and hospital may be subject to lawsuit and liability when a total informed consent is not obtained. Knowledge of state law is essential to assess risks and to determine the rights and responsibilities of each party when unusual forms of treatment can be interpreted as being experimental. Hospitals and other facilities that engage in experimental treatments should have specific, inhouse review boards [ethics committee] to evaluate all aspects of everything innovative. Among the many responsibilities of all concerned is ensuring that appropriate informed consent has been obtained for the purpose of protecting the public, the institution, and the physician where treatment is prescribed [Medical, Legal Lessons, Vol 9, No 1, Pgs 1, 2, Feb. 2001].

Chapter 19

Managed Medicine

Human bondage to the health care ogre is here. Americans may become indentured captives to the socioeconomic morass that confronts the dispensers of medical care. Financial yokes are the immuring restraints that determine the manner in which limited medicosurgical treatment is to be administered.

In an educated affluent society, such as the United States of America claims to be, distributive justice demands that essential medicosurgical care be available to all its citizens. This was the *zeitbeist* during the years of the 20th century. Intrinsic to this primordial shibboleth is the Hippocratic heritage that all human life is sacrosanct. Physicians as essential to the healing profession take a vow (profess) that dedicates them to the preservation of life in all its stages of existence. The sacredness of human life does not imply that any undue influence is to be exerted over medical judgement in its intellectual management of the sick, the comatose, the dying, the elderly, and the irrevocably incapacitated multiple systems injured patient.

Quantitative fixation of expensive, complex therapeutic mechanical apparatus (including those that are necessary for organ transplants, cardiac surgery, microsurgery etc.), monitoring supplex, dialysis equipment, technological complexes, and bioengineering modalities will lead to the rationing of this category of armamentarium. The continual increase numerically in the life expectancy of the geriatric group of citizens will increase the burden of rendering medical care to all citizens. Proportionately the availability of the aforementioned special health equipment, technology, and expertise diminish as the population grows, it will be impossible to satisfy the needs of all those who require medicosurgical assistance as the era of inexhaustible medical facilities approaches a finale. The last day of health care lagniappe is nearing a denouement. No longer is the cornucopia of medicine inexhaustibly plentiful.

Thus indications for inhospital treatment is the target for reform. A reconstruction of the screening criteria for admission will be made with a serious consideration given to economic exigencies. Explanations for requesting inpatient status will be guidelined based upon the following.

1. Justification for admission;
2. Length of stay;
3. Validation of diagnosis;
4. Reasons for admission according to standards of practice in the community;
5. Critical diagnostic/therapeutic services available at the selected hospital;
6. Discharge status; and,
7. Anticipated complications that may prolong hospitalization that have a significant effect on chronic morbidity or impending mortality.

These facts lead to the truism that serious medicomoral problems have arisen that need to be solved. Not to realize the existence of this grave question is to ignore the truth. To disregard the truth, lends credence to ignorance of truth. Pejoration intensifies to the point when those in command are unaware of their ignorance. Limited medical resources are anticipated. As a reality it is not to be ignored or made deprecatory. When rationing of medical services is realized a certain policy will be mandated. This may be founded upon either a "first come first serve" basis or an age cap will be placed on those allowed to receive specialized medicosurgical treatment. Hence any quality or quantitative control mechanism will be *de facto* a health care rationing system.

With the rising sentiment favoring economy in health costs, the financial onus of employing life-sustaining technology for the critically injured, the moribund, and those with chronic diseases can be ignored easily by many without a conflict with conscience. Planned HMO economy has an accentuated fiscal parsimony that clamors for diminished expenditures for health care. Thrift in treating long-term infirmities, especially those of old age, is conducive to the acceptance of euthanasia. The cannily of medicine does not erupt out of the outbursts for penury in health care. Medicine's virtuous asset is caring for the sick/infirm/aged with educated knowledge plus learned experience. This noble heritage may vanish as the Ciceronian pithy quotation *vivere ad summam senectutem*,[1] may not be tenable in this century.

Medical Dilemmas In The 21st Century

As the cost for medicosurgical treatment rises geometrically many social, economic, legal, and moral implications come into view. Limited medical facilities will demand rationing of dialysis, sophisticated state-of-the-art prostheses, pacemakers, organ transplantations, microsurgery, monitoring appliances etc. Hospital beds will be reserved for the deserving in the Cardiac Care Units (C.C.U.). the Intensive Care Units (I.C.U.), and at Burn Centers.

Selectivity of patients by physicians because of the exorbitant spiralling premiums for malpractice insurance has become an ugly necessity (especially for general surgeons, obstetricians, anesthesiologists, and neurological surgeons). To avoid medical malpractice accusations physicians of all genre practice defensive medicine that give rise to excessive costs to patients, insurance carriers, hospitals *et sic ad infinitum*.[2]

Within the confines of the current socioeconomic dilemmas, doctors of medicine are under crushing pressures. These burdens are the result of their own moral inertia which allowed non-medical persons to dictate medical policy. Among the distressing bulwarks that beset the medical profession are the many alternating changes seen in the health care industry as a totality. These variations run the gamut commencing with bioscience education to the financial intricacies of hospital practice, the recruitment of funds for scientific research with the present-day emphasis on cancer, AIDS, and third-party interferences.

Factual appraisal of the unanticipated occurrences in modern medical practice demonstrates that economic stress and strain has become the paramount concern of all its participants. Hospitals seek cost-containment with new sources of revenue. Employed salaried physicians are subjected to lower-cost medical care programs with their appended di-

1. To live to the greatest [longest] old age.
2. and so into infinity

minished reimbursement scales. Doctors in private practice are cognizant of the financial disenchantment surrounding them which has penetrated threateningly their own economic security. Seeking surcease from their extraneous pressures physicians are unionizing themselves. Some prepaid health systems deny patients the right to select physicians of their choice. Other similar health programs provide a list of physicians who agree to the regulations prescribed by the health care contract.

Among the persuasive forces that have altered the previous tranquility in medical practice is an employer's direct acceptance of less expensive means of providing health care for employees. Analogously governmental reductions in the basic fees for medical services has had the same concluding result. With the increasing number of patients enrolling in economically attractive medical care programs, physicians have no alternative but to accept them. The end result is a lesser financial return to the physician with a progressively increasing number of patients he/she is required to treat.

Many physicians fear that with the intensive scrutiny of their activities ever present, they are under a duress that encourages actions with conclusions based on financial considerations rather than on medical knowledge. Incentives such as pecuniary rewards for conserving health care resources can lead to ethical transgressions. Cost-containment may become the sinister temptation leading to moral weakness that disrupts the code of bioethics. In addition, the loss of unfettered personal thinking breeds sycophantic decisions. Hence the selection of a therapeutic regimen may be prejudiced for economic reasons. Loss of intellectual autonomy is conducive to biased actions that are not always consonant with ethical behavior.

These adverse circumstances are reflected in the annual decline in applicants to medical schools plus the diminished academic standing of those college students who do apply for admission. Even with the lowering number of medical school applicants, it is predicted that there will be an oversupply of American physicians in the future. This consensus has an economic impediment of much gravity. Like many physicians of today, those of the future will have to accept a lesser income. Medical graduates of tomorrow can not be lured into this profession as a lucrative financial venture.

Sad it is to relate that a purposeful study unfolds the truism that the business of medicine has become medicine's primary business. When curtailment of financial expenditures for ultimate economy is accentuated over health needs, then medicine's altruistic attempt to reach its historical fulfillment is hampered. The pursuit of economic goals to the detriment of necessary medical diagnostic procedures and/or therapy may lead to bioethical bankruptcy. Solutions to the psychoneurotic economic crunch as a major disturbance to the harmony of rendering medical care is not to be solved impetuously. An impartial evaluation leading to equitable solutions is the *sine qua non* to the ethical fortitude that preserves sanity in the medical profession. Without indulging in a rodomontade[3] it may become a recorded landmark that the physicians of the 21st century will be the last of the traditional lancepesades who followed willingly, voluntarily, and autonomously the precepts of Hippocrates. Concurrently the loss of professional personal individuality in medical practice is the ransom that has been demanded by the societal exigencies that may not produce the same munificent scientific achievements that have benefited past generations.

Many a nemesis on medicine's premises has caused it to shed its chrysalis long ago. This noble science that treats patients artfully is not the doyen of its own domain. Rather it is the chirmless slave of a socioeconomic pendulum over which it has relinquished control unwittingly. Without nicenellyism it can be stated that external authorities have extirpated professionalism out of the health care services. This surreptitious usurpation forebodes a more drastic curtailment of freedom in the practice of medicine and surgery as the years after 2001 roll along with father-time.

Medical knowledge, surgical talent, practical scientific experience are not found on the commodity exchange. These are not saleable assets even in the presence of the rapidly growing commercialism in medical care facilities. Personal acclaim, the acquisition of indigenous wealth was not the motivating force in rendering health care to those in need. May this laudable credo persist in spite of unethical threats to medicosurgical practice because of financial parsimony.

Dedication to serve the sick, the injured, the deformed, the helpless, and the mentally deficient is the well-sung spirit of medicine. This benevolence is founded upon the fiduciary confidence placed on physicians by proper licensing governmental agencies. Because of this trust, governments allow doctors to dissect the human body, cut living tissues,

3. Rodomontade is boasting, bragging, bombastic.

administer powerful drugs, and to use potentially lethal instruments. For other citizens to perform these acts would be a punishable criminal offense. This faith can not be brutalized by ignoring ethical standards for selfish gain in any way whatsoever.

Physicians, admission personnel, triage officers, hospital administrators, and others have become keepers of the keys to the reception room of health care. As such they have a sensitive position that can be stained with moral disaster for themselves and probably for those they are presumed to serve. Contemporaneously they are not to permit the practice of medicine to languish on the vine of professional famine because of intellectual malnutrition resulting from socioeconomic tripotage and coercive economic sources.

When social justice prevails in a strong, elected, duly constituted national government, it behooves the appointed officials to accept certain obligations founded upon their collective duty to the populace. Among these are to furnish their citizens with the security of unrestrained personal movement, to the tranquility of national peace, to an unobstructed access to those avenues that protect public health, and promote the general well-being of its citizens. Cooperating with this *pro bono populo credo*[4] is a legion of bioscientists. Under the shadow of obscurity, they are servants to a human cause as they display inconspicuously and without hubris, a profound sense of anonymity with the highest code of ethical control within the ranks of any recognized profession.

Neglect In Managed Care

The burden of giving ethical treatment under the management of business enterprises is no way different than if the patient is under the private supervision of a solo physician. Personal affinity may be gone but the responsibility to perform professionally and honestly remains.

Managed care incorporates five entities within its prospectus. These are consumer, patients to be treated, providers of therapy, insurers who pay for the care, and the purchasers of the medical/custodial care who are not patients. Excessive insurance carrier interference and negotiators for the less expensive managed care have dehumanized professional medicosurgical therapy and nursing care.

---

4. belief for the good of the people

Added to the above five units can be the input from investors in corporate management of health care and the managerial bureaucrats. Both have the primary concerns to protect and capitalize on the investments made to obtain the greatest return on the purchased shares. Under this pressure ethical considerations are set aside easily as money matters consume most of their time and energies.

Health Care Systems have pre-conceived programs designed to reduce costs according to business criteria. Theoretically the schedules are to increase the quality of daily personal hygienic, nutritional observances, and attention to social well-being. With these domestic overviews access to medicosurgical treatment is to be facilitated. Practicality impedes the fulfillment of all the promises made. Due to economic pressure quality of, and approach to medical care are not attained.

"If increased quality is chosen, reducing cost is abandoned. If reducing cost is chosen, increased quality of health care is sacrificed . . . Managed care consumes 30 percent of the total cost of the managed health care plan to pay for the high-salaried management bureaucracy . . . to reduce health care delivery costs quality may be unintentionally reduced" [Buesseler, 1999].

Neglect of patients under business management is an egregious moral offense. Such negligent vigilance is unconscionable and is in violation of fundamental bioethical codes. In some instances the expenditure designated for medical care is diverted into other depots. Sidetracking money given for a specific use agreed upon by both parties is akin to theft of services to be given. It is usury in disguise of a facility to serve those who are unable to serve themselves. Allocutions against these abuses are like wailing in the wild winter's watered wind.

Chapter 20

Misconduct In Research

Incentives to sly sin are found not only in aphrodisiacs but also in false admiration in wrong persons and places. Hero-worship of actors, athletes, politicians, financial moguls, media personalities, and others of similar vintage is a mirage. So much public attention is devoted to them that it is repetitious, dull, tedious with arousing boredom. Endless exaggerations, superlatives, and applause of this sort are not inspirational. Because insincerity is discernible beneath the thin coating hiding the danger of temptation to follow their examples. Too often the successes, failures, fortunes, and misfortunes of the rich and famous are chronicled exhaustingly as if they are the sources from whence arise the hopes of humanity, dreams of youth, and is life's purpose. When in reality they are the incarnation of impudicity.

Oblique priorities in emulation ignore those more worthy of accolade and praise. Many who are selfless, courageous, and altruistic often are unknown. Underappreciated they labor in silence unheard of, unhonored, innominate living quietly under the shadow of anonymity. Intellectual growth brings change. With each new modification comes challenges and added moral responsibilities. Preconceived ethical plans allow the management of whatever moral questions may arise. Real-world solutions must grow from control of what is not right, incorrect, and false. This is the basic philosophy of research. This instills righteous value into every accomplishment that fortifies unshakably what is produced by intellection in the form of an invention, a discovery, or a written treatise. Into every professional career there lies embedded the seeds of moral hazards. For bioscientists it would be idiocy to fertilize these seeds for any economic or other acquisition. Money is never worth more than brain power which should be directed only by the best inducements. Cynicism of self demoralization is a mockery of virtue, scorns morals and sneers at ethical conduct.

Bioethics fosters bioscientists to provide perspective performance as a demand for the accomplishment of prescribed goals. Only the morally uninformed would detour from this objective for imagined gain. Otherwise marvelous mental machines grow into a menace. The threat of ethical error is found when incautious snap decisions are made.[1] They produce sleeky inflections that give the appearance of an amazing feat. Those who are prone to appear decisive by making a quick decision erode thinking processes which lead to conclusions that are more often wrong than right.

There is more than casual concern that as medicine rolls forth with ever-increasing momentum, technologically it seems to be taking medicomoral leaps backward by quick decision-making. Apparently in some areas bioscience is experiencing moral retrogression with bioethical reversion. Temptation to fame is mutilating the spiritual intangibles which are the treasures of the medicosurgical profession.

For an appropriate assessment of the unbalancing bioscientific issues at the technical and other levels, well-disciplined, updated bioethicists are needed. Without prejudice they can arrive at determined solutions to unfixed answers attached to perplexing bioscientific problems. Thus conclusions reached will be authoritative and comprehensive which will not permit bioscientific misinformation to mislead and beguile even the least educated.

A German publication on non-discursive morality of medical experimentation is quite pertinent to the topic being presented. An excerpt from which is quotable. "One can well understand the beleaguered mentality of many medical experimentalists, as they found themselves in the position of 'enemies of the people' rather than benefactors of mankind" [Elkeles, 1996]. Drawn from a wide range of archival sources, this study by Barbara Elkeles merits serious attention by all concerned with the origins, nature, and causes for ethical abuses, errors in bioscientific research, and misdeeds in clinical medicosurgical practice. It appears the relationship between altered bioethical theories and biomedical practice

---

1. Theoretically, decisions made within 30 seconds or less are faulty.

has become estranged. Modernists in the sciences consign the thought of moral codes to an older world of stagnant-ridden history to which current bioscientific thoughts, words, and actions do not subscribe, assent, and seem not to belong to even partially.

Perhaps due to the broad inclusiveness in the definition of science some mischievous minds deny impure actions of professional behavior as not being pertinent to science. This is erroneous. Merriam-Webster Dictionary describes the scientific method as "principles and procedures for the systematic pursuit of knowledge involving the recognition and formulation of a problem, the collection of data through observation, and experiment, and the formulation and testing of hypotheses." Hence science is not limited to chemistry and physics.

These two hard sciences are included in the wide boundaries of science. Within the range of its scope, any intellectual activity that requires study and method is science. Succinctly knowledge gained through experience is science. Therefore to believe misdeeds devised and/or promulgated *via* intellectualism is not degradation of science is a misconception.

Many issues for solution that researchers have embraced are clear problems for which cloudy answers may be given. Violation of honest investigation is never excusable. In certain areas of research, the eagerness to find answers puts a priority on haste. Waste of time is not to be encouraged. But haste makes waste in different ways—especially when ethical answers are required.

Factual recognition is given to the common knowledge that this century is to be a period of great progress in the biomedical sciences. Excitement fills the air in laboratories. Transference of research products into useful and requested clinical application sometimes is jeopardized by ethical barriers. Clinical investigation by laboratory research provides what are the end-products of molecular biologists, cell biologists, geneticists, immunologists, and bioengineers. Collaboration and interaction has been challenged by bioethicists in specific spheres of investigative application. Subterfuge to deceive an ethical impropriety contributes to criticized misconduct in bioscientific research.

Laboratory and clinical investigations should be pursued in the context of well-defined goals, questions to be answered, and rigorous methodology. Internal and external periodic reviews of the ongoing project to assure the quality and moral compatibility would guarantee its ethical bioscientific acceptance. These noble goals are arrived at by admirable hard-work.

There is no magical yellow-brick road to fame. It is a reward arrived at from industrious mental exertion and physical labor. Fame is an accolade. Notoriety is not. The first is laudable. The second is deplorable. The difference between them is a great divide.[2] Bioscientists, medico-surgical clinicians, and all in health care acquire fame passively by their good deeds. By their ethical performances and moral example they avoid unwanted notoriety.

Deceptive Practices In Bioscience

Ethical aspects of medical practice still find a fundamental basis in the Hippocratic Oath whose core is, *Primum non nocere*.[3] In considering personal dilemmas when confronted with professional obligations, bioscientists must abhor evil actions. Any evil act performed by a physician, a bioscientist, and/or any well-educated person is magnified tremendously. Such persons are expected to know better, to have control over misleading influences, and to have the intellectual strength to ward off temptation.

Practicing physicians/surgeons have been granted an honored place in society by those who seek their help. This privilege gives them a share in the most hidden secrets of many patients. Suddenly a doctor of medicine will be a surrogate priest, minister, rabbi to a sick person and the family. Hence a vocation to study medicine demands special efforts with ancillary stamina that beget humility. Although meekness is a fine character trait, it does not imply wimpishness. A pertinent thought is:

> There is a world of difference
> To all both vital and immense
> Between the good doctor and bad;

---

2. Fame means great reputation and recognition abroad, usually in a favorable sense. It is public esteem, renown, and glory. Fame implies being very widely known. In a broad application it is not specific but implies favorable acceptance. Notoriety is the condition of being known unfavorably. Generally it implies a short-lived publicity based on something unworthy. An equivalent to being infamous is its finality.

3. First, do no harm.

But it is just as true and sad—
Between the good and none at all
The difference is very small.

The threats of professional evil conduct can be exorcised by the adherence to natural principles which grow out of humanity's fundamental creation. To be unethical is intellectual malnutrition that results in moral contabescence. Bioethical absenteeism can become the albatross that weighs heavily on the grandeur that is medicine's cynosure. Simultaneously it can lose its claim as an expert in humanity. Thus physicians will fail in their duty to defend the welfare of the people entrusted to their care. Unchangeable proper ethical conclusions should not be made alterable by nonmedical outside forces. Prudence, reason, and profound sensitivity are the rulers that lead to bioethical stability.

Medical discord founded upon sad experiences has taught that with the passage of time, bioscientific counsellors become wiser. With this thought paramount, it may be written: The maintenance of the highest ethical standards is essential for the salvation of bioscience's dignity and the preservation of moral sanity in its practice.

The history of bioscience is peppered with indiscretions. This appears to be what happened in Nazi Germany under the watchful supervision of hundreds of scientists, physicians, bureaucrats, and eugenic proselytizers. "Comprehending what happened in those twelve years of German history is probably easier if Nazi evil is seen as unmitigated, relentless, untainted by beneficent, or even useful works. Acknowledgment that the Third Reich was progressive in certain matters of public health appears to mitigate the enormity of everything else that happened in its name. Nazi medicine has come to be symbolized by experiments on concentration-camp prisoners as the apotheosis of inhumane and unethical science—and nothing more" [Proctor, 1999].

Nazi Germany had the medical infrastructure and a health-conscious political party with unrestricted police powers. This allowed authoritative control of any growing threat from illnesses, social diseases, and physical imperfections. The preoccupation with bodily defects was reflected in the biased obsession with non-aryans, gypsies, the handicapped, and other individuals who were designated as societal menaces whose impurities were malignancies threatening the health of the state. "Dachau had greenhouses where medicinal plants were grown. Some of the experiments done on prisoners tested herbal remedies" [Proctor, 1999].

"Medical research was corrupted by Nazi ideology. Race-consciousness led some scientists to spuriously dismiss the importance of environmental risk in certain ethnic groups, which were thought to be cancer-resistant. [It goes without saying that whole populations fell entirely outside any concern for their health or welfare.] The campaigns against radiation hazards and tobacco served state interests, namely protection of the national 'germ plasm' and the fertility of German women, who were urged to produce as many aryan offspring as possible. Occupational safety helped to enforce each man's 'moral duty' to work—usually for the good of the state, and ultimately, for its war effort. So, too, with dietary recommendations. One Hitler Youth Manual declared: 'Nutrition is not a private matter!'" [Brown, 1999].

The story of Nazi medical research and German public health policies have eluded the attention of medicolegal historians for various, undisclosed reasons. Science can be value-free. "Passions are often involved in the pushing of science in one direction rather than another for better or for worse . . . Ideology does not fundamentally corrupt scientific inquiry any more than 'good' research guarantees good behavior . . . Nazism has to be seen as more than a demonic caricature, a straw man fabricated to efface the links to other times and places . . . We need to challenge the comfortable notion that Nazi Germany was unique and defies comparison" [Proctor, 1999]. Nazism was to be the banality for good in Germany, but it turned out to be the banality of evil.

Areas Of Maleficence

Nazism will be remembered as synonymous with racism, hatred, immorality, and genocide. The masked forces behind this senseless regime were physician-psychiatrists who violated human rights and dignity in Germany. Unnoticed and undiscovered were they who were the unseen advisers to Hitlerism. Misdeeds and atrocities were founded upon miscited psychology called ideology which is an antigen that immunizes against reason.

German psychiatry[4] made victims who in turn became enemies. The teaching was "Psychiatric science demands empirically that such people

---

4. Psychiatry was a noun devised by Johann Christian Reil in 1808. Prior to that year 'psychic medicine' was used. Psychiatry literally is 'doctor of the

are rendered powerless" [Röder et al, 1995]. "Since its inception, psychiatry had worked for and with the state, and was, in essence, charged with the responsibility of keeping order and setting norms of society demanded by those in power. It rewarded compliance and punished disobedience as a matter of politics, not medicine" [Röder et al, 1995].

Nazi propaganda was the extermination of "life unworthy of living" as victims of oppression were called. Beneath the surface was the incentive that Aryan people needed more room to expand. Hateful propaganda of racial superiority found a commonality with German psychiatrists' degrading, immoral theory of "racial hygiene" and eugenics [Röder et al, 1995]. This relationship of psychiatry with politics is beyond being unethical.

Fraudulent Science

Lessons to be learned are first that extraordinary people should not become so busy that morality would be eliminated from their life. Secondly, medicosurgical research fails to be strong materially, if its performer is weak spiritually. Insidiously an antagonistic confrontation is inevitable between material gain and spiritual debility. These two forces in conflict will engender an internal inadequacy that will destroy any proposed project in the biosciences.

Recognizing the touchstone blessing of academia some research scientists worship the false god of success. In their desire to overcome competition and achieve greatness a devious pathway may be taken to the illusive rainbow of renown. Fading memory recalls some past scientific, dishonest laboratory acts that if undetected could destroy the charisma of medical research.

Some pages in this book bring into focus the discovered ethical infractions by some scientists. These irreverent actions give rise to the inevitable question as to why an educated person stoops to this Icarian, unacceptable deportment. Without justification of these ignoble pursuits, some responses are proposed. A caveat goes with these answers that is

---

soul' derived from the Greek 'psyche' [soul] and iatros [physician]. The first textbook on this subject was written in 1758 by W. Battie with the title, Treatise on Madness.

taken from the tragic drama Julius Caesar (Act iii, Scene 2, Line 80) by William Shakespeare:

> The evil that men do lives after them;
> the good is oft interred with their bones.

Great expectation is not the equivalent to impossible expectation. At times people demand too much from the medical profession and its allied health care purveyors. Hence discord arises which leads to controversy. From controversy often comes an inordinate exaggeration. Gross exaggeration surreptitiously is the progenitor of medical falsehood. Truthful research is the honest pathway to repetitious medical accomplishments that strive to solve the perplexity of overcoming diseases. The *cognatus* of research is the distance the investigator must travel between the problem and the answer. Frequently the distance is incalculable.

In an effort to satisfy the public's craving for newer weapons against disease, deformity, and death medical research is relentless, hourless, and persistent. The research scientist does not have the luxury of philosophical evenings in the winter and rural days in the summer. Research endeavors carry with them turbulent days without surcease. These expended efforts have the approbation only of the person involved in the research process. With successful achievements fellow researchers rejoice, but the silent or constrained approbation of the laity is noticeable. Perhaps this is the differentiating logo between the reasonable person and the unreasonable one. It was George Bernard Shaw who wrote: "The reasonable man adapts himself to the world; the unreasonable man persists in trying to adapt the world to himself."

No need is there to plumb antiquity. But, "In history, as well as now, one encounters individuals who, unsatisfied with social institutions, get the idea to improve the world or, at least, put something new in place of the old . . . They appear in the rôles of leaders of revolutions, founders of political parties, . . . and they make themselves and others unhappy. The incubation phase of the disease is long, often reaching back to childhood" [Richard von Kraft-Ebing, 1892]. These are unfortunate persons who have not learned that "the search for value and meaning is the key to psychological well-being" [Frankl, 1946].

An example is discerned when science assumes a greater than necessary influence over human beings. Imitating false science, accepting its theories without evaluation can lead to fadism and trends that are unethical. Eagerness for change in itself is not morally good if there is ethical disintegration with it. Progressive and so-called humanistic approaches to life may have attractive labels. Beneath which may be subjugation of morality with social decay inevitable.

One of the first signs of this catastrophe is language change. Evil is not named as such. Psychiatric terms camouflage it with euphemistic, innocuous sounding phrases as behavioral disorder, social pathology, personality disorder, sexual addiction etc. Concepts of good and bad behavior, right and wrong, conduct and responsibility have disappeared from the daily used vocabulary. No check is made on the modern socially engineered assault on religion, morality, ethics, and plain honesty. Where has old-fashioned honesty gone? Nothing is ever anybody's fault. Religion is out-of-date. Forgotten is that religion provided the markers for the morality and spirituality which maintained with preservation all civilizations. Religion supplies the exalted inspiration that gives the highest meaning, conforming standards, and steadfast purpose to life.

Misbehavior has been insinuated into every biomedical multi-disciplinary group by attachment to utilitarianism.[5] In a self-serving, calculated eagerness for expediency and practicality the principle of adherence to what is right may be discounted. Pragmatism[6] is temporarily rewarding but is not always effectively workable. Utilitarianism does not entirely have use for utility. When utilitarianism becomes the unreliable standard for arriving at an ethical judgment, a false conclusion may be reached that excuses misbehavior. Although not always so, scandals and maluse of bioscience should be alien to medicine, surgery, and all their specialties.

Scientific medical endeavors are not blasé however dour the task. Even when gloom fills the laboratory, bioscientists should not be dis-

---

5. Utilitarianism is the philosophical doctrine that considers utility as the criterion of action and the useful as good, worthwhile, and preferable. The ethical theory was proposed by Jeremy Bentham and John Stuart Mill that all moral, social, or political action should be directed toward achieving the greatest good for the greatest number of people. Utility is the quality of being useful, i.e., usefulness.

6. Pragmatism is used here as a method, tendency or course of action in social and all other affairs that are characterized by the rejection of theory and precedent with preference given to practical means and expedients.

gruntled. For then a wily mentality is found easily whose latitude favors ambiguity which allows deceit. Evenhandedness is threatened thereby which is the bioethical reprisement without tricky stratagems.

The drive for unique professional recognition is an unbridled desire which is a need to satisfy egotism. Hence a choice should be made not to be discouraged with what has been done properly. Because what is performed with accuracy has been stamped with the brand of honor. Always there should be the thought of the ethical matrix that gives respectable proportions to professional attractiveness. External applause does not pacify internal discord when disturbing dishonor is attached to the acclaim.

Achievements accomplished by memorable past bioscientists were prodigious. The indigenous erudition of each was matchless. Their collective scholarship touched the éliteness of genius when considering the beneficences they gave humanity. Such life-saving contributions merit profound gratitude. Worthiness of praise to each of them is undeniable. The inescapable, relevant truth is that they were honorable and did not deviate from the finest ethical standings. Even if, during their lives, they were not known for genuflective piety.

But they were known for fidelity to responsibility. They knew honor has only one approach. That ethical exploration is not a search expedition to obscure truth or destroy it. Correctness does not allow either marginalization or divergence from the steady course. They knew in advance that ethical standards are not expendable, explorable or negotiable.

Present bioscientists would do well to follow the lead of those colleagues who lived before them. The old and the new are united in the understanding that a clean endeavor leads no assaults on integrity. Even as clearly defined bioscientific explorations lead to right conclusions which are meaningfully helpful. Medical technocrats of dutiful honor when confronting the new technology of bioscience do not focus on any bargaining for either gainful purposes or ambitious reasons. The right way is the only way. Even if the wrong way may be easier, quicker, lucrative or more rewarding professionally. Hesitancy in this sort of mental negotiation is not only a debate between right and wrong, it incorporates the devil as a participant referee and prejudicial umpire. Malfeascence should never drive a biomedical scientist to unearned success. Abnormal ambition is inhospitable to efficient accurate professionalism.

Deviance in medicosurgical practice and bioscientific research does not long endure. No odium can be rationalized into a good based on utilitarianism when malfeasance has taken the spotlight. Expediency has a demerit if it toys with the tendency that renders ethics irrelevant. This occurs when the violation of moral principles is swayed by public opinion polls and popular consensus. Both of which are not concerned with the distinction between right and wrong. Similarly, purposefully planned ambiguity is a camouflage that drives into obscurity ethical questions that remain unanswered.

Historically, medical science is not entirely compatible with the indiscriminate modern world. Very noticeable is the sense of what is acceptable and what is utterly unacceptable when unprincipled, pragmatic judgments underlie moral decisions. The lure of rewards can blind a person's willingness to differentiate between good and evil.

Biomedical researchers in cloning, the genome project, cellular engineering, technologies relating to the origin of human life, and other advanced scientific technology must sustain purity in their motivated activities. Thus will be preserved their historical untarnished credibility. To conserve their pristine character it may become necessary for them to retrace the moral steps of decades long-gone. Returning to former hardcore beliefs as the antidote against the toxic germ of unethical utilitarianism is not retrogression.

Ethical choices in biomedical enterprises are everywhere as the need for decision selection increases with newer research projects. Serious, unprecipitous thought should be given to the need for weighing potential benefits from biomedical technology against innate unethical issues resulting therefrom.

Primal virtue, moral awareness, and responsible accountability are not to be ignored in scientific research. Freedom in science does not license deviation from this obligation. It is not inconceivable for honest, regulatory, ethical criteria to be persuasive in flourishing scientific activities. Illuminating, valued criteria assist in solving disturbing dilemmas. Decisions are facilitated by right reason when perplexing choices are to be made under the tantalizing enticements and rich rewards from temptation to deviate from prescribed ethical criteria. Ambition, propulsion for celebrity status, political, and economic forces must not influence biomedical scientists either adversely or tendentiously. Firm adherence to positive, strong ethical principles teaches how to use acquired knowledge wisely, beneficially, and altruistically.

The powerful, mentally advanced sector of society known as bioscience is neither exempt from temptation nor immune against infectious misconduct. A panel of distinguished psychologists found that a fellow specialist was under the onus of serious scientific misbehavior. The umbra overshadowed his research that "had been highly influential in encouraging the use of stimulant drugs for severely retarded institutionalized children. . . The panel concluded that Dr B did not carry out the described research. He simply invented the results" [Greenberg, 1987].

In California the phenomenal rise of a young medical scientist was the talk of the school of medicine. When he was alleged to have committed extensive research fraud in heart research, it was difficult to believe. An investigation concluded that Dr S reported patient and animal studies which were never performed [Greenberg, 1987].

A Massachusetts research team retracted its reports on a major research discovery which was the finding of a vital molecule in the immune system. When the research could not be duplicated, a doctoral post-graduate student admitted he had faked key results to conceal failure of the experiment [Greenberg, 1987].

At a New York medical centre, a world-famous cardiologist was exposed by a series of charges by a former laboratory colleague. The allegations indicated falsifications. Other accusations were undisclosed because of the ongoing investigation by the National Institutes of Health.

A federally funded research project of $725,000 was voided because the researcher in cardiology produce fabricated data and errors in documentation. The excuse was the hurried pace in the laboratory and the emphasis on productivity [Greenberg, 1987]. A luminary in science, a Nobel laureate said, "All laboratories that produce a large amount of information are in danger of becoming prey to people who wish to publish for their own gain, but that is probably three quarters of the laboratories in the United States" [Benacerraf, 1987].

During the 1950s and early 1960s, the CIA gave psychedelic drugs to hundreds of Americans who were unaware that they were part of the agency's experiments on mind control. In 1972 the experiments were declared useless. The CIA project with psychedelic drugs, called MK Ultra, was instituted when the agency feared the Soviet Union might use LSD as a chemical weapon or that China would perfect brainwashing techniques [Obituary in Wash times, 1999].

These reports suggest that the ethics of laboratory and clinical research have distorted knowledge for the wrong purpose. Little attention has been given to the personal morality of the investigator who has the leadership position, is the ultimate planner, and decision maker. Therefore he is the captain of the ship responsible for the ethical compass of all aboard. His recognition of bioethics and sensitivity to moral values will determine the experiments' route. Self-interest is not to be persuasive in arriving at the ways and means of bioscientific research and clinical investigative practice. Underlying all matters pertinent to biomedicine should be an unalterable, draconian, procrustean commitment to high moral standings as presented in a prescribed code of bioethics. No holder of a professional license to practice medicine and surgery has a right to downgrade and bludgeon bioethics. The same requirement is relevant to bioscientific research.

Applied research bioscience and clinical medicine should be allied for the integrated benefit of humanity. The aim is to aid persons stricken by diseases, injuries, and infirmities. No one, no matter licensure privilege, can claim by depending on scientific competence, that they are free to decide on the ethical destiny of their labor that is tarnished.

Inaccurate and false research can be detrimental to patients, e.g., administering medication that is useless, and others that may have serious side-reactions. Not to mention the millions of dollars wasted on inaccurate research. Inexcusable, faulty, tampered research may lead honest bioscientists downward away from their objectives.

The modern pharmaceutical industry is on the threshold of ethical peril. With the cost of prescription medicines so high critics are many. In the changing economy the pharmatech corporations are tempted in many ways due to their desires to search for new medicines. Differing research and development costs are excuses given for expensive drugs that are beyond the purchase ability of many citizens. Without high prices, these companies maintain they do not recover their costs for continuing research. Danger lurks in pharmaceutical laboratories that profit margins may discount ethical standards when drug prices fall, shortages occur, and rationing is a possibility [Matthews, 2001].

Omar Khayyam [1070-1123] in his doleful lamentation wrote these words appropriately with persuasive, fluent, and graceful, emotional expression.

> Indeed the idols I have loved so long
> Have done my credit in this world much wrong:
> Have drowned my glory in a shallow cup,
> And sold my reputation for a song
>
> Rubaiyat, Stanza 93

Chapter 21

Junk Science

Dictionary definition of junk is lengthy for something that is useless. Anything worn-out or to be discarded because it is valueless is junk. Also it includes material of inferior quality, cheap or shoddy. Intangibly it refers to what is meaningless, fatuous, unbelievable—nonsense. The last definition has been applied to dishonest bioscience. It is sad to state that anything referring to medicine should have a downhill word such as junk applied to it. This makes one crestfallen. Junk science is dishonesty disguised as a discipline.

The mere thought of it awakens the vision of unsentimental, unethical scams tangled with moral torpor as enticing mechanisms that foment conduciveness to blindsided scandal. Purveyors of such inferior merchandise have no nobility of character which is a treasure trove that has few equals. Character has some genetic origin but it is Bessermerized in the stream of life. No exception is given to bioscientists who are exposed to the same elements as every other person residing in the world to be dishonest.

This is a threat in new experiments in which many disciplines will do research together where each should be first among equals. Envy may enter their project that can curtail adherence to high ethical behavior. Electrical engineering, computer science, physiology, and currently unperfected micro-electromechanical systems [MEMS] are cooperating in the development of anatomical parts to be manufactured commercially. The aim is to defeat deafness, overcome paralysis, improve treatment for many diseases [epilepsy, chorea, Parkinsonism etc], and facilitate diagnosis of bacterial/viral agents. Added to these awaited benefices are drug and vaccine therapies that are not available at present. Blindness will be diminished and in some instances may be abolished by chip technology amalgamated with microbiology. There is great expectation for all these anticipated medical benefits to be realized. In the research journey to this medical progress, bioethics must be preserved in a pristine state of prominence.

Unfortunately some learned bioscientists with masterful talent, excellent credentials, and professional stature have succumbed to certain external forces that caused a character deficiency in them. Deviation from what they were taught resulted in unethical performances that were medical spoilage. Some examples of which are to be mentioned.

Purposeful Deception

Decades ago the Krebiozen cancer cure fiasco was a dark blotch on medical history which haunted clinical medicine years after the echo of it was gone. It is the incredible story of a distinguished professor of physiology in Chicago who spent the last twenty-seven years of his life advocating an anti-cancer substance that was curative. The comedy of errors was a humiliation of bioscience.

Other similar blemishes occurred subsequent to the Krebiozen fraud. In Mexico an all-purpose cancer cure was popularized with wide acceptance. Called Laertrile it became the magic potion for those who could afford the cure. Several movie stars from Hollywood went to Mexico to be treated. Their deaths disproved the efficacy of the therapy.

In 1998 a Milanese physician gave an attractive name to an intravenous solution that was a cure for cancer in any region of the human anatomy. The cost for the medication was more than $1,000 per week. Known internationally for its remarkable results, it was manufactured only in Italy and Turkey. Profitable for two years it was condemned by the Italian government.

During the dictatorship of Josef Stalin, a soviet scientist claimed discovery of a new form of water. The features of the aqueous marvel was that it had different thermal properties and vapor pressure that were dissimilar to that of ordinary water. It was called polywater. The discoverer proposed the use of the water to treat diseases which would revolutionize medical therapy. The passage of time disclosed that this water never existed. For his great scientific contribution the Russian Academy of Sciences bestowed upon the researcher an award similar to the Nobel Prize. After the deception was revealed, the award was rescinded.

In New York State a highly publicized medical fraud became the subject of a book that was on the best seller list. The deceit was in research. In order to demonstrate that a skin graft from a black to a white mouse was possible and successful, a researcher painted the so-called transplanted area on the white mouse with a black felt pen. The doctor brought the painted mouse for demonstration to the director of the research institute who had employed him. A committee decided that his conduct was not compatible with the discharge of his responsibilities in the scientific community. He was dismissed from the faculty.

In the 1970s research scientists published their descriptions of various permanent lines of Hodgkins lymphoma cells. The availability of such tumor cells in permanent cultures was a vital need in the study of this class of lymphomas. It was found that the author's work was not documented properly because the researcher tampered with the ultracentrifuge.

During the 1980s when medical malpractice was at its height according to the number of lawsuits filed alleging torts of various degrees, the news media broadcasted that 45,000 out of 400,000 physicians were practicing unethically. Many of them had obtained counterfeited, fraudulent, and similar perverted degrees from non-American medical schools. Others with legal diplomas were practicing unorthodox medicine which was a pseudoscience. No allegations were made against surgical practice, although many accusations were made that tonsillectomies were overdone as a constant source of income economically labeled as "bread and butter" money.

Pseudosciences

Untenable theories, contrived gimmicks, tricky methods that claim to have bioscientific function are pseudosciences. This includes therapy such as balneotherapy whose principle requires submerging in water for curative results. Another pseudoscience is biorhythm which is supposed to predict human behavior [fortune-telling included for the same fee]. The method charts the patient's physical, emotional, and intellectual cycles. Many pseudosciences have generated theories and practices that persist to this day.

Franz Anton Mesmer [1714-1815] proposed mental seduction as a form of therapy for mental disorders. Mesmerism was the precursor to hypnotism. He was acclaimed in Austria even when his professional activities were bizarre. Mesmer maintained that the human body "retains an invisible fluid called ether that is affected by planetary gravitation" [Cover Story, 1999]. A person's health relied on the adequate flow of the fluid which had to be in accord with gravity for good health. Discordant fluid was the cause for ill-health.

Mental and intellectual attributes were interpreted by the study of the face and head. This was phrenology. Franz Joseph Gall [1758-1828] a german physician studied and practiced this science. As a foremost neurophysiologist his reputation was gigantic. Under his leadership phrenology became extremely popular. Gall and his associate [Christoph Spurzheim, 1776-1832] "conducted extensive examinations of the heads of errand boys, inmates, patients, and friends [Hunt, 1993].

An exceedingly provocative novel on psychiatry was inspired by a Vienna physician teaching in London. The stimulus was the result of a much quoted lecture. "Therapeutic Applications of Hypnosis and Suggestion" expressed "a kind of Machiavellian altruism" [Yardley, 1999].

"His thesis was simple: Suggestion—that is, 'the act by which an idea is introduced into the brain and accepted by it'—was the great unsung force in history. It fueled religion. Child-rearing to nation-building were subjected to its power. Bernheim's insight was twofold: first, he proposed that suggestion could be used therapeutically, as a means of treating certain psychogenic disorders; second, that the state of highest suggestibility, what he called credivite, could be induced through hypnosis. Bernheim was espousing an early brand of hypnotherapy, in other words . . . Bernheim advised a more direct approach: identify the most ostensible source of the patient's complaint, induce a hypnotic trance, then suggest a way in which the disorder might be repaired" [Hansen, 1999].

At a busy clinic in London "healing suggestion" is a treatment chosen by many patients. A following of enthusiastic advocates has been a marvelous propaganda machine. Physicians triage the patients very carefully. They "take the cases you know you can treat" [Hansen, 1999]. Success is possible because selectivity disallows overreaching of hypnotic suggestion. Thus these physicians establish "a reputation for effectiveness" so that "patients would come with higher hopes—higher hopes meant greater suggestibility—which meant [they] could afford more challenging cases, enjoy more success, and greater faith" [Hansen, 1999]. Not to mention increasing their revenues.

When scientific misinformation is used in a court of law to seek millions of dollars, it is not only unethical but borders on criminal tactics. A Seattle trial lawyer brought a legal action against a utility company alleging that personal injury resulted from electromagnetic fields. Parents claimed their 5-year-old daughter developed a rare type of kidney cancer from improperly protected electric wires from which came electromagnetic emanations.

The attorney tried to persuade the jury [without success] that electromagnetic fields cause cancer. "He had two widely reported scientific papers to support his conclusion. . . The two papers were published two years before the first lawsuit went to trial. One of the papers appeared in the Annals of the New York Academy of Sciences, the other in FEBS Letters, which is published by the Federation of European Biochemical Societies" [Perkins, 1999].

"The author of both papers was a cell biologist. His research concluded that electromagnetic fields exert a biological effect that leads to a variety of illnesses, including childhood leukemia.

That was all trial lawyers needed to beat a hasty path to the courthouse. And that's all 'public interest' groups needed to hound power companies around the country to move electric lines, to install shielding, or to bury new power lines in the ground (at a cost of more than $1 billion a year, according to government estimates).

"As it turns out, all the scary stories about electromagnetic fields causing cancer, all the lawsuits seeking millions of dollars in damages from electric companies, were based on a false premise. The author has been exposed as a scientific fraud.

"Indeed, the federal Office of Research Integrity, an arm of the U.S. Department of Health and Human Services, found the author engaged in scientific misconduct in biomedical research by falsifying and fabricating data and claims about the purported cellular effects of electric and magnetic fields.

"This finding by the integrity office, published in the Federal Register, is consistent with earlier findings by the Lawrence Berkeley lab, which took a hard look at EMF research back in 1995 after a whistleblower challenged his results. Lab investigators surmised that the cell biologist unscrupulously discarded data that did not fit his conclusion.

"Indeed, practically every major study of electromagnetic fields published since 1992 has contradicted the scientist's conclusion that power lines cause cancer. Perhaps the most authoritative of these studies was completed two years ago by the National Cancer Institute.

"What motivated the scientist to doctor his research results, to mislead the public into believing that power lines cause cancer? At least one longtime skeptic of the EMF-cancer link, a University of Maryland physics professor told the New York Times that the kind of junk science promoted is not altogether uncommon for the field, which seems to attract crusaders out to demonize certain industries.

"But there is also a huge financial incentive for junk scientists. Indeed, on the basis of fraudulent EMF research, one scientist managed to score $3.3 million in federal grants from the National Institutes of Health, the Energy Department, and the Pentagon.

"That's why junk science is such a growth industry in this country. Scientists have a tremendous financial incentive to hype some putative public health threat—whether it be asbestos in schools and office buildings, pesticide traces in foods, or electromagnetic fields from power lines.

"Moreover, some scientists have an unholy alliance with trial lawyers, who use their research, no matter how questionable, as pretexts for multimillion-dollar personal-injury lawsuits (sometimes paying scientists generous consulting fees to tell a jury how, say, EMF can cause leukemia in 5-year-old little girls)" [Perkins, 1999].

Manufactured results in scientific research are a gross violation of ethics. It is degradation beyond measure which is an insult to intelligence, a moral travesty that is an enigma to conscience.

Another instance of misuse of science, in this particular instance for punitive reasons was at a federal government agency in 1999. "With little public notice, the EPA time and again has used slipshod science to justify new anti-pollution rules, then defended the rules to the hilt, even if that defense came at the expense of its own scientists.

"The latest example: a gasoline additive mandated by the Environmental Protection Agency poses a health risk, according to a blue-ribbon panel. The agency accepted the findings and said it will find an alternative to the additive.

"But the report did not contain new research. The panel just collected studies long available to the EPA. The agency either was too busy cheerleading the fuel additive to examine that research seriously or willfully ignored it.

"The EPA apparently has yet to learn that sound environmental rules require sound science" [Pierce, 1999]. No intended good intention can give approval to any research fabrication, false therapy, administration of *placebo* medication as curative, and deceptive appliances in the biosciences.

There are times what may appear ludicrous and seems to be inappropriate to science may have value. Merit may eventuate in what initially may be looked upon as fatuous and highly improbable. A situational side-bar in point is the research studies that may turn vegetables into vaccines.

At the University of Virginia there is a greenhouse. On the entrance door is a sign. "This greenhouse contains genetically engineered plants. Do not remove any plants from the greenhouse.'" These are tobacco plants being grown to study how and if they can be used in medicine.

"They are part of a study exploring how to turn common vegetables, such as tomatoes and carrots, into edible vaccines that could wipe out a major killer of children in developing countries. This pioneering research is also laying the groundwork for edible vaccines to fight viruses that cause the flu, or maybe even AIDS.

"Funded with a $3.3 million, five-year grant from the National Institutes of Health, the study is focusing on creating a low-cost vaccine to prevent thousands of children from dying each year from a waterborne parasitic amoeba that causes amebiasis. The goal is to turn plants into manufacturers of a foreign protein that would prevent the parasitic amoeba from killing cells in the large intestine.

"Many more years of research will be needed, though, before an edible vaccine made from a common vegetable becomes a reality. Research to make edible vaccines began only a couple of years ago. So far, only one human trial with potatoes has been done.

"No vaccine currently exists for any parasitic disease. An edible vaccine has more promise than one injected through muscle. Intramuscular vaccines are not effective at stimulating an immune response against an infection in the bowels" [Casey, 1999].

Hence this research in botany is to be encouraged and not considered in the category of false science. The application of plants in scientific studies have a wonderful heritage in the genetic work of Gregor Mendel

[1822-1884], the clinical use of the foxglove plant by William Withering [1741-1799], and many other pioneers.[1]

Ethical conduct and honest scientific research walk together soignéely hand in hand without fearing either threats of moral destruction or death of their studied enterprises. Authentic Judeo-Christian-Muslim consciences integrate each other into credible, joyous normalcy of professional endeavors. All three religions are compatible in their unity. For every scientist of whatever denomination, their faith instills in them that there is divinity in their vocations.

Hence bioscientists derive their ability, willingness, and readiness to serve humanity through the gift of knowledge which they have received, accepted, and bear with immeasurable patience. This crucial rôle is the unfissured rock upon which is built the scientific format and moral fortitude of modern, biological medicine in the third millennium. Such dedication to bioscience is a reflection of the caring love of the Good Samaritan.

Credible scientific research has demonstrated it is a dynamic force in health-enhancing value that can increase the quality of life and extend longevity. However the lack of enforcement of normal bioethical standards is a serious impediment to the continuance of these benefits. False claims on the basis of poorly documented recommendations can be deleterious to health. This misfortune is not remedied easily when bioethical codes are not evoked even after the event. These incidents are implemented and defended by scientists who, with full knowledge aforethought, do not evaluate data which has not been monitored bioethically.

Withholding self-imposed and/or peer judgement is a grievous fault. Cautionary surveillance is an obligation that should prevent ethical dan-

---

1. Mendelism is the principle of heredity formulated by Gregor Johann Mendel. Referred to as Mendel's laws consisting of three sections: Law of Segregation, Law of Independent Combination, and the Law of Dominance.

An important therapeutic advancement was William Withering's discovery of the use of foxglove [digitalis] in cases of edema due to congestive heart failure. The plant was possessed by a family of Shropshire farmers. Withering traced their success to the use of a mixture containing foxglove. By assiduous observation he established the proper method for the administration of digitalis [dosage determination]. In addition he demonstrated peripheral and pulmonary edema were not primary diseases but could be due to cardiac failure. His *Account* of the *Foxglove*, published in 1785, is his masterpiece.

gers in research. Intense bioethical oversight is not first on the agenda of most research bioscientists. By avoidance they work under an aura that does not include moral alertness and keen ethical awareness. Flagrant violations of ethical codes is an outright abuse of the privileges given to those with a doctoral degree in a scientific specialty. Too many of whom accept the creed that any solution to a premised research endeavor must be delivered however flawed it might be.

On the contrary, ethical based bioscience fosters admirable well-being that is a mutual reinforcement for researchers that increases the motivation for greater productivity of merit. Moreover it develops patience in research which diminishes any impatience. This allows facile acceptance of manageable ethical restrictions. A new tractate and clarity of thinking are required to instill bioethics as the keeper of conscience in all scientists. With this will come down the false flag of autonomy in science that sustains the agenda that everything science can do is permissible.

Bioscientists have no allegiance to ethical authority which is not even a moiety in their specified professional lives. For this reason, among others, the predictable outcome of scientific initiatives are not always met with either roaring approval or maximum denunciation. Under destructive or constructive criticism the contamination of immoral infection is not disclosed. Ethical beliefs are not promoted privately. They are more easily avoided when generalized. Invariably this subject becomes embedded into the fabric of public life where it disappears in the everchanging, progressive, sophisticated culture.

With all this antagonism, security is found in past history whose lessons teach that morality and ethics survive. In the sphere of the bioscientific community there is no strong preoccupation with ethics in the competition for success and its appended rewards. Even when it importunes social justice and the disenchantment it brings to the non-scientific population. Widespread dedication to a cause among bioscientists does not advocate ignoring virtuous behavior. No scientist of every category should either fear or deny the injection of ethics into the active scientific community.

Chapter 22

Fraudulent Publications

Personal instincts demand more and more success. The added advantage of words in print, even if they are supposititious, is a medium that communicates success to colleagues. Language stands behind the human mental development which speaks for the originator. This news of success travels. Becoming archival history, it is preserved after the author is gone. Hence the impetus to be read in print is difficult to resist and is recessive in few bioscientists. Perilous is the vacuity of internal denial of any malintention during the literary production. Interior maneuvers of the mind that dominate conscience can sidetrack ethics leading to a collapse whose self-made wreckage is scandalous.

Many opinions have been presented as new ideas which find their way into printed journals. Sometimes a new idea is a composite of two or more older ones molded into one forming a collage that is accepted for publication. Empowered with this uncanny ability, some authors rearrange and add to ancient publications with magical recomposition that has a new appeal.

Power of the printed page is nothing without a moral intellect behind it. Misplaced writings that bring about malevolent conclusions which may produce harm is deviltry. Without centralized, personal control the beneficial effectiveness of unmonitored bioscientific endeavors—including writings—are unworthy of the acclaim given by peer reviewers deficient in adequate scrutiny. This is negligent professional vigilance.

With either faded or failed ethical intent, the intellect can recycle what the past recorded long ago. Cloaked in new apparel, the old thought may go unrecognized even by the expertised. Deception can be so conceived and so written that even the specialist is deceived. Connived, near-fanatic devotion to falsity has its devotees. Disguised deception can permeate scientific societies easily even at the expense of ethical opponents. Few ghost writers are made to suffer censure and opprobrium.

Competition in the savage race to be first may blind a bioscientist to ethical diktats. Public awards, political acceptance, glamour of glory can trump ethics. Dedicated bioscientists do not have to be unethically dishonest to reach stardom in the constellation of recorded professional achievements. They do not follow an unproven adage of "publish or perish" even if it means faking it. Fraudulent science is never permissible.

Torrential rivalry for monumental rewards is fertile soil for the growth of illicit, irresistible impulse to engage in wrongdoing. "Ethical sogginess is no rarity in science . . . Young physicians seem to predominate among the culprits of fraud cases, a distinction that is attributed to the post-medical-school catch-up that they must play against straightforward PhDs, who begin research careers as graduate students right after college" [Greenberg, 1987].

Another ethical pitfall is to facilitate the route to publication by adding to the authorship departmental colleagues [especially the chairperson] who may be a member of the editorial board of a bioscientific journal. The non-contributor does not refuse even with full knowledge that he/she made no substantive contribution to, knowledge of, and either read or knew the validity of the contents contained in the research paper.

Reporting scientific writings to verify research or clinical observations for reading in professional journals will be deposited in libraries. This does not acknowledge that dishonesty is uncongenial to didacticism. Moreover false statements send honest scientists down false trails to error. All these imperfections may go undetected and are not marked by librarians.

Illustrative Examples

A well-known professor of medicine at a highly respected medical school was censured for plagiarizing twenty-four percent of a chapter in a previously published medical textbook which was not his own. An ethics committee concluded he displayed "grossly negligent scholarship." The doctor's explanation was that he was so engrossed in his new position as chairman of the department of internal medicine that he did not get around to making sure permission had been granted to use some material he borrowed for the new textbook he was preparing.

In 1991 a Nobel Prize-winning molecular biologist retracted a published paper when allegations of fraud were made. An influential scientific article bearing his name as a co-author had fraudulent data that was an embarrassment to the university of which he was president. His published research "purported to make a critical contribution to understanding the immune system. The report prepared by the Office of Scientific Integrity [OSI] of the National Institutes of Health, listed numerous instances in which it concluded that one of the co-authors falsified and manufactured data" [Galdwell, 1991].

Much publicity was given to a published pedophilia report that was founded on opinion not scientific study. "The American Psychological Association did an abrupt about-face on an article it published about pedophilia . . . The report, which appeared in an APA scholarly journal, suggested sex between children and adults is not necessarily harmful and that, if the children were willing participants, such sexual relationships should be labeled in scientifically neutral terms . . . The chief executive officer of the APA acknowledged inconsistencies . . . that should have caused us to evaluate the article based on its potential for misinforming the public policy process. This is something we failed to do . . . The article provoked angry public reaction . . . One of the misinterpretations was that the article could be used in court briefs to justify or condone pedophilia" [Duin, 1999].

This publication in an authoritative journal as the official voice of a national psychological association is more than misleading. It could have been used in a court of law as persuasive evidence. Additionally it sanctions immorality, and gives the impression that an immature child can give consent to an evil act thus defending it as consensual. A compounding fault rests with the editors who failed in their duty to screen manuscripts thoroughly. Any supposed study "that urges psychologists not to assume that sex between non-related adults and minors is an abusive act is irresponsible, and in my opinion unjustified" [DeLay, 1999].

A different kind of ethical embarrassment can arise in reference to editorial policies of medical journals. This was demonstrated when a prestigious medical journal's eminent editor resigned his post. The senior editor of the magazine founded in 1812 is highly regarded by American physicians. The dispute between editor and ownership was the use of the magazine's distinguished name to sell consumer newsletters and other publications. When launching new magazines and advertising them they were stated to be the same publishers of the respected medical journal. The editor opposed "tying the journal's reputation to consumer health letters and other magazines that have no real connection to the medical journal's standards or editing" [Boston, 1999]. This philosophical difference is not entirely an innocent disagreement. If the new publications are separate and distinct from the medical journal, and the latter has no editorial attachment to the new publications then the name of the medical journal should not be associated with them. Naming the ownership as the publishers of the new literature would be proper and fortify the structural reliability of the publications because the owner is a state medical society. Any misguided ethical strategy would make the new publications deceptive. Such actions are morally unsanitary.

Methods Of Misleading

Whenever human morality is mute and philosophic ethics is tongue-tied, falsity is fortified as it becomes loquacious. The resulting, rigorous rhetoric supports invalid pretenses in sound and writing that can have unforeseen, unintended inauspicious consequences. Cheating in scientific writing is one of these non-predictable end-products. Fraud is the convenient denominator for such scientific misconduct.

Legally fraud is criminal deception or the use of false representation intended to benefit the deceiver. Bioscientists who cheat knowingly, willingly, and actively with full consent of free-will have committed a major sin. Falsification, invention of, and tampering with research data is not excluded but included. Some bioscientists try to mitigate the event by not strengthening it with lies remaining silent, and not responding to questions with straight answers. This eliminates fraud in its strictest sense as benefit from the misdeed is denied.

Another denial of fraudulent wrongdoing is when the false writing is not used to obtain financial support from public or governmental agencies, and private sources. Fraud is committed when on the basis of false data the scientist is trying to secure a research position, to prove that public funds have been used properly, to convince grantors of research money, or the general public that a certain procedure, equipment or drug is acceptable and safe. When the motivation of fraud is to obtain grants, it is well to recall past history. Some are born to greatness, some inherit it, but most have to achieve it by industrious effort.

Charles Babbage [1792-1871] a mathematician and contributing inventor to the first calculator listed the cheating ways applied to research reports. He stressed four methods that he discerned. These are listed alphabetically and not as to frequency of usage.

1. Cooking is choosing only the data that suits the researcher to prove the point being investigated and studied. This means the elimination of negative results.
2. Forging is recording observations never made or seen, experiments never carried out, citations of non-existent manuscripts, and outright plagiarism or lies.
3. Fudging is the rearranging of data to fortify a proposal, experiment, or an aim to be proven.
4. Trimming is the manipulation of data to look better. Also called massaging data which includes amplification, declaring the use of more animals than were used, and the calculated number of controls were less than stated.

Violation of Ethical Norms In Writing

Editors who formulate policies for the acceptance of manuscripts for publication in their journals must have integrity, a high caliber of morality, unquestionable ethical criteria, literary skills, and vocabulary choice that is scholarly admirable. Mediocrity in bioscientific writings does not add to the biomedical profession. Contrarily it degrades it. Simplicity in words does not always convey the message authoritatively. Since the reader is an educated person, the vocabulary used should be equal to that intellect. A baroque style of writing is not to be erudite only in their field. As intellectual leaders they are highly honored. Equivalence to which requires the use of spoken and written words that are not simple, ordinary, lack luster, and promote only lackadaisical thinking.

There is no easy answer to what constitutes the ideal editor for bioscientific publications. What is known are the issues editors generally confront. These are mainly alerts to which they must give undivided attention. Number one is the submission of the same writing by authors to more than one publication. Changing the title over the same material does not make it something new or different. This is a maneuver that adds to the author's bibliography of contributions but diminishes honesty, credibility, and ethical standing. Only an editor or peer reviewer who is acquainted with the subject can detect the surreptitious duplication. When a manuscript is submitted to several journals at the same time, there is no detection of the duplicity.

Another ethical trespass is outright fabrications that have to be retracted *via* editorial route. This causes much encephalalgia among the editor's staffers. The absence of corroborative data from other periodicals does not always give rise to any suspicion. No index is available to make certain that something is awry.

Another questionable ethical practice in journalism relates to an excessive number of authors on a manuscript. Nothing indicates the true author from the supernumeraries. There is no separation of the work-producing author from those who are less productive and others who are non-productive investigators. Much of the author padding is to increase the number of each author's publications or to assist a colleague to obtain an academic promotion. Long lists of publications in a dossier can be a determining factor in acquiring a higher position.

A reasonable number of authors of a single manuscript is an empirical question. In an unnamed specialty journal an article had 10 authors most of whom resided in different states and were teaching at non-associated medical centres. Difficulty arises in trying to believe they all participated in producing the not-too-gigantic report. Experience teaches that no more than two or three researchers actually do the work. This may include the collection with analysis of the assembled and researched data.

Usually it is verifiable that one person composes the format and writes the manuscript. Several others will read the manuscript for corrections and/or additions without any contribution to the essential matter contained therein. It would be more appropriate ethically to cite the editorial assistance as an acknowledge critique and not as co-authorship. Imposing a limit on the number of authors would not be unreasonable. It would eliminate unjustified authorship with ethical enrichment of bioscientific literature.

A third issue involves the relationship of scientific journals with lay publications. Reference is made to scientific authors who send their unrequested reprints to newspapers, health magazines, and other non-professional publications in the hope of free publicity for themselves. Under the guise of an altruistic desire to educate the laity, many authors spread their reprints generously. The public can be persuaded by inadequate reports when lay appeal outweighs scientific accuracy. Good science is the benchmark by which scientific productivity is measured. Whether the subject published has lay appeal or not is immaterial.

Sensationalism in bioscientific efforts are not compatible with its classical history. Editors have a moral obligation to protect the laity from questionable science. As well as not to allow faulty publications to give the impression that science can deliver more than the printed data allow. Inaccurate scientific writings raise false hope and erode scientific credibility. No manuscript should be published that may raise false hope in a person afflicted with a particular disease [Palumbo, 1987].

As a fourth issue attention is focused on the imperative of appropriate use of statistical methods. Statistics can be manipulated to serve a preconceived purpose. Improper, designed correlation of statistics with falsified data is both misinformation and disinformation. It is an overzealous artifact to use statistics without any review of the data by the research team. Movable statistics attempt to give data validity which is not warranted.

"Unfortunately, reviewers seldom peruse data and its analysis carefully to point out flagrant misuse of statistics and the potential for selection bias. It is the editor's responsibility to ensure that the biases in a study and the analysis of the data are carefully reviewed to avoid errors in interpretation that may be misleading and overstating the results of the data" [Palumbo, 1987]. The editor's connate right is an ethical duty to ferret out intellectual misconduct and to condemn it without hesitancy.

"To be an editor of a scientific journal is not only a challenge but also a public trust. The editor must be dedicated to identifying good science and sharing it with the scientific and lay communities in a responsible way. In recognizing and discharging this responsibility, the editor promotes and promulgates scientific information of the highest quality" [Palumbo, 1987].

Concludingly, an editor of solid worth to scientific literature has a motto: *Servabo fidem, sic igitur ad astra* [I shall serve [keep] the faith, thus [we shall reach] the stars [immortality]. Lofty ethical ideals in scientific writing must be preserved. If due care is not taken to conserve what is right, medical and bioscientific literature will decay into scribbled persiflage.

Chapter 23

Laboratory Approach To Humanity

A critical assembly of philosophers, theologians, bioscientists, and engineers is concerned about the uncontrolled large-scale laboratory interference in human physiology and the unrestricted accessibility to its facilities. Biotechnology has excitement without any added ethical anxiety of its coupling with the value-laden morality inchoate to reproduction, birth, and death. This genetically engineered wedding can be an illicit marriage.

Despite its increasing attractiveness, laboratory bioscience has spread confusion as to the exact place and extent of its research. Theorization and experimentation appear to be uncontrollable. The social consequences of biomedical innovation are commencing to appear. "Between life and commerce" bioscience sees no difference [Bud, 1993].

Within the current climate of frenzied scientific investigations, every aspect of life to death of the human embryo to the weary geriatric body is under scrutiny. Like ancient tales of geographical explorations, accounts of biomedical research inspires, thrills, and frightens—often like primeval hostility. Situations arise which are tests of normalized bioethics.

Ethics has been a recognized, privileged area for philosophical study, reflection, and conclusions. Without gross exaggeration there is currently a marked inflation of published writings on this timely subject. Some features of contemporary ethical discourses confuse the uninitiated. Rhetorical statements and written commentaries seem to be more existential than bioethical.

The misappropriation to self-legislate is disguised as autonomy. Freewill as a gift of individual independence can mislead into the labyrinth of "spurious principles of morality" so ably stated by Kant.[1] With an unnatural, false foundation any beginning built upon it, is capable of demonstrating natural forms of activities that can be disseminated without medicomoral testing. Pseudo-justification for research activities of questionable ethical content are published by university faculty members and philosophers. Thus are created unreliable absolutes of ethical imperatives which are doubtful with the continuance of relativism prevailing pervasively.

When any scientist becomes subservient to ethical misconduct he is submitting to immoral behavior. Ethics and morality are germane twins. Infringement of one magnetizes the other into a firm attachment most difficult to disengage. Both may indicate a misgovernance of conscience leading to a voluntary subscription to spiritual anarchy. Contrariwise adherence to high bioethical standards is a reserve force. It assists in the exploration to solution, issues that enable scientists to arrive at medicomoral decisions in questionable scientific areas where intellectual hesitancy has stymied ethical progress in a positive direction.

Medical advancements and decision-making, at times, can be in conflict with bioethics. Statistical studies have been made that indicate when a patient decides not to consent to a procedure [laboratory or otherwise] that decision may not be honored by the health-care provider. Under constitutional, statutory, and common-law, the right to refuse is protected. Courts have awarded money damages against health-care providers under various tort theories. Also the rights of patients and next of kin have been upheld with dismissal of claims for payment of unwanted procedures. Lawsuits for the wrongful administration of treatment etc have both an ethical and legal component. Careful concern is necessary when certain therapeutic modalities and laboratory procedures are to be instituted.

Reducing humanity to a series of problems to be solved in the bioscientific laboratory would mean the end of human freedom. Technical feasibility has taken precedence over every law of science even when wisdom is against it. For the sake of humanity as created beings bio-

---

1. Immanuel Kant [1724-1804] was born and died in Königsberg, Prussia. The philosophy of Kant is called variously the critical philosophy, criticism, transcendentalism, or transcendental idealism. Quotation is from paragraph 88 of Kant's The Fundamental Principles of the Metaphysics of ethics.

science must listen to moralists who object to laboratory procedures that go beyond normalcy favoring the unreal and the unnecessary.

Loving, devotional, and procreational good intentions do not exculpate laboratory scientists whose misapprehension places human beings on the same level as inanimate things. Forms of procreative techniques performed in laboratories incipiently are morally wrong as a threat to humanity's reproductive function. In artificial procreation the conceived is produced, not generated. Bioscientific laboratories now produce persons. "[M]an enters the universe of being through a relation that at its inception does not put him in real reciprocity with other persons" when produced in the laboratory [Caffarra, 1998].

Value of Life

Laboratory transgressions against human dignity have paralyzed restraining opposition. Tampering with human life has become the self-assumed right of laboratory-confined bioscientists. With their new medical research tools human tissue placed in laboratory animals will produce hybrids for the study of diseases.

"In a series of bold experiments, scientists have created laboratory mice with tiny human organ structures—lungs, intestines, pancreases, lymph nodes, thymuses, livers and immune systems. The purpose is to study the viruses of human diseases in living human tissues.

"The animals, whose organ tissues are derived from those of human fetuses, provide a singular opportunity to gauge the effectiveness of various antiviral drugs. The mice have been successfully infected with the AIDS virus and with two cancer viruses that cause leukemia. The organ structures are not miniature carbon copies of adult organs but contain complete structural subunits of each organ and carry out the organ's normal functions in duplicate with the mouse's own.

"Because human fetal tissues are being implanted into animals and not humans, the investigators are not subject to the Federal ban on the use of such tissues in medical research. The ban, imposed by the Department of Health and Human Services, was intended to prevent women from having abortions for the sake of donating fetal tissue to people, but the regulations make no mention of mice.

"To create mice with human immune systems, bioscientists take the thymus, liver, and lymph nodes from human fetuses less than 22 weeks old and divides them into hundreds of pieces, each about the size of a grain of rice.

"Using a microscope, they implant a piece of each organ under the kidneys of young mice. Within days, the mouse's blood vessels move into the human tissue, nourishing it and encouraging it to grow. In a month or two, the human organs are the size of blueberries and are able to engender the cells of the immune system" [Blakeslee, 1990].

"Last month, newspapers reported two legal disputes involving new reproductive methods. The first [Davis v. Davis] was a battle for custody of seven frozen embryos, conceived by in vitro fertilization two years ago. A lower court had referred to them as 'children in vitro,' and granted them full protection under the law. The Tennessee Court of Appeals gave joint custody to the parents, who divorced shortly after the embryos were created. Since they do not agree on the disposition of the embryos, it would seem that the 'children in vitro' are destined to enjoy their legal protection in the freezer indefinitely.

"The second case [Johnson v. Calvert and Calvert] involves three parents of the same baby. One of the two women was unable to become pregnant because she had had a hysterectomy. She and her husband conceived an embryo by in vitro fertilization and hired the other woman to carry it to term. The woman who gave birth to the baby is unwilling to relinquish it. The California Superior Court, in a modern version of King Solomon's approach, threatened to send the newborn to a foster home if the three parents could not agree. The genetic parents were willing for this to happen, but not the woman who gave birth to the baby; she relinquished temporary custody to the genetic parents.

"I relate these strange tales not just to astonish, but because they illustrate many of the problems engendered by our new forms of reproductive technology and the uses to which they are put. I do not propose to offer solutions to the problems; indeed, some of them seem to me to be virtually insoluble. I intend instead to describe the context in which the problems arise and thus, I hope, to provide as balanced a view of them as possible.

"For millenniums, there was only one way to get pregnant. That was not without its problems, of course, but society had plenty of time to devise ways of dealing with them. Now, we are faced with a proliferation of new reproductive methods, often involving more than two people, which present unprecedented and complex legal, ethical, and social problems" [Angell, 1990].

These unethical processes are not always successful. "The majority of egg cohorts evidently possess the potential to produce a pregnancy, but cryopreservation of human embryos significantly reduces their capacity for implantation . . . two-thirds of the frozen and thawed embryos in our study lost their potential to establish a pregnancy . . . In the absence of more reliable ways to predict the potential of a given embryo for pregnancy, the morphologic features of the blastomeres could be taken as a possible guideline. Unless there are at least two or three morphologically sound embryos available for fresh transfer, we recommend no embryos be allocated to cryopreservation" [Levran, Dor et al, 1990]. It may be stated that all is not well scientifically which increases the bioethical criticism of the pregnancy potential of human oocytes that are affected by cryopreservation.

Good intention does not minimize an unethical act. Exemplified is oocyte donation to extend the reproductive potential for women over forty. Preliminary results imply that the endometrium in women 40 years-of-age and over retains the physiologic ability to respond to gonadal steroids, providing receptive anatomy for embryo implantation and gestation. This probability may be a scientific contribution to obstetrics, but it is an infringement on medical ethics.

"As many as 10 percent of women have ovarian failure by 40 years of age, and until recently these women were considered to be hopelessly infertile. With aging, diminished fertility is believed to occur principally as a result of oocyte senescence, but it could also be due to resistance to implantation of the embryo in the endometrium. After implantation, the loss of pregnancy is also increased in women over 40, presumably as a result of a combination of detrimental changes in aging oocytes and the endometrium.

"The incidence of genetic anomalies in the offspring of women undergoing in vitro fertilization and embryo transfer is not different from that in the population at large. Whether the incidence of such anomalies in this older group of women with ovarian failure will resemble that of the younger donors who provide the gametes or that of their own age group is a matter of speculation. The increased incidence of anomalies in the offspring of older women in general may be due to either the older gametes or lack of rejection of abnormal conceptuses by the endometrium of older women. Similarly, the rate of miscarriage in these older women is not yet known, but results suggest that it is not different from that of younger women in the general population.

"The rates of pregnancy with donated oocytes in women with ovarian failure who were 40 or older approximated that in younger women in the same program, demonstrating that receptivity to embryo implantation can be maintained if not enhanced by hormone replacement therapy in such older women. The probability of randomly achieving pregnancy in women with ovarian failure in this age group with any other existing method is extremely low. Since women in this age group with functioning ovaries are considered appropriate candidates for infertility treatment, it seems appropriate that those without ovarian function should also be allowed a chance to experience pregnancy if they desire it" [Sauer et al, 1990]. Benevolent altruism is not the palmyra palm that shades protectingly the font of immorality from which flows bioethical insults.

False motherhood received a crushing blow in Germany when the Bonn Parliament introduced severe ethical rules on genetic engineering. A law was passed banning surrogate motherhood, genetic manipulation, and the use of a dead man's semen to produce a child. This is described as one of the strictest such laws in the world.

"The law bans women from being used to carry children for childless couples and allows so-called 'test tube babies' only when the egg used comes from the woman who is to have the baby. The surrogate mother herself would not be punished, but doctors performing the in-vitro fertilization will face up to three years in jail.

"The German law bans research into human embryos or manipulation of human genes, setting jail terms of up to five years for anyone fabricating clones or hybrids of animals and people. Anyone using the semen of a dead man to impregnate a woman or creating an embryo without the donors' knowledge faces a sentence of up to three years in jail" [Reuters, 1990].

Another sensitive topic for ethical evaluation is the use of aborted fetal cells in the manufacture of rubella vaccines. Reports from England and the United States have instigated objections from anti-abortion organizations. Students have refused to participate in an English school program to vaccinate children against rubella [German measles] because the vaccine was derived from aborted babies. The same method of vaccine manufacture is pursued in the USA. This dilemma is compounded by the knowledge that vaccine alternatives exist in the United States but not in the United Kingdom. Rubella vaccine from chicken egg cultures is available. But it is less reliable and has serious allergic side-effects [Roberge, 1999].

The right-of-refusal has appropriate foundation. Using tissue from aborted babies is tainted with cannibalism. But the grievous objection is that the ingredients of the vaccine are obtained from a direct, voluntary abortion that kills an unborn baby *Ex malo bonum non sequitur* (no good can come out of evil).

Artificiality in bioscience is an interference with mother nature. Once started it will not cease as eager scientists are in the *milieu* of perpetual motion for ideas to secure a trophy niche in the museum of the great and glorious names in medicine. On the horizon in research laboratories will be seen bizarre experiments with manufactured titles that are not printed in published medical dictionaries. Some of these new titles will center on specific, unsolved diseases and bioartificial organ replacement. New sources for tissue will be under a title such as xeno and allografts. Proposals for xenotransplantation for immuno-isolation devices will be highlighted. Other subjects considered on the laboratory program are genetically modified cells, new biomaterials, and other technology oriented themes [Hunckeler et al, 1998]. With each advancement, there may be another bioethical berm to cross.

Genetic Fantasy

Socioeconomic status is a forceful motivator for the acquisition of good health, an attractive body, beautiful face, and secure longevity by any available means. Mechanisms that assist in satisfying these desires are sought after with a passion. So it has become factual that genetics is the scientific oracle of Delphi with Mount Olympus not far behind to dispense the miracles foretold and sought after with earnest eagerness.

Science fiction is fantasizing a future society in which advanced genetic technology will enable parents to select many of the characteristics of their offspring. This cafeteria-like access to the genome would allow breeding of human beings for beauty, physical, and mental superiority nearing perfection. Future generations are to be a population composed mostly of genetically engineered citizens—a superrace. "The Human Genome Project and the knowledge it brings could take us closer to this goal or move us strongly in the other direction by deeply undermining the core assumption of equality on which our society is based" [Mehlman, Botkin, 1998].

Testing For Gender

What scientists can do is not necessarily moral. All the modern medical advances collectively have not explained many human anxieties. Knowing in advance the gender of a baby before birth is an uncertainty. However the joy of knowing it at the time of delivery balances the pre-birth solicitude. The surprise of gender may not always satisfy the egotism of a parent. A healthy baby is the desire. No concern should be given as to whether it is a boy or a girl. Gender is not a congenital anomaly.

"Five good reasons support the view that prenatal diagnosis for gender choice is ethically wrong. Three are ethical reasons that apply today:

1. Gender is not a disease. Prenatal diagnosis greatly helps parents with a higher risk of genetic disease. But such tests ought to be done only for medical reasons based on real genetic risks. Gender choice does not qualify as a serious, medical reason.
2. Gender selection violates the principle of male-female equality. Imagine explaining to your "selected" child why he or she ought to be fair to the opposite sex. Feel hypocritical? It's due to violation of the equality principle.
3. Abortion for unwanted gender can not be justified. Abortion is a serious moral issue. Abortion of a normal fetus for gender alone trivializes the seriousness of abortion.

The last two reasons are to protect the future of medical genetics and to avoid any precedents for eugenics. A medical geneticist is a specialist in the relationship between heredity and disease. The importance of medical genetics grows with each new genetic discovery applied to human health. Geneticists are part of many complex ethical problems because they counsel parents and families.

"Most people believe a line should be drawn in the use of genetic knowledge. On the right side is use of genetic knowledge for real diseases that cause lifelong suffering or early death. On the wrong side is use of knowledge to make normal children taller, smarter, or thinner. To be male or female is normal, isn't it? So, this trend points to a precedent for eugenics, a danger sign[2] in medical genetics' future" [Fletcher, 1987].

"The reality of sex selection has brought out concern over the possible imbalance in the sex ratio. Polls showed a preference for a first-born male. Sociologists, demographers, bioethicists, and reporters voice concern over the 'impending' male preference now that technology can change a desired choice into reality.

"We of the modern world frequently get caught up in our own hype. Successes in electronics and computers have given us the impression that comparable results should be forthcoming in medicine. Organ transplants, artificial hearts, test-tube babies, and the like get considerable media attention. Even though the media report these as breakthroughs, the number and successes are few. To develop a system whereby the human female can conceive from a sex-preselected sperm is no small test indeed" [Ericsson, 1987].

"Human experience, going back centuries, teaches that when a new technology becomes available, it will be used. There is no reason to suppose the new knowledge that permits parents to decide the sex of their children will be any different. One way or another, those who want that ability badly enough will find doctors to help them.

"True, there are serious potential problems. In China, where families are encouraged to have only one baby, many couples whose first-

---

2. Amniocentesis is a morally indifferent undertaking. It is of great value in managing the pregnancies of women who have become sensitized to Rh positive cells. By injecting Rh negative women with Rhogam, highly concentrated Rh antibodies, when they are at risk from exposure to Rh positive cells, they can be prevented from becoming sensitized themselves.

Amniocentesis has other uses that are of great benefit to the preborn child. The most frequent indication for this helpful use of the technique occurs during the last 3 months of pregnancy when the mother is experiencing medical problems which are a threat to herself and the baby. An example is severe hypertension. The obstetrician may elect to deliver the infant several weeks before the due date to be certain the baby can survive outside the womb. To ensure that the baby can survive outside the womb the obstetrician will order an amniocentesis and have the fluid analyzed for evidence of lung maturity before accomplishing the delivery. Amniocentesis has been blackened and called many degrading names. While studies were being performed by amniocentesis, simultaneously, efforts are made in chromosome and gene research [Colliton, 1992].

born was a girl have used infanticide to get rid of the unwanted child and then tried to get a boy the next time. That, too, is a means of choosing the sex of children.

"As a result, china's present generation of children has a significant excess of boys over girls. That, China's leaders realize, guarantees serious problems as these children reach maturity. The relative scarcity of young women a decade or so from now will increase their value, while the relative surplus of boys will decrease the average value of young men. Excess numbers of males also encourages homosexuality.

"The public needs to be better informed about the likely consequences of large-scale use of medical sex determination—assuming most families using this technique will want boys. Natural sex selection, without human intervention, provides equilibrium. About 5% more boys than girls are born. But boys are weaker than girls; more males than females die in infancy and childhood, and roughly equal numbers of young men and young women come to maturity, facilitating the pairing up of the sexes to create families.

"Unfortunately, rational arguments may be inadequate to discourage excessive utilization of medical techniques to decide the sex of babies. But price also has a rôle in deciding how often a medical technique is employed. So authorities ought to make sure that sex determination is provided only by physicians who charge very high prices. And this service should not be covered by any form of health insurance, governmental or private. The combination of a better-informed public and high prices ought to be adequate to assure that while sex determination of babies is available, it will be used by few" [Schwartz, 1987].

"Has respect for human life degenerated to such a degree that some now find it acceptable to destroy an innocent unborn baby's life simply because the baby is of the wrong sex? Due to advances in technology, pregnant women are now able to determine the sex of their developing babies earlier than ever before. If they decide 'it' is not what they prefer, they can choose the ultimate form of planning parenthood by choosing to kill their unborn child. What's next? Should we kill the unborn child because she has brown eyes instead of blue, red hair instead of blond, because she's black instead of white?

"But many militant feminists argue that this practice must be allowed in order to preserve full freedom of choice. Unfortunately, it is becoming more widespread. It is the ultimate technological abuse. Such advances should be used for compassionate solutions for real problems—

not the destruction of an innocent human life simply because the parents want a little boy instead of a little girl.

"The Supreme Court's 1973 decision did not require women to even give reasons why they choose abortion. They were just given the right to abort. Almost every survey has shown that, when given a choice, a couple would prefer having a boy rather than a girl. This should say something to women who have fought so hard for 'reproductive rights.' Their right to abort is being turned against them, being used more and more to kill healthy unborn girls just because they are females.

"Tests such as amniocentesis and chorionic villus sampling are being used increasingly for sex selection. These tests, originally used to detect congenital or other medical problems in the preborn baby for purposes of treatment, are now being used to discriminate fatally against those with physical or mental handicaps. For many parents, it is not enough to have a perfectly healthy child. Now they must 'choose' even the baby's sex by this lethal method. The attitude toward human life, tragically, is becoming such that a pregnant woman who discovers her preborn baby does not measure up to her elitist standards of physical and mental perfection—or sex—now may simply dispose of the baby and try again.

"Are we willing to accept the innocent unborn child as something equivalent to store-bought goods that can be disposed of if defective? It is time to stop this lethal discrimination and change the laws to restore the protection, dignity, and respect each new human boy or girl deserves, whether born or preborn [James, 1987].

Biotechnologies Relating To Origin Of Life

Complex moral questions face those involved in health care, preventive medicine, and physiological improvement of biological functions. Some laboratory activities concocted as fantasies have become real to the extent that it makes many ethicists recoil with horror. Without emotional reaction, logical reflection favors a negative conclusion on much of what is being done in the technological interference with human life.

Medical researchers and bioscientists should be careful before initiating the first step in a laboratory project. Once the direction is established and undertaken, the destination must be given adequate attention. Continuance of the project must be considered early and the right of withdrawal must be included in any contractual obligation or grant restrictions. Having been decided the direction chosen may be impossible to change.

"The road to the separation between procreation and the act of conjugal love has been taken, the possibility of arresting the series of applications that stem from it is out of the question. It is therefore extremely difficult to prevent people from using procreation and the human being thereby 'produced' according to convenience or caprice. When we denounced this danger in 1978 the response from the secular world was that *abusus non tollit usum*. But the fact is that that first step was already an abuse and of such portent that it made all subsequent abuses possible.

"Thus experimentation was carried out on excess embryos, on the freezing and later use of surplus embryos, on the production of embryos directly intended as material for biological experiments over and above their occasional use in *in vitro* fertilization. Then there is the use of embryos for tissue transfers, for pre-implantation diagnosis for purposes of selection, then sex selection and now cloning. It was all as predictable as the water rushing over a cliff that becomes a waterfall: of course, once it has started to cascade down the cliff it does not stop half way. If one wants to stop this cascading or the advance of the biotechnology train, it is necessary to return to the source, to the initial station, and to re-establish there the 'natural' process which is the inseparable unity of love and life, of spousal union and procreation.

"Yet another consideration from a secular thinker, J. Testart who defines artificial procreation as the preferred way and the long dreamed-of means for what he calls the biocracy or biotechnocracy of man over man for the purpose of eugenics. This is what he says: 'Biomedical interference in procreation implies the greatest possible control over product quality. In all perverse naïvete it entails a eugenic concept of the world that is imposed without an official debate. It sets in motion an irreversible and insidious life-control mechanism, which will find better expression with the development of the new technologies'" [J. Testart, Le désir du gène, Paris 1993, p. 122]. The same author draws the consequences: the human species becomes multioviparous because of artificial procreation techniques, genetics become discriminatory, society becomes competitive, and persons intolerant.

"The attempts and hypotheses for obtaining a human being without any connection with sexuality, through 'twin fission', cloning, and parthenogenesis, are to be considered contrary to the moral law since they are in opposition to the dignity both of human procreation and the conjugal union.

"But there is a further consideration to be made: these more or less experimental practices introduced by artificial procreation imply another negative factor of an anthropological and ethical nature, which is perhaps the most serious of all: the denial of the fully human dignity of the human being from the first moment of fertilization" [Sgreccia, 1993].

"A further consideration concerns legislation rather the lack of it. Never as at the end of twentieth century has the law been subject to such a variety of influences, and it now seems to be giving way to those of biotechnocracy. International norms have left prenatal life without effective protection; national laws have permitted abortion and now, how will we manage to arrest the course of eugenics and biocracy or biotechnocracy? Consistency is required in law, just as it is in people. It is now time to move on from the study of bioethics to that of bio-law, but a place to stand is necessary, just as it was for Archimedes. The foothold is recognition of the full human dignity of the newly conceived child. Either the right to life and to dignity also belongs to the newly conceived, or we lose our own dignity with him and legislation itself loses humanity" [Sgreccia, 1993].

False enlightenment on mechanical intrusion in originating life fails to accept that the unplanted embryo has no eternal destiny but should be treated as a human person.

Familiar Methods

The many ways, means, and techniques relating to mechanical fertilization are not acceptable as the teaching of bioethical guardians of the medical sciences. Knowing about them reveals the reasons for this non-approval. The laboratory dehumanizes procreation. Biotechnology allows people to become parents but they are not total fathers and mothers.

Because the artificial origin of the life is from these procedures: artificial insemination, *in vitro* fertilization, gamete intra-fallopian [tube] transfer, low tubal ovum transfer, embryo banks, surrogate motherhood, postmortem insemination, and interspecies fertilization. All these systems do not respect the dignity of the human person. Eliminating the goals of marriage the child is a product, a commodity purchased. Without love that joins parents and child disputed parentage always is a threat. Artificiality in procreation questions the moral goodness of the act. "An act is good only if the end is good, the means are good, and the intention is good" [St. Thomas Aquinas, 1225-1274].

Tersely expressed the modalities of human life manufacturing are the following.

1. Artificial insemination in which sperm harvested by onanism is introduced mechanically into the uterus of the future mother. Sperm is taken from the husband, obtained from a third party, or a sperm bank.
2. *In vitro* fertilization uses ova harvested from the mother by laparoscopy. They are fertilized by sperm of the intended father. The process is completed on a petri dish. The embryos are then grown in test tubes for 14 to 17 days when one is implanted into the recipient's uterus. The others are frozen, used for experimentation, preserved in case of failure to replace the first one, or discarded. Combinations of egg and sperm are four in number indicating the husband's sperm may not always be used with the wife's ovum. Outside donors may supply ova and/or sperm. The chance for success of this procedure is 50 percent. Pro-life advocates oppose *in vitro* fertilization.
3. Embryo transfer is the implantation into the uterus of an embryo produced in the laboratory or an embryo that was conceived naturally and removed from the natural mother's uterus. This is termed artificial inovulation.
4. Gamete intra-fallopian transfer involves the extraction of an ovum/ova from the ovary, placing it near sperm cells *via* a catheter, then inserting both in the natural mother's uterus. Sperm is collected by means of a perforated condom.
5. Low tubal ovum transfer [LTOT] is a method of transferring ova from the ovary without passage through the fallopian tube. It is used to overcome blockage of the tube/tubes.
6. Embryo banks are long-term storage depots for extra embryos gathered for *in vitro* fertilization which can be implanted in the natural mother, surrogate, or a stranger.
7. Surrogate motherhood is carrying an embryo/fetus/child in the uterus of a woman to term, then giving it to a couple [or

single parent] who has contracted to pay her for the service rendered. The possible methods for initiating surrogacy are: artificial insemination of surrogate with the sperm of the husband, *in vitro* fertilization with embryo transfer using ovum of wife and sperm of husband, *in vitro* fertilization using donor ovum and husband's sperm, *in vitro* fertilization using donor ovum and donor sperm.

8. Postmortem insemination uses frozen sperm to inseminate the wife after the death of the husband or using sperm obtained after death at autopsy.
9. Interspecies fertilization is grotesque but has been done in many laboratories throughout the world. Cross species fertilization was publicized in 1979 with apes. Current biological researchers do studies on hamster eggs fertilized with human sperm. Most interspecies fertilization procedures are done by veterinarians, zoologists, and embryologists.

These artificial machinations have deleterious psychic effects that are discussed rarely in public. Psychiatrists do not breach the confidentiality of the physician-patient relationship. However mental trauma is not absent in those "parents" who have participated in one of these processes. Just as little is said or written about the psychological disturbances in women following abortion. Both situations treat children as commodities which is a disrespect for their personhoods.

This rudeness lowers human esteem facilitating devaluation of life. Viewing a person as an object that can be bartered discounts the divine participation in the life-origin process. Producing life artificially is permission to some people that life can be destroyed when it becomes useless. This false concept ignores the autonomy and the personhood of the child so conceived as there is no protection to safeguard it. Neither is there any protection given to the newborn nor any given in his/her behalf by the pseudo-parents or courts-of-law.

On the color scale of reputation bioscientists should be lily-white. This pristine image should not be altered even by the most disgruntled. Despite periodic weaknesses to stray, the fundamental ethical policy to do what is proper should not be fimbriated. The more sensible-minded bioscientists are, the less vulnerable are they to any hacking of bioethics.

A synthesis of precise bioscientific performance with monitored, custom-made, morally configured bioethics is a devotion to the profession as a quality worthy of safe-keeping. With this background well-established, when bioscientists look at their future work projects, they will know exactly which way to go. They will not waste time plotting competitive strategy. Better use of which can be applied to the delivery of solutions that bring real strength to bioscience. Healthy research atmospheres flourish in this ambiance. Good ideas originate in clear minds predisposed to unyielding, exalted bioethics. Such forcefulness of clearly thoughtout, rational wisdom, and courageous moral thinking can counteract the disruptive amoral influences in medical science and biotechnology.

Anatomical Defects After Biotechnology

With vain-glory there is denial of imperfection. It is no different with biotechnologists. The tumult of praise drowns out all negatives. Defects unpublicized detract from sincerity, accuracy, and truth in bioscience.

The news in 1997 that embryologist Ian Wilmut had cloned a sheep by reprogramming one of its somatic cells to act as the nucleus of an egg was universally startling. Many greeted the announcement with disdain, others were horrified. "But for every good-looking lamb and calf conceived in a laboratory dish, a confounding number of animals come out oversized, malformed or are not born at all" [Law, 1999].

"The problems are so persistent in artificially reproduced and genetically engineered animals that some scientists are devoting their full attention to what they call Large Offspring Syndrome.

Today, animal cloning, if not quite commonplace, no longer is spectacular. Dolly was followed by more sheep clones, cattle clones, and mice clones. But the chances of producing healthy young offspring from cloning and other reproductive techniques involving genetic manipulation are still quite low, 10 percent at best. Now scientists want to know: Why doesn't it work more often?

"Besides being big, some of the abnormal calves have other problems: cleft palates, difficulty breathing, low oxygen levels in their blood, retarded ability to stand and suckle. One calf nicknamed Goofy was born with a disproportionately small head and hooves, long body, and big joints.

"Even if researchers don't fiddle with the genes of their experimental offspring, the animals may have strange development. The calves in the UC-Davis study are merely products of in-vitro fertilization, a procedure in which sperm and eggs are combined in petri dishes to produce embryos that are then transferred into cows' wombs.

"Just because it hasn't happened in people doesn't mean it won't. The prospect of hidden health problems troubles a veterinary researcher in reproduction at the Royal Veterinary Agricultural University in Denmark. 'The main problem, to me, is the subtle differences that nobody wants to admit to" [Law, 1999].

"Britain extended a ban on human cloning and said an advisory group would be set up to assess the benefits and risks of the technology. The Government said it would have to consider whether to allow cloning research to improve treatment for serious diseases. Cloning of human embryos for reproduction or research is forbidden but a panel of experts had recommended that curbs be eased to allow research on embryos to create cloned tissue or organs or treatment for disease. The Government had been expected to follow their lead" [Reuters, NY from UK, 1999].

Incomplete disclosure on laboratory input on the origin of human life has eliminated the birth anomalies that may occur. The most common one is supernumerary fingers—especially of the thumb.[3] Biotechnology in procreation is dysfunctional and ethically unacceptable. The procedures should be opposed by medical authorities, disapproved by theologians, and condemned legally worldwide. Behind the biotechnical scene exists only an indistinct silhouette ethics that is not vulcanized by tested truth.

Not to disclose failure and complications in research adds one more ethical ruin to a profession that is fast becoming rich in odium. Scientific ventures have no boundaries. Bioethical restrictions are powerless to slow down the jaggernaut propulsion. Not even fermented skepticism and criticism can brake the speed. Now the possibility of human cloning is not startling because of the facility with which fetal cells are cloned [Wade, 1998].

If only fetal cells are the source for clones, how are they obtained? Who is to be cloned? How are human beings for cloning to be selected? Many more questions will be asked. Moral permissibility is withheld. Technical availability does not grant bioethical approval.

Modern eager research enthusiasts whose purest motive, supposedly, is dedication to an altruistic goal persists even if it means corrosion

---

3. Pyloric stenosis has been reported in boy babies.

of normal scruples. Rejecting all ethical obstacles the pursuit by any means is defended with warlike words. Their strong motivation has been reduced to a single ideology which to them is sacrosanct.

However loathsome and bizarre in the absence of a stringent conscience some of the best bioscientists do some terrible things. Keeping faith with ethical norms is admirable, unfortunately the scientific community is losing those members who are faithful to them. The ranks of these warriors are becoming thin. To fight the battle against unethical practices needs more than one lone soldier, it takes a cavalry. Only those trained in bioethics can rescue this spirit of morality from oblivion. But the cavalry does not come to the rescue unless the call for help is sounded. This is the way to bring back the moral treasure trove which is bioscience's wealth.

Chapter 24

Incomplete Research Before Human Use

What is done in haste may be repented at leisure. Insufficiency in the research process may destroy the promise of some benefit in medicine. An experimental vaccine for a retrovirus that causes diarrhea in infants and children was awaited with much hope by pediatricians because it was to be more effective than the available vaccine.

When twenty babies developed an intestinal obstruction due to intussusception after taking the oral vaccine, its use was suspended. "Further research is needed before the experimental vaccine, known as 89-12, could be marketed. Licensing, if it ever comes, would not be for at least three years because the critical third and largest stage of testing has not begun" [Altman, 1999]

"The Centers for Disease Control and Prevention called for suspending the use of Rotashield because the agency had received reports of babies who had developed a painful blockage of the bowel. Epidemiologists for the centers are investigating the link between the vaccine and the bowel obstruction. There were 32 reported intussusception cases; in 27 the bowel obstruction began three to seven days after the babies received Rotashield, officials of the centers, a Federal agency in Atlanta, said.

"The suspension is viewed as a prudent public health measure. But it has been embarrassing for the Government because Rotashield was developed at the National Institutes of Health, a Federal agency in Bethesda, Md., before it was licensed. Also, centers officials promoted the vaccine even before the F.D.A. licensed it."

"Rotashield's future could have 'dramatic' implications for the expanded tests that are needed for the 89-12 vaccine. If Rotashield is taken off the market permanently, then scientists testing rotavirus vaccines in the United States could do it much easier because we could use a placebo group, which can not be done ethically if there is a licensed vaccine and the effectiveness is more apparent with a placebo group" [Altman, 1999].

Responsible Bioscience

At the intersection of medicine and initiative bioscientists find great satisfaction without either fear of or concern for ethical distortion. For example cancer care under private auspices leads the way in a promising treatment. Called "autologous peripheral stem-cell transplant" it rivals costlier and the difficulty to find donors for bone marrow transplants [Sanders, 1999]. The main targets for therapy are Hodgkins disease, non-Hodgkins lymphoma, and acute myelogenous leukemia. By using "growth factor" medication stem-cell production is increased in the blood by extracting them from the patient concentrated, stored, and reinjected after chemotherapy. "The stem-cell harvesting and the high-dose chemo can be done on an outpatient basis" [Sanders, 1999].

To help men infected with HIV to have a safe path toward fatherhood bioscientists are trying to be helpful. The technique is called sperm washing. "A process that separates sperm from seminal fluid for artificial insemination, sperm washing has been used for two decades in the United States for male infertility . . . researchers are experimenting with it in an attempt to isolate sperm from [the virus] that carries HIV" [Frazier, 1999].

There are ethical and legal objections to this practice, which began in Europe in 1992. In the United States it is risky. Bioethicists disapprove when the sperm are obtained by onanism. Laws in Florida and California forbid transferring HIV-contaminated blood or human tissue from one person to another.

"Like most other assisted reproductive technologies, sperm washing is virtually unregulated. It is outside the authority of the federal Food and Drug Administration, which regulates drugs and medical devices but not medical procedures. The federal Centers for Disease Control and Prevention issued a warning in 1990 against using the procedure with HIV-positive men, because the CDC found that the washing did not always eliminate the virus. But the agency has no regulatory powers. There is still an element of risk for mother and child, since doctors are unable to say for sure that sperm washing completely cleanses the sperm of HIV, even when the level of the virus is undetectable" [Frazier, 1999]. Scientific acceptance of sperm purification is being held in abeyance as bioethical approval is denied.

A New York based geneticist *via* computer search of the medical literature on baldness led her to Pakistan researchers who had discovered people in a remote village with an inherited baldness disorder. This led to the identification of the first human gene ever linked to hair loss. The genetic defect causes only the rare condition found in Pakistan and not the common type of alopecia. "The newly identified gene[1] appears to play a crucial rôle in the formation of hair . . . understanding its function might help scientists devise better ways to prevent and treat various forms of baldness" [Grady, 1998]. This is laudable genetic research without any bioethical impediment.

Medieval Latin's *laboratorium* meant a workshop. A laboratory is exactly so with much frustration that rebounds in an urgency to accomplish what was constructed mentally. The plan does not always materialize into an objective reality. Therefore completion of a new biomedical task well-done gives a majestic aura to the accomplisher worthy of multilayered acclaim. Success animates the mind being repetitive with each numbered, favorable outcome.

Contrarily lack of productivity brings miserable, melancholic stasis. Defeat in bioscientific endeavors engenders an increasing dispirit, subclinical anger, and inarticulated sadness. Recuperation from the disappointment often requires a great amount of spirited encouragement, intellectual coaxing, salutary pensiveness, and occasionally nursing of an exhausted body. Only with renewed recrudescence is there a return to deep thought and rapt concentration.

Without advancement in a laboratory project, and faced with abject failure, the investigating bioscientist is easily disenchanted. When intellectually stifled productivity is pinioned. The bioscientist and the labora-

1. Discovered by Dr. Angela Christiano, Columbia-Presbyterian Medical Centre, narrowed the search for the gene to a region on chromosome 8, one of the 23 paired threadlike strips [filaments] of genetic material found in nearly all human cells.

tory staff are pilloried internally by burdening wretchedness. When difficulties appear insuperable, perseverance, and prayers open the laboratory door through which enters a burst of inspirational optimism.

Only those who have been there know the bewilderment. Mental torture brings a derisive scorn that does not exist but is felt. An unsolved scientific mystery appears with a renewed purpose to solve it. By training the bioscientist does not stray from the desire, will, and determination to find a solution. Patience rewards the initiated. Historical purview fails to record patience on the mute memorials to distinguished scientists.

Surgical Replacement Of Body Parts

Progress in technology has allowed the use of natural and manufactured materials to treat patients who in former years had to reshape their lives as they attempted to adapt to anatomical losses. Inanimate material has been used to manufacture joints which are functional. Highly technical materials like titanium alloys, powerful composite of carbon fibers pressed into a matrix of resin, and strong polyethylene are used in replacing joints. Orthopedic skill fits the artificial joints comfortably in the residual bones [Canby, 1989].

Degenerative arthritis of incapacitating severity in major joints is overcome by replacement surgery. Porous cobalt-chrome coating on the implants permits strong bonding with bone. Old cumbersome prostheses after forearm loss are gone. New ones of carbon composites use computer chips to send impulses from upper-arm muscles to new fingers [Canby, 1989].

Yearly estimates are that in the United States 150,000 hip replacements and 125,000 knee replacements are performed. These implants are approved by the Food and Drug Administration. This surgery is the least in number when compared to the thousands of surgical operations performed in rebuilding the human body from head to toes. To mention a few are demineralized bone in the mandible, dacron blood vessels, collagen nasal implants, skin grafting, dacron tendons, Jarrick heart valves, and others including organ transplantations.

Spare parts surgery has beneficial status in the victory march of bioengineering. No ethical criticism has been hurled against the manufacture of these materials. When human anatomy is used in experiments, care must be taken as to the method whereby they are obtained. Consent for removal of cornea and other anatomic structures is permissible and has no negative moral effects. There is no ethical contradiction to donation of organs after death provided that they are removed when death has been certified.

Bad publicity has occurred in this area when sales representatives participated in the surgical replacement of knees and joints. Their excuses were that they were demonstrating the proper procedure to be followed for the optimum results of their products. In New York several lawsuits took place because of this transgression. The orthopedic surgeons involved were sued for medical malpractice and the salesmen were arrested for practicing surgery without a license.[2] Both surgeons were sued for not obtaining consent from the patient as well as being charged with deception, false pretenses, and ghost surgery. Morally, all violated basic medical ethics.

Artificial and transplantation of organs are standard surgical procedures that have been a means of alleviating suffering and prolonging

---

2. When the authorized state governing body is satisfied that the person under evaluation is competent in a specified field of health endeavor, a license or certificate of registry is granted with certain restrictions. The document issued may or may not indicate that certain restricted covenants are collaterally attached to the issuance of the said license or certificate. State laws contain rules and regulations concerning the confines within which the licensee may act in rendering medical or allied services to the general public. Thus it is that from the moment physicians are granted a license to practice medicine and surgery they become tethered to the laws of the state. This right of control over medical services rendered to the general public [citizens of the state] finds a basis on the Roman law, *Jus Promovendi* [capacity residing in one person of controlling with the assent and assistance of the state, the actions of another person]. It is from this that the power of the state obtains a fettered control over medical practice. Since the concern of the state is the advancement of the general public [the citizenry] the completed sentence upon which the state bases a regulatory authority is, *Jus Promovendi Pro Bono Populi*. The translation is "The right to advance for the good of the people [the public]." Upon this statement rests the theoretical foundation for the existence of all governmental strata which derives it's power from the people for the benefit of the people. The voluntary action of the people to conform to the precepts of the laws promulgated by the state is called justice. Thus *Jus Promovendi* finds its politico-social reciprocal obligation in the formative *Lex Romana* [Roman law] (Cowell, 1948).

life. Added to those already listed are auditory prostheses, cochlear prosthesis, implants, microcomputer driven implants, and auditory nerve stimulators. Eyesight has been aided by a silicon retina—although not perfected. Worthy of mention are automated drug delivery implants for pain relief, insulin delivery, and as an asset in the treatment of chronic illnesses. Cardiac pacemakers and cardioverters have proven their value. All these contributions to health care are examples of responsible bioscience assisted by medical engineers. Research efforts of this distinction have no ethical detraction and are representative models for scientists to emulate wholeheartedly.

Chapter 25

Reuse Of Disposable Medical Equipment

Medicosurgical equipment manufactured after one-time use is not to be cleansed and used on a second patient. This is morally wrong and can be perilous legally. Cost-containment has tempted many hospital administrators to allow reuse of disposable equipment. This action ignores the manufacturer's warning against second-use, and resterilization. Labels on disposable items warn against reuse.

"Without much federal oversight against devicemakers' advice and in the absence of any industry standards, hospitals take the gadgets, apply toxic chemicals and high temperatures to clean and sterilize them, then use the instruments on other patients. The little-noticed practice covers upwards of 1 million devices each year, a small share of all disposables and an everyday result of the cost-cutting pressures of managed care. It is becoming so commonplace that a burgeoning 'reprocessing' industry has emerged to serve the hospitals that do it—despite a dearth of hard scientific evidence indicating whether it is safe.

"This has sparked a subterranean debate that few people in the medical industry are eager to air in public. Hospitals defend the practice as prudent and harmless. Devicemakers generally refuse to discuss the matter publicly, but some of them are quietly lobbying the Food & Drug Administration to take a harder line on 'reprocessors'" [Weinberg, 1999].

The most frequently encountered, highly invasive repeatedly used items are reported to be the following, according to the Association of Disposable Device Manufacturers who oppose reprocessing.

Commonly recycled disposables	Use
Electrophysiology catheters	Cardiac testing
Sequential compression devices	Improving circulation
Biopsy forceps	Removing tissue samples
Pulse oxymeter sensors	Testing blood oxygen level
Laparoscopic instruments	Minimally invasive surgery
Balloon catheters	Dilating coronary arteries
Drills, bits, blades	Orthopedic surgery
ERCP catheters	Removing gallstones

[Weinberg, 1999].

Product Liability

Recycling of one-time use equipment, after cleansing by whatever means, can damage it in an unseen way. When reused it can break, leak, infect, and cause other damage to a patient. Breakage of disposable equipment has been known to occur leaving a foreign body in the patient. This is a basis for medical negligence which in a court of law is an almost assured verdict in favor of the patient-plaintiff. Demonstration of the foreign particle by xray and its actuality after removal is the persuading evidence. This is supported by the legal doctrine, *res ipsa loquitur* [the thing speaks for itself].

Although it is not the manufacturer's fault, no witness is found easily to testify the product was reused against the advice stated on the label. Responsibility is thrown back to the maker of the instrument under the established law of product liability. The misuse of disposable equipment is unethical, legal allegations of negligence passed on to the nonculpable manufacturer is immoral.

Nonetheless the law of product liability is available for those who elect to use it. "Product liability refers to the legal liability of manufacturers and sellers to compensate buyers, users, and even bystanders, for damages or injuries suffered because of defects in goods purchased. This is a tort which makes a manufacturer liable if his product has a defective condition that makes it unreasonably dangerous to the user or consumer. [Cobbins vs. General Accident, Fire, and Life Assurance Corp., 3 Illinois App. 3d 379, 279 NE 2d 443, 446" in Black's Law Dictionary, Sixth Edition].

"Although the ultimate responsibility for injury or damage in a products liability case most frequently rests with the manufacturer, liability may also be imposed upon a retailer, occasionally upon a wholesaler, middleman, a bailor[1] or lessor,[2] and infrequently upon a party wholly outside the manufacturing and distributing process, such as a certifier. This ultimate responsibility may be imposed by an action by the plaintiff against the manufacturer directly, or by a claim for indemnification, asserted by way of a cross-claim or third party claim by the retailer or wholesaler, or others who might be held liable for the injury caused by the defective product. Under modern principles of products liability, and with the elimination of privity[3] requirements in most instances recovery is no longer limited to the purchaser of the product, or even to a user, but may extend to the non-user; the bystander who is injured or damaged by a defective product, for example" [Black's Law Dictionary, Sixth Edition].

---

1. Bailor is the party who delivers goods to another.
2. Lessor is one who grants a lease. One who rents property to another.
3. Privity is the mutual or successive relationship to the same rights of property. In its broadest sense, privity is defined as mutual or successive relationship to the same right of property, or such an identification or interest of one person with another as to represent the same legal right.

Chapter 26

Endorsement And Prescribing Drugs

An added moral tripotage concerning which physicians may be tested centers about the relationship of medical practitioners to drugs in its multifarious applications, acquisitions, or promotions. Under the aegis of the law which grants to certain educated people the legal right to prescribe and/or to dispense medications, a physician/surgeon may be caught in the web of ethical indiscretion. By prescribing indiscriminatingly restricted narcotic, sedative, analgesic, soporific, tranquilizing and/or mood elevating drugs physicians are deviating from indoctrinated, professional inherited Hippocratic responsibility.

Doctors of medicine may be motivated to devious behavior in order to please a social, political, theatrical, or journalistic patient of prominence. Either the good or detached propelling intention does not militate against the unprofessional tainted action. Under all circumstances and in all situations, be they either adverse or perverse, true professionalism must be observed and preserved. The circle of medical elegant excellence does not grow in the soil of moral turpitude but flourishes in the garden of honored, standardizing virtue.

From another viewpoint on this subject, thought must be given to the ethical conduct of those engaged in promoting the usage of certain drugs manufactured by indigenous pharmaceutical corporations. There may arise from this objective constructive criticism in the probability that a conflict of interest may arise when continuing medical education programs are sponsored by manufacturers of drugs. Corporations issue invitations to attend free seminars at annual medical meetings. Complementary dinners, receptions, samples, and souvenirs are given to physicians. Journals are handed out at meetings with generic titles but underlying information does not deny that the aim has a uniform, specific purpose of advertising and promoting a single therapeutic agent.

Whatever is done by physicians in clinical practice must be to help patients. This is the obligation they accepted when they grasped that hard-earned doctorate. New drugs, new therapies, new approaches to medicine must be evaluated carefully and physicians are not to be brainwashed by sentimental enthusiasm. To do this may cause more harm than is realized.

Too often pharmaceutical firms have relentless promotional efforts that are convincing. The motive is a financial one. Advertisements are inexorably linked to increasing income. Nothing else matters to them. Thus drug firms promote their products for unapproved use. "A ruling by a U.S. District Judge allows drug makers to give doctors copies of published medical studies that highlight the use of their drugs for diseases not approved by the Food and Drug Administration. The FDA had sought to severely restrict drug companies from doing that for fear the companies would tell doctors only the benefits of their drugs, while leaving out the risks.

"This is a major victory for drug companies. Drug companies traditionally have been limited in what they can say about their medicines, beyond the specific uses approved by the FDA. However, doctors can prescribe FDA-approved drugs for any use they deem proper. As a result, drug companies can make money from patients taking drugs for unapproved uses. A Judge ruled that the Food and Drug Modernization Act illegally restricts the free speech of drug companies. He termed government arguments defending the limits 'preposterous'" [Judge Lambeth, 1999].

These are days that bring out strong initiatives which introduce many new items into science. Especially is this noted in discussions on genetics and cancer. Among these are functional medical applications to disorders of gene expression which aim at the maximizing of genetic potential and the advancement of studies in xenobiotics [toxic chemicals in environment and food, byproducts not properly detoxified and eliminated]. Another is nutritional and cancer prevention through photochemicals. These prospects are based upon an understanding proposed that "plant-based diet confers many health advantages and how substances from plants may be effective in the prevention of specific cancers" [American Institute for Cancer Research, 1999].

Many novel strategic and experimental designs are in progress that have not been perfected, thereby lack approval. Caution is advised in their use and promotion. It is unethical to use what is unproven and wrong to prescribe for a patient with a deadly disease anything that instills in those who are ill a false hope of a magical cure from something unknown. An ancient adage to remember is

Be not the first by whom the new is tried,
Nor yet the last to set the old aside.

Moral Implications In Prescribing

Page-turning volumes have been written on legitimate use of medication, traffic in illicit habit-forming drugs, new medicine for old diseases, how the drug lords do business including the black cocaine tactic.[1] The litany of items pertinent to drugs is endless. Drug companies add to the list constantly. They have made their reputations on solid science and controlled studies in the past decades. Many bioscientist question if these standards prevail nowadays.

A world-known German drug company is selling a concoction of Ginkgo and B vitamins that purport to help support memory and increase mental concentration. There is no scientific evidence that this vitamin boost or Ginkgo improves memory in healthy people. "But science, it seems, can not be allowed to stand in the way of a hot consumer trend. The market for herbal medicines is worth $4 billion a year in U.S.A. This is the drawing-card that seduces companies historically rich in scientific accomplishments to abandon fine reputations to sell dubious

1. Columbian drug smugglers have developed a black cocaine that defies detection by drug-sniffing dogs and standard chemical tests. Known as *coca negra* it is a mixture of cocaine, iron dust, and charcoal. When the black cocaine reaches its destination, it is separated with a simple solvent like acetone or ether. Columbia, Peru, and Bolivia are the principal source countries for coca, from which cocaine is made. Mexico has built empires that smuggle tons of South American cocaine. Drug related deaths in the USA are about 14,000 annually and social, health, police, and criminal cost is more that 110 billion dollars [Seper, 1999].

remedies with full knowledge that the product is synonymous with toxicity and danger" [Forbes, 1999].

Knowingly to prescribe anything therapeutically unreliable is to attract the wrath of critics. It is the brand of being unethical to enforce pharmaceutical inaccuracies in gullible patients. Distasteful to morality is prescribing what is useless. Untested ingredients may be harmful. This is moral anathema.

Many specific examples are available that demonstrate the folly of relatively quick results which bring uncautious enthusiasm for a therapeutic drug. Especially is this true of drugs used against cancer. The drug Taxol is one that was advanced for so-called adjuvant therapy after breast removal followed by radiation. Not explained adequately was one factor that was not expressed satisfactorily concerning women patients. Those "with so-called estrogen receptor positive types of breast cancer did not show any benefit from Taxol . . . Roughly half of breast cancers are estrogen receptor positive, though the percentage is different for pre-menopausal and post-menopausal women" [Pollack, 1998]. Full knowledge of a drugs deficiencies is necessary to be an ethical physician.

Independent thinking has promoted the cause of marijuana as a potential medication. It may have medical benefits for patients with advanced forms of cancer and AIDS, but many serious health problems may result from smoking the drug. A major question to be answered is whether medicinal use is encouraging substance abuse or will it lead to taking harder addictive drugs?

"Marijuana is used to treat diseases ranging from glaucoma to multiple sclerosis, migraine, Parkinsonism, and Huntington's disease. [A White House] report found little data to show the drug was an effective treatment for those conditions. . . Marijuana's potential as medicine is seriously undermined by the fact that people smoke it, thereby increasing their chance of cancer, lung damage, and problems with pregnancies. The marijuana leaf contains more tar than tobacco, along with many other potential cancer-causing agents" [Larson, 1999]. It appears the intended medical cure equals the disease. These many critical warnings are not conducive to ethical approbation of marijuana usage. In addition there are psychological effects, such as euphoria, anxiety reduction, and drowsiness that may precipitate additional complications.

Temptation to be better in any human endeavor never changes. Vanity hungers for greatness. Its intrinsic motivation is a reptilian, rueless, ruthless rue. Succumbing to temptation leads to a maleficent response in some form no matter how it is measured quantitatively and camouflaged qualitatively.

Reference is made to performance-enhancing drugs, including the banned substance erythropoietin which increases red blood cell levels [Italian Olympic Committee, 1999]. Another performance stimulator is Viagra which recalls to memory that it is a modern drug used for an ancient purpose.

"The sad thing about the male sex drug Viagra, as Cicero and other Greek and Roman thinkers would have argued, is not that it helps people to make whoopee—ancients were not noticeable for their reluctance to make whoopee—but that it encourages dependency. If there was one thing an ancient male feared, it was dependence. The man who could not be master of himself might as well be a slave or, even worse, a woman. Not exactly a chat-show way of looking at the world.

"In his treatise De Senectute ('On Old Age', 44 BC), Cicero, the Roman politician and philosopher, argues that blind lust 'clouds a man's judgment, obstructs his capacity for reasoning and dulls his intelligence' and that one of the pleasures of old age is that, while it is not wholly deficient in sensual pleasures, it does not miss them—and so can not be said to lack them. Consequently, the weakening of temptation to indulge in them, far from supplying an excuse to inveigh against old age, is a reason for offering old age hearty congratulations. Cicero goes on to point out that, when an Athenian thinker (Epicurus) asserted that pleasure was the standard by which everything should be judged, the Roman reaction was to pray that their Greek enemies embraced this doctrine—they would be a walk-over.

"Cicero continues in the vein of the Preacher, that to every thing there is a season, and a time to every purpose under the heaven. 'Boys have their own typical pursuits, but adolescents do not hanker after them because they have their own interests. These in their turn cease to attract mature grown-ups because they too have their special interests—for which, when their time comes, the old feel no desire since they again, finally, have interests peculiar to themselves. Then, like earlier occupations, these activities fall away; and when that happens, a man has had enough of life and it is time to die.'

"In this most servile of ages, when dependence on resources impersonal to oneself has never been greater—especially those provided by government and media like television—Viagra is yet another invitation to self-enslavement. The tragic poet Sophocles, asked in advanced old age how he felt about sex, famously replied, 'I am delighted to be free from it, like a slave from a savage and tyrannical master.' No chat shows for him" [Jones, 1998].

The Chilean bishop, Most Reverend Tomas Gonzalez, explained the moral implications of Viagra. He did this after Chilean health authorities approved the distribution of the anti-impotence drug. Bishop Gonzalez is the Chilean Bishop's Conference's expert in Canon Law and Moral Theology. He explained to the public that the use of the pill has no new moral implications.

"The traditional teaching of the Church regarding sexuality within marriage applies to this drug," said Bishop Gonzalez, explaining that Viagra is "morally neutral and can be used for good or evil." "Within marriage, Viagra can provide a scientific and speedy response to the concrete problem of sexual impotence, thus becoming a morally acceptable means for the fulfillment of one of the main goals of marriage, which is procreation," the bishop said. "In this context, the use of the pill requires the other conditions that have always been needed in a healthy marriage: love, mutual respect, and communication." He added, "When Viagra is used as a tool to obtain sexual satisfaction as the only end and regardless of the conditions that makes sexual intercourse morally good, it becomes as bad as the intention of the user." The bishop said that Viagra should not awake more admiration or mystery than any other medicine that helps improve some human functions. "Nevertheless it probably does so because it is related to sexuality, an issue that our society frequently wraps in malice or mystery" [Gonzalez, 1998]. Viagra has been sold legally in Chile since September 1, 1998. Chile has become—after Argentina—the second South American country to legalize the pill.

The manufacturer of Viagra issued a special warning about its meteoric product. It was to desist from giving nitroglycerin to person's taking Viagra for impotency. "The Viagra label already has a warning that it should not be used by those taking organic nitrates like nitroglycerin, which is primarily used to treat angina—chest pain caused by clogged arteries. In a statement yesterday, the drug maker cautioned against inappropriate use.

"Viagra, which is easier to use than other impotence remedies on the market, became one of the best-selling United States drugs after its introduction [April, 1998]. Using Viagra and nitrates together can lead to large and sudden drops in blood pressure" [Bloomberg, 1998].

To administer and/or prescribe Viagra and other drugs classified as being anti-impotency without knowing the cause of it, is empirical posology unworthy of the ethical physician. Professional competency includes moral correctness which requires the physician to seek the etiology of this insufficiency. Thought must be given, therefore, to constitutional and neurological diseases that are known to cause impotency. Treating the cause for impotency may eliminate it and thereby the necessity for its treatment. Consideration is required to eliminate psychosomatic impotency which occurs more often than is realized.

These same ethical dicta are applicable to other prescribed impotency remedies. Among these are cantharides [Spanish fly] and Yohimbine. The first is a toxic preparation from crushed, dried bodies of the beetle known by its entomologic name as *cantharis vesicatoria*. It has been used as a counterirritant that produces skin blisters. As an aphrodisiac its *modus operandi* is to irritate the urethra stimulating the mucosal lining which results in engorgement. Yohimbine is a poisonous alkaloid, derived from the bark of a tree whose arboreal designation is *Corynanthe yohimbe*. Used formerly as an aphrodisiac. Its original medical value was as a local anesthetic and mydriatic [to dilate pupil of the eye]. These preparations have no place in the armamentarium of the clinical, ethical bioscientist.

Abortion opponents are opposed to the abortifacient drug RU-486. This French abortion pill has been approved by the Federal Drug Administration. Unanswered are the additional possibilities that this drug may have deleterious effects on the women who take it. A US senator "raised the prospect of legislation [against RU-486] . . . Anti-abortion activists have long sought to block [use] of RU-486, which was found effective in ending pregnancies . . . The drug has been manufactured by a French company since 1981 and is widely prescribed in Europe" [Goldreich, 1998].

With the issue of abortion constantly in view as a sanctioning of killing the innocent, to use RU-486 as an abortion adjunct is a grievous immoral offense against humanity that is grossly unethical. The ancient precedents of medicine abhor unnatural practices and historically has fought against them. Resistance to bioethical transgressions renews that precious esteem which is the bioscientific inheritance and has been strengthened by its embrace of immovable morality.

Non-medical Use Of Drugs

Although politicians speak about their good efforts in diminishing drug addiction, it is a falsity. If many of the claims made are to be admitted as true, some difficulties arise in the field of philosophical psychology with repercussions in epistemology when called into question their basic trustworthiness.

Maluse of drugs may lead to addiction very insidiously. Drugs overcome will-power to resist them. The transitory pleasure is the allure which is detrimental to the body and the mind. "The extremely difficult question of the dependability of our noetic[2] powers and their aberrations under the influence of these pharmacologically active substances seems especially to have been neglected" [Waters, 1975].

Physicians who treat drug addicts privately, those institutionalized, in half-way houses, and/or as ambulatory outpatients have very serious moral responsibilities. Many programs merely substitute one drug for another without indepth examination of the patient physically and psychologically.

Drugs distort personality in a manner that thinking is contorted as well. Acts committed under the influence often are found excusable because of a physician's testimony. Such witnesses are aware "that certain kinds of drugs, known as hallucinogens produce in the user a general effect which is to sharpen the senses to a supernormal degree of awareness" [Watts, 1962]. "[T]here is a difference in principle between sharpening perceptions with an external instrument, such as a microscope, and sharpening it with an internal instrument, such as one of these drugs" [Watts, 1971].

Attending physicians must use their professional talent to extract patients from attachment to drugs not merely to be the mediums through which the addict continues his misperceptions. Continuance of this habit diminishes the power of knowing external reality, so that extramental falsity becomes reality to the addicted. "For not only are the powers of sense, knowledge, and understanding then unreliable, but judgment, dependent as it is upon the whole noetic apparatus, is likewise defective when the mind is called into action. This uncertainty of reliability attach-

---

2. The Greek word *noesis* means of, relating to, originating in, or apprehended in the intellect.

ing predicates to a subject would be accomplished by a like uncertainty concerning reasoning since each conclusion depends upon the reliability of its premises" [Walters, 1975].

The ethical responsibility of physicians is to discourage non-medical use of drugs. If addicts are under a physician's care, he/she is obliged to combat the addiction according to modern standards. No amount of begging by the addict that the drug is needed for survival should persuade the physician to do anything unethical. The influence of drugs is a sensitive power that tampers with the internal panorama recorded by the conscience. So that, to the addict what is magnificent, is to a clearer viewer ordinary, even below par, and valueless. For much of what passes as brilliant to the addict subject, under sober circumstances the same person will recognize its mediocrity [Milbauer, 1970].

The eagerness with which many people of all social strata seek the drug experience has reached epidemic proportions. It has created an imaginative world for these users that perpetuates the abuse with loss of any personal consideration of the self-destruction being produced. "For not only does the object, stimulating the external powers, play its part in determining the experience, but through the higher internal senses other influences become operative. Imagination, associating images as thus influenced, causes the subject to view as certain and real what is perceived" [Pollard, 1965]. Chronic addiction arrives at a time when the veracity of intellectual knowledge is obtunded according to the mental performance of the drug user.

Psychophysical changes increase with great deviations can develop while a physician is treating an addict. Moral responsibility and ethical demands require that the physician recognize these symptoms and to take proper precautions against their pejorization into disordered judgment which easily leads to seeking an escape from daily living [Hans Selye, 1960]. This narrowing of the mind is a delectation of emotive powers to which normalcy is unaccustomed.

All these probabilities weigh heavily on the moral stature, integrity, and ethical consciousness of bioscientists involved with inappropriate use of drugs. When sacred morality is wounded by the poisoned darts of impious activities that injure bioethics, silence and indifference must not be the vogue. All that is needed for the triumph of evil medical practice is for good doctors to remain silent. Outrageous, unethical behavior pertinent to the non-medical use of drugs is an offensive contempt for professionalism. As a subheading under morality, bioethical imperfections break down faith in the medical sciences. When vicious infractions of ethical standards take place, doctors of medicine are splattered with mud. Contrarily, the importance of being earnest in the fulfillment of ethical codes is the benchmark of incommensurable excellence in bioscientific research, medicosurgical, and clinical practice. Furthermore it expresses the intellectual acumen of bioscientists in poiesis with their philosophy and moral theology.

Medication Errors, Side Effects, And Patient Safety

There is a moral commitment to the public that by virtue of a license to practice medicine and surgery a physician has vowed to perform certain duties and adhere to certain principles of conduct. Acceptance of the written license is a lawful act to which the state board expects the physician to abide by as a contractual relationship. Among these obligatory dicta is the prescribing of drugs with full knowledge of their proper usage, dosage, toxicity, side effects, and other necessary precautions.

Notwithstanding these *caveats* physicians do make mistakes. They are not abreast with all the pharmacologic improvements that are produced. For example, "according to a 1997 study by the Centers for Disease Control and Prevention, half of all doctors treat ulcers merely with antisecretory agents to combat stomach acid" as treatment of choice for peptic ulcers [Ross, 1999].

"Heart attack survivors should get beta-blockers to cut their blood pressure, beginning right in the hospital. This policy is based on massive studies and endorsed by national medical organizations. Yet doctors prescribe beta-blockers to only one in three patients. Heart attack patients should also start on aspirin within two days of hospitalization, yet 40% do not.

"Angiotensin converting enzyme (ACE) inhibitors, which lower blood pressure and reduce the burden on the heart, are also underprescribed. High blood pressure is undertreated. 'Only 70% of people with hypertension are detected, and that's not so much the physicians' fault,' says the director of preventive cardiology at Massachusetts General Hospital and Harvard Medical School. 'But only 55% are treated, and only 25% are treated to the proper goal, and that is the physicians' fault.'

"Doctors also often fail to push cholesterol-lowering pills. A doctor may start a patient on a low dose of an anticholesterol drug, and when the patient doesn't come back for an adjustment, that dose becomes permanent. Why don't doctors make the effort to see the patient again and adjust the dose? Probably because of a wrong assumption: that the drug won't make much of a difference.

"Juvenile diabetes patients—who require insulin injections from the day of diagnosis—should test their blood sugar at least four times a day and inject insulin at least three times to keep blood sugar as close to normal as possible and thus lessen the risk of complications like kidney failure and blindness. This therapy has long been accepted by specialists, and it received rock solid support from a huge trial published in 1993. Yet most doctors still prescribe only one or two shots a day. When a major advance in medicine occurs, it takes about ten years to change the way doctors practice," says an endocrinologist at the University of Washington. Only 40% of juvenile diabetes patients get three or more shots a day.

"Asthma patients with moderate or severe cases should inhale steroids to fight the inflammation, but most don't. The Head of the Institute for Asthma & Allergy in Washington, D.C., says that 25% to 30% of asthmatics are on steroids, half as many as should be. Last year about 5,600 people died from asthma attacks. Doctors are leery of steroids because these powerful drugs have serious side effects when used for the long-term treatment of rheumatoid arthritis and other autoimmune diseases. But in asthma treatments the drug doesn't leak much beyond the target organ, the lungs. So doctors should prescribe steroids a little more liberally.

"Morphine is underprescribed for dying patients. Trained to be careful not to let postoperative patients become addicted to narcotics, doctors are too timid in using it among people for whom addiction is hardly a worry. Half of dying patients suffer from very severe pain, according to a study by The Robert Wood Johnson Foundation.

"Infections caught in the hospital cause an estimated 77,000 deaths a year. Many are surely caused by bad hygiene, as attested to in a study by the Centers for Disease Control & Prevention finding that 14% to 59% of doctors and 24% to 45% of nurses did not wash their hands between patient visits. I suspect those numbers are even higher, states the former director of public health in New Orleans, now in private practice as an internist. In 1993 medical students staked out the toilets at a convention of infectious disease specialists. They found that only 68% of 498 doctors washed their hands. Why the lax attitude? 'Antibiotics,' is the reply. We've grown complacent. If this study had been done 50 years ago, it would have found very different behavior.

"Depression is grossly underdiagnosed, says the head of Kaiser Permanente's Care Management Institute in Oakland, Calif. A questionnaire asking whether patients have had trouble sleeping, whether they cry a lot, whether they lack energy and so forth, can tease out most cases. 'It's simple, but underused.'

"Data mix-ups caused not by individual but by collective incompetence cause most medical errors committed inside hospitals. Last year a computer consultant in Mentor, Ohio, sweated bullets by the bedside of his grandson who was hospitalized with leg pains. 'My wife and I'd be sitting there and the orthopedic team would march in and ask us what had been done today.' 'The infectious disease people would ask later what the surgeons did. If there was a paper record, nobody consulted it. We had become the conduits of information.'

"One way to avoid such snafus is by requiring doctors to enter observations and orders in a hospitalwide database, such as the wireless system that recently went live at the Montefiore Medical Center in New York City. The system forces physicians to make the entries themselves, not leave the work to nurses. The database flags possible drug interactions and reminds doctors to follow certain guidelines. Hospital recordkeeping leaves a lot to be desired. One study showed that out of hundreds of written requests by very sick people that they not be kept on life support, just 22 proved accessible to doctors.

"What are we to make of this litany of medical folly? The chief executive of the Kaiser Foundation Health Plan & Hospitals, attributes just about all of it to system failure, rather than to individual doctors who don't do their homework" [Ross, 1999].

In helping with the drug theme, physicians are susceptible without resistance to false and misleading propaganda information on drugs by the manufacturers thereof. An example in point was disclosed in the legal entanglements of the pioneer maker of oral contraceptives. The manufacturing firm did not give physicians their known knowledge on the adverse effects of the hormonal medication on animal livers. The pathologic finding was hepatomegaly due to benign growths (cysts). Without an understanding of the side-effects of drugs no physician can practice his/her profession with honor. Not to advise a patient of the possible harmful reactions of prescribed drugs is to be culpable of *medicina mala in pectore*[3] as well as being exposed to the threat of medical malpractice.

As written previously culpability falls on drug maleffects in breast cancer therapy. The brief-lived popularity of Taxol blinded prescribers to its possible toxicity. "Taxol, generically known as paclitaxel is made from the yew tree [genus Taxus]. Because it is already approved for use in advanced breast cancer and ovarian cancer, doctors used it for early-stage disease. . . Side effects included lower white blood-cell count and a numbness in the hands and feet that can make it difficult to perform tasks like buttoning a shirt" [Pollack, 1998].

Those who prescribe drugs must know the complications, allergic reaction to them, and any other effect the medication may cause. This is the ethical obligation to the patient and innate to medical responsibility. Always doing what is right ethically is how physicians define themselves.

When a new arthritis drug was introduced it was a national sensation. Surpassing the popularity of the impotency medication as the "fastest-selling new drug ever". Called Celebrex it "promises pain relief with fewer stomach problems than other drugs. Unlike Viagra, patients take it every day and it is usually covered by insurance . . . Celebrex is one of the arthritis drugs supposedly to be free from stomach irritation.

"Celebrex was the first in a class of new arthritis drugs called cox-2 inhibitors, which target an enzyme called cyclo-oxegenase-2 that causes inflammation. Unlike earlier drugs, cox-2 inhibitors don't act against a second enzyme, cyclo-oxegenase-1, which protects the stomach lining.

"Ulcers, stomach bleeding and other gastrointestinal side effects are a major problem with many painkillers, such as ibuprofen or aspirin, causing an estimated 16,500 deaths a year. While tests show that cox-2 inhibitors may cause fewer ulcers than other drugs, the Food and Drug Administration still required the same warning about side effects on Celebrex's label as the older drugs. The manufacturer is conducting further tests to confirm that Celebrex is safer" [Galewitz, 1999].

Eight months after the introduction of Celebrex federal regulators reported receiving 95 complaints of errors by physicians and pharmacists dispensing the anti-arthritis drug. "They say the health profession-

---

3. Bad medical practice in the heart: meaning undisclosed.

als are confusing it with the similar-sounding Celexa, a depression treatment, and Cerebryx, an anti-seizure drug. Pharmacists say most of the mix-ups occur because they are unable to read the doctor's handwriting on the prescription" [Galewitz, 1999]. Medical experience in prescription-writing indicates that reported errors are only a fractional of the actual number of mistakes that occur because the reporting system is voluntary and physicians/pharmacists are embarrassed to admit their errors. But ethical requirements demand care in drug handling in every way.

Here again is the occasion when excessive enthusiasm for a new medication sets aside mention to warn against side-effects. No matter how minor a drug defect may be it is not to be avoided as a warning to the consumer. To do this with knowledge aforethought is professional irresponsibility and is ethically forbidden.

Dereliction of duty accrues to any medicosurgical practitioner who deviates from the standards of health care norms that are known or should be known to all persons who treat the sick, the injured, the infirm, or the deformed. Each physician is accountable to his/her patient. Contemporaneously the medical profession as an entity is responsible to the general public *via* its institutions and the self-imposed regulatory mechanisms it may adopt independent of governmental impositions. The ethical association of medicine with patients and with society is more intricate today than in past years because of the progressively changing social ambiance into which all of us have been thrust.

Chapter 27

Refusal To Treat

Years ago a thoracic surgeon was viewed with askance when he refused to operate upon a patient with AIDS. In a past generation, twice removed from the current one, the surgeons had fear of contracting syphilis through unintentional wounds while performing surgery. Surgeons and physicians shied away from luetic patients. However they did not shun their professional responsibilities to them. Personal knowledge verifies that two New York surgeons were infected with syphilis from patients upon whom they were performing an intra-abdominal operation. An accidental scalpel wound was the entry site for the spirochete. Even with a laboratory report proving syphilis most surgeons do not hesitate to do their duty even if there is no guarantee of payment. Tradition has established well the moral imposition to treat all patients even a miserable harlot with AIDS, syphilis, and other sexually transmitted diseases.

In a well-written book on bioethics, the author does not mention AIDS as a pathosociopolitical concern and no reference to a physician/surgeon's obligation to treat such patients as an intrinsic obligatory factor of bioethics [Caplan, 1997]. Avoidance of this issue verifies that: "The primary reason bioethics seems so hard and to some simply impossible is that we have lost faith in our ability to see others as our brothers . . . who need our help much as we will someday need theirs" [Caplan, 1997].

The living testimony to the quality of medicosurgical patient care involves the doctor and the patient in the mutual process of a "shared humanity" [Cleaveland, 1998]. For physicians there is: "The duty to work for a just and moral society is no less than our obligation to learn and to practice excellent medicine" [Cleaveland, 1998]. Thus physicians contribute to this hoped-for moral society by adherence to superb bioethics that are impeccable. Physicians, thereby will occupy a sacred place in shared humanity.

Physicians have turned away from treating patients with a rare disease concerning which little is known. To eradicate the ignorance, a conference was held at the National Institutes of Health in April 1999. Temporarily the illness studied was called, Malodor Syndrome, because no name was given to this undiagnosed disease.

"This first scientific conference on one of the most unusual of 6,000 rare diseases: fish malodor syndrome is also known as trimethylaminuria. In the disorder, digestive enzymes fail to break down trimethylamine, a substance that in high concentrations makes the breath, sweat and urine smell like rotting fish or other offensive things. A description of the disease typically provokes jokes and laughter, but it doesn't take long to see that it inflicts profound harm not only on the patients but also on their families and co-workers. And the disease may include other serious symptoms that have yet to be proved, such as depression and seizures.

"In 1997, scientists identified a gene that marks the disease, proving it is a hereditary condition. However, researchers presented data showing that it also can be caused by damage to the liver from hepatitis A or other diseases.

"A London neuropsychiatrist said 0.1 percent to 1 percent of the population suffers from the disorder, depending on the country. In the United States, that would be hundreds of thousands of patients, virtually none of whom have been identified" [Goldstein, 1999]. Honorable physicians do not deny treatment to patients with arcane diseases. If they do, society will ostracize them like pariahs. As they did to lepers.

Obligation To Public Health

Within the context of bioethics is the moral obligation of physicians to be concerned with and assist in the betterment of public health. Cooperation with disease control public agencies is a personal obligation of physicians. Those diseases that cause epidemics demand assistance from individual physicians. The current health care scare concerns tuberculosis which has returned to haunt public health officials. AIDS has not disappeared, and sexually transmitted diseases have not reached a plateau.

The public health danger has increased because of multiple drug resistant organisms that thrive like they did in the pre-antibiotic era. Collectively and individually physicians must assist in, as well as contribute to bringing under control ravage, epidemic-producing diseases. And to give their expertise to eliminate multiple drug resistant illnesses.

The medical authorities realize that prompt action is necessary to contain the spread of these diseases. Physician input and research efforts are required to solve this overwhelming public-approaching disaster. This is more than a societal-political concern. It is one that touches on world health. Every health care provider has a moral urgency to help overcome impediments to normal health. As well as to encourage the implementation of practical programs against the spread of diseases. Specific to each physician is the ethical requisite to report to the proper civilian authorities all their encounters with communicable diseases.

Tort of Outrage

Since the late 1970s there have been lawsuits against physicians based on pleadings by plaintiffs predicated on the tort of outrage [Hirsh, 1978]. To establish the allegation four elements must be proved. These are:

1. The wrongdoer's conduct was intentional or reckless;
2. The conduct was outrageous and intolerable in that it offended against generally accepted standards of decency and morality;
3. There was a causal connection between the wrongdoer's action and the emotional distress resulting therefrom; and
4. The emotional distress was severe [Hirsch, 1978].

"Using the tort of 'outrage' as a basis for malpractice claims appears to be tied to two trends in the law" [Prosser, 1966]. The first is that a physician has the professional responsibility to identify any reasonably foreseeable harmful situations. The second is the expansion of liability for emotional injuries. Generally, it is no longer necessary to prove physical injuries to recover for emotional harm, as it was in the past.

"In a 1971 case, the Oregon Supreme Court ruled that a mother could recover for emotional distress caused by a physician who refused to treat her baby who had been critically injured in an auto accident. He initially refused to examine the unconscious child, saying there was nothing wrong with her. After the mother and grandmother pleaded with him, he performed a negligent evaluation and examination and in an outrageous manner refused to treat the child, who by this time had vomited a considerable amount. In addition, he subjected the child, mother, and grandmother (who were also injured) to inhuman treatment. He made them stay outside in the snow and cold rather than in the office for a significant period awaiting the arrival of the child's father" [Rockhill, 1971].

"In another case, the Washington Supreme Court ruled that a husband could sue for medical malpractice because physicians and a hospital had failed to provide medical treatment for his wife, who had terminal cancer with extensive metastases. The husband claimed extreme emotional suffering because the defendants, under outrageous circumstances and exceeding the bounds of decency, abandoned his wife and refused to treat her despite her dire condition. The court ruled that the plaintiff had a legitimate cause of action in 'outrage' for his own mental suffering while having to watch his wife die untreated" [Grimsby, 1975].

"The Court of Appeals of Tennessee in 1975 held that under the tort of outrage punitive damages could be allowed in addition to compensatory damages. The plaintiffs had sued because the hospital failed to dispose of their deceased child's body as promised. Instead, the hospital stored the premature infant's body in a jar of formaldehyde. Six weeks later when the mother asked the whereabouts of the body, a nurse handed her the jar containing the shriveled body. As a result, the parents, particularly the mother, suffered prolonged and severe emotional distress. An appellate court held the hospital was liable for outrageous conduct" [Johnson, 1975].

"In a New Jersey case, the trial court ruled that the tort of outrage was not a viable basis for a suit against a hospital. In that case, parents claimed the hospital's employees failed to telephone them when their child died. When they came to the hospital, they learned their child had died, but the body could not be found for several weeks. The presiding judge ruled that the four requirements for the tort of outrage had not been satisfied. On appeal, the higher court held that the hospital's failure to inform the parents promptly of their baby's death and its inability to locate the body for three weeks resulted in intense, prolonged, and unrelentless emotional anguish. Reversing the decision the trial court sent the case back for further proceedings based on tort of outrage" [Muniz, 1977].

Liability of physicians for negligence has expanded over the past thirty years. Consistent with this legal philosophy, the tort of outrage has been invoked and increased as another cause of action in malpractice lawsuits against health care providers. The best prophylaxis against allegations of outrageous conduct is strict adherence to stainless bioethics as the best policy for bioscientists.

The Greek word *arete* sums up the desirable entities for a complete professional life. Difficult to translate in one word, its definition is virtue and excellence appended to which are skill, prowess, courage, nobility, honor, and effective self-control. Succinctly it is honesty applied to impeccable morality which is the spinal column supporting the body of a worthwhile civilization.

Chapter 28

Respect For Patient's Autonomy

Questionable ethical conduct of physicians skyrocketed into unbridled controversy in 1975. Media madness over the care of Karen Quinlan was a holiday for journalists. When the furor over Karen subsided another media uproar was heard about eighty year-old Brother Fox. This Marist brother was in coma. The superior of the order had to petition the court on Long Island for a discontinuance of the life-sustaining apparatus. The holy brother died before a decision was reached.

Other headlines that blazoned the non-medical journals and newspapers were Baby Jane Doe with multiple birth defects, and more recently the Finn legal controversy that involved the Governor of Virginia. The bizarrity of the latter warrants reviewing it briefly.

"An attorney for Finn, who was awarded $48,000 by state lawmakers for legal expenses in her prolonged right-to-die dispute with Gov. James S. Gilmore III now says the state may owe his client 'hundreds of thousands of dollars' more because of the governor's intervention in the highly charged case. Just when Gilmore thought he had put behind him the knottiest political controversy of his tenure by authorizing the $48,000 payment to Finn, whose husband, Hugh, died in a Manassas nursing home in October, her attorney has raised the stakes. Gilmore's press secretary confirmed today that Finn's attorney has written the governor asking her for more than $100,000 to end the dispute. No money has been paid thus far.

"The saga of Hugh Finn, a Louisville broadcaster catastrophically injured in a 1995 auto accident, captured the nation's attention last summer. When Michele Finn asked doctors to withhold food and liquids from her brain-damaged husband, Gilmore, at the urging of Hugh Finn's parents and some of his siblings, went to court to keep him alive. Gilmore's eleventh-hour intervention was blocked, first by a Prince William County judge and then by the Virginia Supreme Court. Finn, 44, died in the Manassas facility Oct. 9, eight days after his feeding tube was removed" [Baker, 1999].

Too often the non-medical media is over-zealous in either being for or against an issue. Their reports become distorted thereby by exaggeration, oversimplification or misinformation. Even if the printed report is circumspect, it is highly sensationalized even on the editorial page [Angell et al, 1994]. The way "a scientific result is framed can greatly affect its impact" [Angell et al, 1994].

Past and present uncertainties bring about strange behavior in those caught in the web of dubiety. "In contrast to the general public, physicians have learned to live with uncertainty" [Linenthal, 1995]. "Medicine is a science of uncertainty and an art of probability" [Mumford, 1970]. This is not considered in an evaluation of the fascinating revelry the media, and newspapers seem to enjoy about matters medical. It may be that the differences in their viewpoints is derived from their non-medical intellectual perspective. Thus it is that confidence in physicians is not the same and/or equal to the confidence people have in the press. "For magazines, television, and newspapers have taken stories that deserve modest attention and blown them up to hyperbolic proportions" [Lewis, 1994]. Physicians must always be on the alert not to give information that can be interpreted as unethical conduct.

Medical ethics is considerate of guardianship guidelines for those who are incapable of trustworthy decisions regarding themselves. Currently, as in the past, medical therapy decisions for patients who are unable to think or render an opinion for themselves have to rely upon others to assume this burden. Thus family members or the treating physicians are the deciding source for this initiative. Recently the tendency to give court-appointed guardians authority over the medical and/or economic affairs of incompetent persons has increased. Simultaneously professional and lay interest in the enactment/reform of guardianship laws and policies has been accentuated with persistency [Jonsen, 1987] [Lynn, 1987].

Competency

A competent person in respect to making a decision as to treatment to be given to him/her has had various opined descriptions. The basic difficulty in arriving at one definition for different patients is the attitude toward therapy which vacillates according to personal values, religious belief, family burdens, financial status, and social standing. All these considerations are of moral significance to the patient as an autonomous decision-maker. The judiciary generally does not interfere with a competent patient's voluntary choice of health care.

Legal decisions as to medicosurgical treatment are made when psychological proof of incompetency is presented to a court. This is a necessary condition for justified paternalistic interference with the patient's chosen decision [Buchanan, 1989]. Competency is malleable when it relates to judgment process, misunderstanding of the end-results of treatment, and especially incapacity to care for self. These and other thoughts confuse a patient whose indecision may be misinterpreted as incompetency. "This is not to say that it is unjustified to call for closer scrutiny of serious choices than of trivial ones. But everyone needs to be clear about why this is sound. It is sound for reasons of policy, of utility, of the exercise of social judgment, rather than because these choices are intrinsically more difficult to make in a competent fashion [Freedman, 1981].

Mentally ill patients are considered incompetent until proof to the contrary is forthcoming from a certified psychiatrist. Capacity for rational thought is not adequate [Gaylin, 1975]. Patients with psychiatric illnesses have not been looked upon favorably by civil society. Even today it might be said that the moral status of the mentally ill continues to be compromised by involuntary commitment [Farr, 1999]. By law society categorizes patients either as competent or incompetent. This ensures protection for those who are sick and competent to render their own decisions. Similarly those who lack this capacity are protected from their own misjudgments. "We must constantly strive to sift through the complexities of each individual situation and maximize the patient's self-determination in the framework of protection" [Farr, 1999].

A medicolegal clarification of involuntary hospitalization is appropriate. The term civil commitment refers to the state-sanctioned, involuntary hospitalization of mentally disordered individuals who are thought to need treatment, care or incapacitation because of self-harming or antisocial tendencies. Like the criminal justice system, the civil commitment process authorizes institutionalization of an individual because of behavior deemed unacceptable to the community. Criminal law is based upon the state's authority to protect the community, and while it may seek to rehabilitate offenders, it serves other purposes such as retribution and deterrence. The grounds for civil commitment, however, are designed to focus on the needs of the individual—not society. While the criminal system may be triggered only in response to a behavior that needs punishment, civil commitment is supposed to prevent a future occurrence.

"Also, while convicted offenders may be somewhat uncertain as to when they will be released, the scope of their sentence is established by law. With civil commitment, however, most jurisdictions impose no limits on the cumulative length of time (i.e., the number of commitments) an individual may be hospitalized, although the length of each discrete stay is usually limited" [Guilford, 1996].

"Persons are said to be legally competent if they are able to make rational decisions based upon relevant facts. Competent persons assume legal rôles in society and are held responsible for their jural actions therein. . . Denial is a common psychological mechanism employed by seriously ill patients . . . the first moral question that arises is whether, as in the law, competency regarding medical decisions should be reviewed as based upon mental capacity. Ethicists [Buchanan, Brock] have suggested it should. . . This last criterion ensures that the choice made is the one likely to be adhered to throughout a course of treatment, and it also speaks to the moral significance of the patient as autonomous decision-maker" [Farr, 1999].

Autonomy is the quality of being self-governing. It includes self-determination, independence, and being the autopilot of one's own destiny. Medical autonomy is a patient's right to privacy, self-guidance, and arriving at a decision for medicosurgical treatment. Every competent person because of free-will has a moral right to autonomy. Which must be respected as an ethical obligation placed upon those health care professionals in attendance.

When a patient is unable to give reasons for choices, "rationality may be demonstrated through other measures such as how the person has lived prior to hospitalization" [Freedman, 1981]. The moral question regarding autonomy resides in the mental capacity to exercise it freely and unencumberedly. This is acknowledgment that all persons "who have the capacity to make their own treatment decisions retain the freedom to do so, and those who lack such capacity are protected from their own misjudgments" [Farr, 1999].

Bioethics On Trial

The test of bioethical strength occurs under many conditions and in multiple situations. The burden increases when medical decisions must be made for another person—especially an incompetent patient. Caring for patients under the stress of dire health needs, the physician must not relinquish or alter any standard of moral perfection no matter how powerful the persuasion to be led astray by consultants and relatives of the patient. Bioethical insights must be keen, firm, and without ambivalence. Absolute ethical probity eliminates theorizing as it accepts therapeutic limitations. Agonizing over a thought-out conclusion reached honestly is not to be a misadventure. Deconstruction of ethical models should not take place, but remain the best of their kinds even when they are in disagreement with a surrounding consensus. No abandonment of ideal ethics is to occur for the satisfaction of a large quantity of discordant opinions.

Preoccupation with the vigorous attacks on age-old standards of medical perfection have brought forth a moral struggle. The combatants are those who are strict adherents and others who interpret ethical restrictions loosely and on a one-to-one basis. Bioethics was born out of the womb of medicine. It is proper that it has the validity to answer medicosurgical questions on morality. This is its bestowal from its progenitor.

In bygone years medicine as a professional entity did not concern itself with business, economics, and money. Modern times "recognize that economics is an integral part of the calculus of medical ethics. It has been fashionable in the past to believe that medical ethics must be divorced from the vulgarity of money, but today nothing could be further from the truth. Medical ethics and medical economics are as close as two sides of the same coin. For every ethical position there is an economic consequence: for every economic constraint there is an ethical choice. Secondly, since health care is a system, in fact a system of systems, a full appreciation of its ethical underpinnings requires enlarging the traditional philosophical domain of ethics to include an understanding of concepts more familiar to students of ecology than of the humanities. For instance, an ecological approach reminds us that all parts of the system are intricately interdependent, that there is an unending competition for limited resources, that diversity is usually a virtue, and that sustainability is an imperative" [Atchley, 1999].

"The ecologist and philosopher Aldo Leopold was probably the first to articulate the ecological dimension of ethics. He wrote in 1949: "An ethic, ecologically, is a limitation on freedom of action in the struggle for existence. An ethic, philosophically, is a differentiation of social from anti-social conduct" [Leopold, 1949]. Future threats exist that economic factors can undermine the stability of bioethics.

Physician Patient Relevance

Physicians and patients are interconnected by confidence and trust that should not be disparaged by an imbalanced barrage of non-medical policy reformers. Although it has become fashionable in some quarters to argue that patients, relatives, and surrogates ought to be able to make such serious decisions on their own, they should have access to seasoned knowledge pertinent to the medical status presented. Human non-scientific knowledge is not equal to understanding the real side of a patient's illness. This is a fertile source for faulty comprehension that can certify reliability in decision-making. Therefore a physician is the medium that balances bioethical norms with autonomous freedom to decide. Generally physicians respect, fortify, and uphold society's and medicine's moral order. Even as society, medicine, and the law support patient's autonomy in selecting to live a full life, they must sustain the best of each.

Authors of books, tomes, other writings, and lecturers have not given adequate attention and regard for the opinions based on experience of physicians/surgeons who attend the patients for whom an ethical decision is needed. As an example in reference to ordinary versus extraordinary care, the attending doctor who knows the patient is familiar with the illness. Diagnosis of which with the modern methods available can identify almost all the usual diseases. If the underlying disease, injury, and/or pathophysiological state is not discoverable with defining exactitude, a tentative diagnosis is formulated.

Practicality that is sanctioned bioethically is when it is known that a patient has metastatic carcinoma, to institute heroic, extraordinary measures is foolhardy. The same may be written about other incurable diseases, brain injuries [lacerations of the cerebrum], devastating trauma to the spinal cord, and advanced degenerative neurological diseases.

Every human being must accept the inescapable fact of his/her mortality. Everyone must die. When the reality of death is accepted, the ethical obligation of those in attendance professionally must see to the comfort of the patient including freedom from pain. No moral obligation is incurred to institute extraordinary measures that may prolong life. Mature people of medicine know the prognosis of serious illnesses and injuries. They know what to do in accordance with the finest tradition of their profession. Physicians have learned through long centuries of rugged experience that "Ignorance is healed by learning: individualism is healed by loving."

Bioethics is not a theoretical creation of myths systematized into an artificial language to dictate the behavior of biological scientists. More profoundly and specifically professional moral conduct is a conscious, thought-out reflection of the binding relationship between God and those worthy to be called physicians. The truthful bioethical entity is a verification with reiteration of the responsibility owed to the author of creation. Ethical deportment in a learned profession acknowledges truth that transcends everything else in scientific pursuits. Bioscientists are not able always to confirm everything. Especially is this realized if they seek to authenticate the infinite, eternal divine reality which is beyond finite and temporal perception.

One of the greatest problems of this and past centuries has been and continues to be the continuous, systematic elimination of all references to God in the sciences, education, and the formation of our on-going culture. The great disciplines of medicine, law, education, sociology, psychology, and others are in need of recognizing God, His existence, and His laws. With this recognition will come the spiritual dimension of the human person and the relationship to God that flows from this binding union.

Without this perspective any endeavor attempting to serve the needs of people will fall short of intended objectives. Unfortunately, such shortsightedness is evident in the field of psychology today. As well as elsewhere in the intellectual society of science. The mission of all learned people is to go beyond training other candidates in science to be highly qualified in their specialties. They must introduce neophytes to the value of God in their work and to instill in them the moral obligation they have to reconcile science to divine law that adds to the treasury of all sciences individually and collectively [Cronquist, 2001].

Limitation of comprehension is an humbling, stabilizing force even in the most erudite bioscientist. Thus it is recalled that the measure of a human being's influence on the course of intellectual history is inversely proportional to the degree to which his name resounds with positive acclaim among the common people. Hence medical heritage has outlined that bioscientists labor long and intensively not for public affection, rewards, and titles but to contribute something that benefits humanity.

With full awareness of all their obligations, physicians have concluded that under certain circumstances, positive actions are sanctioned. All eyes focus on the bioethical demand to achieve a uniform conclusion pertinent to life-support for certain patients in coma, with advanced diseases, cancer, etc. Most discussions add to the confusion rather than to assuage the discord. Amelioration of the disputes has not eventuated either by conservative reasoning or destandardization. Legal redress has made physicians sometimes timid in their expressions, either in spoken or written words, on this delicate subject. No matter which side of the discussion is taken, some non-medical group is offended. The final conclusion must be reached by clinical physicians and surgeons who have learned by experience, possess proper unbiased judgement, and had practical encounters with patients who were critically ill, dying, and in coma.

With these concerns as prerequisites the following opinions are expressed on the pursuit of ordinary versus extraordinary medicosurgical therapy. These litanized dicta derived from medicosurgical experience are legally protective, medically sound, ethically proper, and neither conservative nor impetuous in origin.

1. Do not institute life-support systems if medicosurgical judgement concludes that such methods will be ineffective;
2. Once started artificial systems should not be discontinued without legal advice and consent from the patient or his/her legal guardian until law equates discontinuation with absence of the life-support apparatus;
3. Before altering/discontinuing therapy of an extraordinary category obtain a written statement from the bioethical committee of the hospital indicating that discontinuance of treat-

ment is in accord with their rules, regulations, and ethical guidelines;

4. Medical care includes feeding and maintenance of hydration until the patient is unable to digest, absorb, and assimilate food and water;
5. Gavage feeding through a jejunostomy, gastrostomy, transcutaneous gastroscopy, or indwelling gastric rubber tube to the stage of physiological ineptitude is not proper;
6. Hospital documents of unusual nature should be witnessed by the charge nurse, and hospital administrator whose signatures should be notarized;
7. Patients, who are physically able, should sign their own consents, writing in their own handwriting: "I have read the above and I understand it"; and,
8. Physicians/surgeons have a moral obligation to render basic, beneficial medical care, not to prolong the act of dying with heroic therapy.

Neither ordinary nor extraordinary care includes medical experimentation, use of untested drugs, activity contrary to nature (human experiments), or improperly arrived at decisions (genocide, group sterilization). Neither ordinary treatment nor extraordinary care includes euthanasia as being acceptable.

Medicine has been defined as an art and a science or as a group of sciences. It is a knowledgeable profession whose members are proficient in their calling and have practical experience in the artful application of their scientific learning. People of medicine are expected to do all they can ethically to treat diseases, injuries, and deformities. They are not guarantors of immortality.

Chapter 29

Advocagenic And Iatrogenic Illnesses

The social pathology of the century just passed has outstripped all of its predecessors in concocted chicanery, distortion of speech, diffusion of misinformation, and abuse of power. Into the outstanding professions of law and medicine the same sinister disgrace has entered serpentinely and sometimes by a manipulative, mental slolom.[1] These newer unethical modalities add more consequences to the myriad of those preexisting. Externally presented as innocuous, internally devastating like the Svengali[2] malice of deteriorated morality. In law this spontaneous combustion of evil is termed advocagenic, a lawyer's contribution to a client's emotionalism and behavior.

The connection of law to medicine in this situation was the side-effect of the lucrative awards in medical malpractice litigation. Attorneys' fees increase with the richer monetary verdicts. But even while many states are trying to eliminate and/or scale down certain classes of claims, many health care givers end up paying huge awards for non-economic damages, punitive damages, and other liabilities that are difficult to predict—as well as—often impossible to insure against. Many lawsuits are triggered by lawyers by their advocacies.

---

1. Slolom is ski term meaning to follow a zigzag course.
2. Refers to a person who dominates another, usually with selfish or sinister motives. Svengali was the evil hypnotist in the novel *Trilby* [1894] by George DuMaurier [1834-1896].

Advocagenic illness is a new name for an old phenomenon [Lynch et al, 1998]. It is the direct contribution of attorneys to emotional and behavioral conditions they cause to occur when their actions tend "to elicit, support, and encourage inappropriate attitudes and maladaptive behavior" [Mayers, 1994]. "There is no accepted term—much less diagnostic criteria or treatment strategies—for physicians to apply consistently when assessing the rôle of an attorney whose counsel may alter a patient's symptoms [for a gainful reason]. An accepted term—proposed [is] advocagenetic" [Lynch et al, 1998].

The term describes any situation in which a counselor-at-law performs an act similar to an iatrogenic action which is defined as "resulting from, or in the course of professional activities of a physician or surgeon; often used to imply autosuggestion resulting from a physician's discussion, examination, questions or suggestions" [Stedman's Med. Dictionary]. Iatrogenic also includes response to medical or surgical treatment, induced by the treatment itself, usually used for unfavorable responses [Stedman, 1995]. Included is injury to a patient during surgery.

Similar in mechanism to iatrogenic, advocagenic describes the association of symptoms etc. to suggestion and/or actions that are either intentional or effected unwittingly. Therefore, the decided upon definition of an advocagenic condition or illness is: "Denoting response to legal counsel or the legal system, induced or magnified by the counsel or system itself; usually used for unfavorable responses" [Lynch, 1998].

A synonym for advocagenesis is dikanicogenic disease which is morbidity fostered by lawyers because of an impending legal experience. The etymology of the word is from the Greek noun *dikanikos* for lawyer. The prime factors in dikanicogenic disease are the level of motivation and the effect of trauma on personality. Understandably, when disability involves a reward for the patient and his counsellor, the desire for improvement is curbed. The climate of our time is such that quick money is eagerly sought after without any reservation. An encouragement is the exaggerated value the patient places on either a personal injury or illness. Even after a satisfactory court settlement, no dramatic recovery from the injury or illness may eventuate. It becomes a fixation not easily dismissed by the patient. The retention of a disability or symptoms of an illness offers a great deal of ego satisfaction and fortification to a person who, under ordinary circumstances, does not get much attention from other people. "The external social response to the disability may far outweigh its financial potential" [Hirschfield et al, 1963].

Usually advocagenic influences conflict with medical opinion and treatment but not diagnosis. An unsatisfactory medicosurgical result is the causal encouraged impetus leading to litigation. An observation of note is the periodicity of symptoms whose recurrences are related to and run parallel to the prolonged legal action. "Despite ample evidence of the effects of litigation on patient's progress and outcome, there is no term previously used to describe this medicolegal connivance.

"The legal profession has few tools for understanding or dealing with the phenomenon of advocagenic illness. The law typically has focused only on areas where a client or attorney has acted in bad faith. In reference to the client, this includes malingering which is not of little significance" [Lynch, 1998]. As regards attorneys, the law may provide penalties for suborning perjured testimony, for barratry,[3] and for "conduct involving dishonesty, fraud, deceit, and/or misrepresentation" [Wisconsin Rules, 1998].

A limitation of invoking the advocagenic concept is that advocagenic illness may occur even where all involved parties are acting in good faith. "Far more important than bad actors in explaining the phenomenon, is a legal system that, like all systems, is perfectly designed to achieve exactly the results it gets" [Berwick, 1995]. "Since more severe and permanent damage leads to increased rewards, a powerful incentive is created that makes advocogenic illnesses virtually inevitable" [Lynch, 1998]. Advocagenesis is mentioned only to condemn it as unethical.

Medical Component: Iatrogenesis

Progress in all things has its impediments. Along its choppy way many produce injuries of all classifications. Medicine is no exception. Errors can be conjured up in the vivid imagination which feigns illnesses that are nonexistent and/or exaggerate symptoms that are minimum into a complex syndrome. Medical mistakes occur that are involuntary. But they are not excusable when they occur because of the causer's irresponsible wantonness.

---

3. The offense of exciting or stirring up quarrels or groundless lawsuits.

Any iatrogenic disease resulting from a deliberate medical act and/or willful intellectual disregard of the obvious is blindness to bioethical responsibility. Iatrogenesis is neither an anodyne for ineptitude nor an ointment for immorality. Both are not propitious prospectives for professional excellence. Contrarily these acts argue for culpable conduct for which physicians/surgeons are accountable in conscience and to be weighed in the scale of Themis.[4]

Iatrogenic disease is a term derived from the Greek word for physician, *iatros*. This process is invisible initially. Eventually it discloses itself by symptoms and observation. In a modern interpretation it signifies physician-induced. Occasionally medical journals contain an article on this subject. As an example, "Iatrogenic Cataract" was the title of a report of a side effect by the long-term use of a corticosteroid [Albanese, 1963]. The cataract resulted from the administration of medication by a physician. Hence the term iatrogenic disease, meaning it was physician-induced.

It is no drollery when a patient without any skilled mental conjecture misjudges a physician's performance. For example, a cardiologist examining a patient's heart with a stethoscope may listen for a longer period of time than is usual. The patient may think it is an indication that heart disease is present. This belief prevails even if the physician has uttered no word.

Much mental illness in the geriatric patient is man-made. Many of these can be avoided and prevented if their origins are recognized as being due to frustration, inadequacies, and misplacement in societal ambiance. Elderly people forced into uselessness, and loneliness soon lose self-expression which is supplanted by false illnesses in order to capture attention. This is especially noticed in geriatric patients who are institutionalized. Such facts do not defy psychological recognition.

Iatrogenic medicine has a two-fold etiology. One source is when instilled by a physician and the other when manufactured by the patient. Irrespective of the origin site, the afflicted individuals have a condition that is real to them. Physicians must identify the situation accurately to separate the psychosomatic from an organic disease. Failure to do so

---

4. Themis, goddess of justice, holds balanced scales and a sword. Her eyes are closed. She is blindfolded to demonstrate her impartiality and propinquity for equal rights under the law—moral equity.

may result in a misdiagnosis. If therapy is prescribed, it will be ineffective but may produce an avoidable complication which is iatrogenic in itself and tinged with negligence—medical malpractice. Iatrogenic illness is another area where physicians may be ensnarled in lawsuits which are avoidable.

Drug-Induced Illnesses

A rare study made by French physicians centered on the rôle of iatrogenic disease in admissions to an intensive care unit. All studied patients admitted to the multidisciplinary unit were segregated from others if they had an iatrogenic disease. Resulting from therapeutic and/or technical errors the iatrogenic complications were deemed avoidable. Included were iatrogenic diseases that resulted in response to a drug. Among the 325 patients admitted during one year, 41 [12.6%] were hospitalized because of iatrogenic disease which counted eight fatalities [Trunet et al, 1980].

"These studies indicate that the prevalence of drug reactions leading to hospitalization in medical wards was 1.8% in a retrospective study" [Auzepy, 1979]. The purpose of these studies was to determine the proportion of admissions from iatrogenic diseases, to evaluate their severity, and to estimate what portion of admissions were avoidable. Drug-induced illnesses were the major consideration. "The cause-and-effect relationship between the drug and an adverse reaction was defined strictly. This emphasized that the reaction was not explainable by the known characteristics of the patient's clinical state" [Trunet et al, 1980].

"The drug-induced illnesses were subdivided into adverse drug reactions and therapeutic errors. An adverse drug reaction was any response to a drug that was noxious, unintended, and that occurred at recommended doses" [Karch et al, 1975]. Therapeutic errors were defined as overdosage, therapeutic contraindications, therapeutic antagonism, or inappropriate route of administration. Infectious iatrogenic disease was proven by bacteriologic criteria. Mechanical iatrogenic injuries had similar requisites. Technical errors in medical or surgical acts were established by anatomic criteria [Karch et al, 1975].

In assessing an iatrogenic disease the establishment of a cause-and-effect relationship between the medical action and the reaction was needed [Jick, 1977]. Drug-induced illness was based upon criteria established by others [Karch and Lasagn, 1975]. With these as guidelines a high prevalence of iatrogenic diseases was discovered. The high degree is explained by the concentration of the patients in a hospital. This represented iatrogenic diseases acquired during hospitalization. A series of separate studies show that 53 percent of adverse reactions were determined to be unpreventable. This percentage represents the risk-benefit ration of treatment compared with the natural history of the illnesses [Weston, 1968], [Pauker et al, 1975], [Tallarida et al, 1979].

Many studies indicate a high number of iatrogenic diseases with a parallel proportion of avoidable therapeutic and technical errors. This is a situation that requires an educational effort aimed at the elimination of the correctable causes for iatrogenic diseases. This is mandatory as a bioethical *onus* to eliminate falling through the thin cerecloth that protects physicians and surgeons.

Ill-winds may blow upon the medicosurgical profession. But their sails are strong to bring them across the tempest-tossed turbulent sea. The Bioethical strength of their purpose is the secret weapon that is their great defense against all anfractious perils. An adopted apothegm for physicians that gives consolation is:

> "When Earth's last picture is painted and the tubes
> are twisted and dried,
> When the oldest colors have faded, and
> youngest critic has died,
> We shall rest, and, faith we shall need it
> lie down for an eon or two,
> Till the Master of all Good Workmen
> shall put us to work anew."[5]

---

5. First four lines of *L'envoi To The Seven Seas* published in 1892 under the title of *When Earth's Last Picture* is painted by Rudolph Kipling [1865-1936] the English author of *Fuzzy Wuzzy*, *Danny Deever*, *Mandalay*, *The Light That Failed* etc.

Chapter 30

Spoliation Of Medical Evidence

Current professional conduct is a series of events not necessarily occurring sequentially but in accordance with economic needs, sociopolitical urgencies, and other mundane factors. Consonant with persons of a given propensity, defense of their actions is expressed in universal comments and with specific reasons. Thus arises ambiguity that is conducive to a lamentable decline in traditional, historical norms. Which standards were not oblivious to the upholding merits of those virtues now considered exiguous. These old models were the source of spiritual strength which has been forsaken. Not tolerated or respected the discursive friendship with ethics is vanishing.

Intellectual paralysis threatens the entire system of ethics thanks to government appointees, elected officials, and the dominance of political correctness. Motivated by a novel, social philosophy preference is given to numerical equality over competency. The result is that the most venerable qualifications of purity that demand abstention from evil is watered down assiduously as being unsophisticated. Ethical pronouncements and brave anti-immoral rhetoric does not curdle those opinion-makers who do not teach allegiance to sublime ethics. To them bioethics is an anachronism.

Bioethics' sorry picture is riddled with misplaced diction in some scientific places. With hectoring attitudes certain bioscientists sneer at moral stability. Unwary colleagues are vulnerable to their poisonous propaganda. Despoliation of bioethics is supposititious tearing down of medicine's moral grace. With such adverse force the salutary effect of morality on professional morale disappears.

Irreverent Expert Witness In Malpractice Litigation

The haceity of physicians' personal moral integrity precludes subvention from irresponsible extraneous sources. Arising from within the human educated conscience, morality is molded by multiple societal encounters that require ethical solutions. Decision-making relies upon intellectual conclusions founded upon good or bad experiences. Honor and righteousness should prevail since it is commensurate with proper dignified deportment. Arriving at a meritorious decision is equated with directional human behavior that leads to goodness, virtue, wisdom, and spiritual sublimation. Individual propriety is a celestial distinction attributed to God himself.

Foreseeing the future, greater moral yokes will be thrust upon the medical profession. Newer ethical problems will arise inevitably with the passing of the dawn of the 21st century. The increase in population, desmological changes, other unseen social upheavals, and numerous medicolegal questions will arise for which answers must be sought. One moral question to be answered by physicians will remain unchanged, i.e., to testify or not to testify against a professional colleague?

Almost every law journal advertises the availability of physicians to be medical experts, to evaluate personal injury claims, or to provide testimony at depositions and/or trials. The crisis created by medical malpractice litigation has enticed many physicians, surgeons, and subspecialists to become repetitive medical experts or medicolegal consultants to the legal profession. No cause of action for medical negligence can be pursued successfully without the testimony of an indispensable expert medical witness. One exception to this rule is if the cause of action is founded upon the principle of *res ipsa loquitur*.[1]

From the medical expert witness' viewpoint his/her court appearance has become a financial bonanza. Thus the persuasive factor in arriving at a decision to testify against a fellow-practitioner often is the monetary gain. To be worthy of the fee paid, the medical witness for the plaintiff must testify in court that the defendant physician's acts or omissions were substantial or significant departures from the current acceptable standards of the medicosurgical practitioner at the time treatment/

1. The thing speaks for itself.

care was given or the diagnostic procedures were performed. The medical witness must support the allegation that the said departures were the proximate cause, or the initiating causative factor in a concatenation of events leading to the injuries allegedly sustained.

The value of the medical expert witness is formidable in persuading a jury to render a verdict in favor of the plaintiff-patient. Average jurors will be sympathetic to a plaintiff with a grave personal injury whose attorney presents a talented medical expert witness whose credibility is obvious. A jury of citizens evaluating a serious injury will be generous in awarding damages when liability is proven. This sentiment prevails "even if the long-term result is to make every health-care shortfall a compensable event. This approaches a legal principle of strict liability, that is, culpability for any harm regardless of intention, act, or omission" [Gibbs, 1986].

The group of physicians/surgeons who are frequent court testifiers are identifiable. With the passage of time they become recognized as plaintiffs' witnesses. Many in this category are retired private practitioners or a professor emeritus from medical academia. Those with a former professorial rank continue their self-conceived doctrine that they are the means of elevating the medical standards in the United States. By testifying in court they perpetuate this effort founded upon their emeritus status while simultaneously receiving an income for services rendered. Some writers have called these witnesses "hired guns" [Gibbs, 1986].

Other medical expert witnesses are in active practice, semiretired, or retired teachers from medical schools who have their own opinions on acceptable medical procedures. They look upon the defendant-physician as one of their students who must be taught medicine/surgery properly. "They are perceived as 'lovable radicals.' No respectable minority of their peers can give credence to their concept and yet none can disprove what they say" [Gibbs, 1986]. Potentially lethal in their effects on medicosurgical practice because of their high professional recognition some expert witnesses are authoritative to the extreme. Only the future will reveal if their influence was better or worse for the medical profession. Their statements in court do create new standards of health care founded upon their personal concepts, theories, and opinions. These dicta become recorded precedents in successful litigation against doctors, hospitals, as well as other health care providers.

Another class of medical witness is looked upon as an entrepreneur whose paper credentials are ominous. They are specialty board certified, have academic stature, or staff appointments at prestigious hospitals, plus many publications in the medical literature. With this sort of professional background they have no difficulty being accepted as medical experts supplying instant expertise for a fee. There is no scarcity of medical expert witnesses in malpractice litigation. Most are known as professional testifiers who have found a lucrative source of revenue in the legal forum where they speak against fellow physicians. If profit is their motive with a wanton disregard of the merits of each malpractice action, then they are practicing unethically.

Medical history records that this sort of thing has existed and continues to manifest itself behind hidden shadows. Disguised as benevolence it appears to be overt altruism. Immoral slings and unethical arrows of outrageous misfortune have struck a lethal blow against the pristine honor of physicians. The discipline of medicine lies mortally wounded on the battlefields of impugning governmental restrictions and specious, frivolous legal allegations. Former beachmarks of competence, compassion, and consideration have been relegated into antiquity. No longer do patients see in their physicians these three Cs.

Doctors of Medicine find themselves between the Scylla and Charybdis of what they know should be done versus following the easier pathway of expediency. When in doubt it would not be harmful for them to remember the classic prayer of St. Thomas Aquinas in the thirteenth century:

> Lord grant me the serenity to accept those things that I am unable to change, the courage to change those that I can, and the wisdom to know the difference [Stockhammer, 1965].

External socioeconomic exigencies may propel some people of medicine to stray from proper moral behavior. Distractions of this caliber lead to dilettantism. It is a fitful state of mind sometimes capable of intense energetic efforts in the wrong direction. A main feature of the dilettante is an indigenous impartiality that erupts from mental inertia. Dilettantism creates only momentary effects that are admired temporarily by observers. With an appraisal that truly evaluates dilettantes it is found that their visible efforts are incapable of turning such exertions into practicalities that are beneficial.

If moral timidity is present, a physician can be seduced by the lure of lucre. Coming days will demand endless hours of discussion to seek the solutions to the rising number of moral problems that will eventuate concerning medicosurgical propriety. When prompted by ambition, ephemeral success, financial gain or other impure motivations to stray from the path of goodness, a truism worthy of recollection is the ninth poetic stanza of a flawless, literary masterpiece.

> The boast of Heraldry, the pomp of Power,
> And all that beauty, all that wealth e'er gave,
> Await alike th'inevitable hour:
> The paths of glory lead but to the grave.[2]

In a former era morality, ethics, proper behavior, familial, and social obligations were within the assigned realm of religion. Scientists shunned these topics entirely or gave minimal attention to them as being alien to their professional vocation. The dint of ever-changing modern social complexities has made it necessary for bioscientists and medicosurgical practitioners to confront moral problems. No longer can they turn their backs on bioethical questions by ignoring them categorically. If they do, physicians/surgeons will be capitulating to other people thereby eliminating an intellectual, influential input which can assist in molding the ultimate formulary that eventually will be the adopted bioethical standards of tomorrow.

More and more theologians of all faiths are promulgating the need for advising their educational authorities to include bioethics in the seminary curriculum as well as making it a requisite course for continuing theological education, accreditation, and for advanced divinity degrees. The essential need for goodness in physicians, surgeons, and all those who render health care is the *sine qua non* for professional sanity, salvation, and success. Doctors of medicine as the guiding teachers of their subordinates, assistants, ancillary personnel, and as first among equals must be above reproach like Calpurnia, Caesar's wife.

When after sufficient mental reflection, plus the full consent of the will, a physician performs an unethical professional act, he/she can not exculpate himself/herself from the appended burden of moral responsibility. For a doctor the calmant of a troubled conscience is not the invocation of the sophisticated philosophic dictum: "*actus meus invitus factus, non est meus actus*."[3]

---

2. Elergy Written in a Country Church-Yard by Thomas Gray [1716-1771].
3. My act performed unwillingly (against my will) is not my act.

As a propaedeutical allegory, it is well to recall to fading memories that good begets good even as evil produces more evil *et sic ad infinitum*.[4] This propageable remembrance contains the bywords that guide humanity away from ethical cacothanasia. Men and women of medicine should chant in cadent unison: *Magna est veritas et praevalet*.[5]

Alteration, Loss Of Evidence

The law of evidence notes that the loss, destruction, or significant alteration of evidence is spoliation of evidence. This is not accepted universally. So that it may be done without fear of legal consequences. In some states a trend is noted in medical malpractice to acknowledge that tampering with evidence is a tort [Cal. Supreme Ct re Cedars-Sinai 1998].

In this California case it was claimed a child had a birth injury. "After the defendant [hospital] was unable to produce certain records including the fetal monitoring strips, the plaintiff filed an amended complaint adding a cause of action for intentional spoliation of evidence and demanding punitive damages. . . The defendant appealed [which was denied]" [Buckner, 1999].

The rejection by the California Supreme Court was based upon the denial of a previous court decision specifically disapproving of the Smith decision fifteen years prior to its own. "The court reasoned that although the intentional spoilation of evidence was to be condemned, that fact alone was not sufficient to justify creating tort liability" [Buckner, 1999]. "However, the court did recognize that there were adequate evidentiary, discovery, criminal, and bar sanctions in existence to deter and to punish spoliation of evidence" [Wigmore, 1940].

It is the moral obligation accepted universally that physicians must keep adequate records of their patients. When confronted with a lawsuit for medical negligence it is ethically impermissible to alter these records in any manner. It is dishonest to declare either part or all of the record is lost when it is not. The ethical misconduct persists even if the law regarding altered, lost or destroyed medical records is still in deliberation.

"A frequent type of complaint filed with State Disciplinary Boards involves medical records. The Board's regulations require that a physi-

---

4. And so unbounded (into infinity).
5. Great is truth and it will prevail.

cian maintain a medical record for each patient adequate to enable proper diagnosis and treatment. These records must be maintained for a minimum of 3-7 years, according to different states, from the date of the last patient encounter which may be only a telephone or mail contact. A physician must provide a patient, or, upon a patient's request, another physician or another specifically authorized person, with the following:

1. A summary which includes all relevant data of that portion of the patient's medical record which is in the physician's possession or a copy of the entire record or any portion of it which is in the physician's possession. It is within the physician's discretion to determine whether to make available a summary or a copy of the entire medical record.
2. A copy of any previously completed report required for third party reimbursement.

A physician may charge a reasonable fee for the expense of providing records. However, the physician can not require prior payment of bills involved as a condition for making records available. The medical record does not have to be provided if the physician, in the reasonable exercise of his or her professional judgment, believes the provision of records would adversely affect the patient's health. However, in such a case, the physician must make the material available to another responsible person designated by the patient."[6]

---

6. Based upon Board of Registration in Medicine, Commonwealth of Massachusetts Newsletter, Vol I, No 1, Pgs 1-2, April 1996. Address of Board Ten West St, 2nd Floor, Boston, Mass, 02111

Chapter 31

Medical Commercialism

With all the money-matters aimed at the medical profession, doctors are in a quagmire of uncertainty. The allure of socioeconomic stability among the learned has become a flimsy propulsion to either ignore or dissociate from ethical norms which should be proudly upheld by an educated society. During the past twenty-five years the ethical conduct of physicians, bioscientists, and health-care providers has skyrocketed into unbridled controversy.

Added to the disputes is the misevaluations in biomedical research. Experts in the field disagree on the value of individual and/or private research efforts when compared to group, government, and/or university sponsored research efforts. Which type is preferable seems unimportant when compared to the more immediate concern over business encroachment into the bioscientific laboratory. The greatest asset in research endeavors is the talent of the researchers which in the world of business can be purchased.

There is an acute temptation for bioscientists to sell the products of their natural intellectual endowments. Many are anxious to grow rich on the present and coming biotechnology, and medical genetic revolution. Medical and scientific discoveries are fortune-making opportunities to which everyone is alerted. In this gold-rush, ethical concerns are shifted aside as many values have become blurred footnotes.

It will be documented that some bioscientific experiments will soar to meteoric heights perhaps dimming the great accomplishments of the 20th century. Those mired in current medical technology may find that they are irrelevant to the future of the biosciences. With change comes ethical intransigencies that will not be solved easily.

With this progress the ever-present fear is that the practice of clinical medicine will become more competitive, less personal, and more like a modern business than an old-fashioned profession. This probability will increase the frequency of contractual relations and financial arrangements between clinical investigators and industry. Economists consider this a proper alliance that is advantageous to physicians because they "hold a monopoly on the right to expose people to potentially dangerous drugs and devices, and since the profits from approved drugs and devices can be considerable, large amounts of capital may be invested in their development" [Rodwin, 1993]. Self-restraint by bioscientists could reduce the public's objection to this arrangement in which money is considered an inappropriate inducement to participate in legitimate research-related activities.

"It has been argued that industry sponsors should exercise restraint in the way they compensate investigators. The sponsor should pay investigators for services performed in connection with a particular subject whether or not the sponsored researcher actually completes the study. Payment by service rather than by subject avoids presenting the investigator with one incentive to pressure subjects not to disenroll. This is important not only in terms of respect for subject autonomy, but also because it lessens the likelihood that subjects who could benefit from standard treatment or from no treatment at all will for this reason be urged to continue in an experimental arm and run afoul of any inherent risks it entails" [Shimm, 1993].

"An important issue that will surely receive increasing attention in the research and regulatory communities is whether investigators should disclose to subjects certain details of their funding arrangements. Ethically, consent requirements in general are more stringent in a research setting than they are in routine clinical practice; potential conflicts of interest are excellent candidates for disclosure and such potential conflicts are more than theoretical. There is evidence that outcomes of clinical trials favoring a new therapy are related to funding by a pharmaceutical company to a statistically significant degree. Of 31 trials favoring traditional therapy, only four (13%) were supported by a drug company, while of 78 trials that favored a new therapy, 33 (43%) were supported by a pharmaceutical firm" [Davidson, 1986].

"Discussion of consent to research has not usually included information about funding sources, and indeed so long as the subject's interests are not jeopardized there does not seem to be any good reason to disclose such information. Nevertheless, that there may be changing attitudes on this subject is reflected in both statutory and case law. A California statute requires that an experimental subject be informed of the source of an investigator's funding for a study. A Supreme Court decision in California's Moore case further suggests that this could be the wave of the future. In Moore, a patient's tissues were used for commercial research without his knowledge or permission. The resulting immortal cell line proved to be a lucrative product. Although the court did not conclude that the patient had the right to a portion of the profits, it did find that potential commercial gain could create a conflict of interest for the investigator that might affect his medical judgment and that must be disclosed to the patient" [Moore, 1990]. Present experience suggests that consent forms for industry-sponsored research usually disclose the funding source. Disclosure may be taken as an obligation of the investigator in the future, in which case it may be included in the consent form as part of a statement of potential conflicts of interest" [Moreno, 1996].

"It is likely that in the coming years new rules will be applied to industry-sponsored research so as to avoid conflicts of interest. It is important to appreciate that such rules do not assume that most researchers permit financial considerations to influence their judgment. Rather, the goals are to deter those few who might be influenced, even unconsciously, and to reassure the public about the integrity of the research enterprise" [Thompson, 1993].

As of these fleeting moments, present-day bioscientists stand in continuity with the old medical covenants. New ventures on the horizon can never dislodge it as a rich inheritance and highlight of medical history. From this imperishable seed will grow the foreshadowed, unbelievable, remarkable medical events of the future. Current bioscientists are the nuclei of the awaited, unborn scholars who will make great strides in the redemption from illness of all humanity. May they accomplish this without transgressing their traditional bioethical genetic transmission.

The number of physicians participating in biological research has tripled during the last decade. Every subdivision of medicine has a doctor of medicine working side-by-side with Ph.Ds as they delve into unexplored realms of the bioscientific unknown. Elective research studies are at an all-time high. Such emphasis indicates its vital importance as a supplement aid in medical progress. Research aims at allowing patients access to undisclosed therapy and novel methods of treatment previously unavailable. Researchers will introduce innovations to patient care that are life-saving and alternatives to present medications minus side-effects and allergic reactions. Selectively, investigative bioscientists are dedicated, in the majority, to compassionate usage of their inventions and discoveries.

Academia Goes Into Business

No longer money shy, universities are selling the fruits produced in their laboratories. In former years private industry reaped the harvest of lucrative research by university and college faculty members. Campus-spawned ventures have converted scientific research products into marketable goods. This was unthinkable before 1980 when the mission was to transfer research technology into benefits for the public good, rather than to make money.

The aweing presence of luminous modern medical technologies does not give bioscientists permission to abdicate moral responsibilities. Commercialism in medicine easily becomes primary when it forgets bioethics. The more exploitative intellectual property becomes the less attention is given to bioethics. There seems to be no abstemious tendency in the financial race that is tinged with profiteering and bioethical insufficiency.

Profit motives are leading some scientists astray. Professors of research and universities patent everything from genes to vaccines, and most scientists rely on grants from industry, in addition to federal support. Many researchers have a vested interest in the research contemplated or done. These interests include "owning a patent directly related to the published work; being a major stockholder or executive in a company with commercial interests tied to the research; or serving on the board of directors of such a company. Only one of the 268 articles studied included a disclosure statement. . . In 1995, the National Institutes of Health adopted regulations obliging researchers who get federal funds to reveal their financial interests in companies to their universities" [Zalewski, 1997].

"Scientists and editors now confront an even more troubling phenomenon: industry's manhandling of manuscripts during the period before publication. Scientists who receive industry funding typically agree to keep their research results confidential until any possible patents are secured. Firms naturally want to examine a researcher's data before publication and it appears they often use the opportunity to suggest, or even demand, alternative ways to frame data. Recently, four of the major authors of a study of a hypertension medication quit to protest pressure along those lines from the drug's Swiss manufacturer" [Zalewski, 1997].

"In an era of unprecedented technological development, freely shared knowledge is becoming an endangered species. American politicians and pundits still spout platitudes about how public education and public access to information are the bedrock of a democratic society. But reality belies the rhetoric. These days, hospitals are battling with investigators over the right to control new treatments, universities are hauling faculty members into court to establish who will profit from their research, and genetic engineering firms are fighting over proprietary rights to techniques and materials. And private claims to formerly public information are appearing not only in medicine and biomedical science, but also in agriculture, software development, and many other fields" [Schulman, 1999]. Ownership of knowledge is not ownership of tangible property. It must be shared for the benefit of all humanity. This is derived from its very essence. Knowledge held in secret helps no person not even the originator of the gained thought. Except perhaps to enrich the inventor or discoverer in some clandestine fashion. Privatization of knowledge becomes a hidden asset that perhaps could stem many inequities that erode what could have been a good life.

Academic Capitalism

Many high-profile universities are business partners. Others have formed their own corporations that manufacture the products made in university laboratories. Not all schools are comfortable with their business connections. The reason is faculty members fear that business considerations, not scholarship, could drive decisions about what research to encourage and influence who deserves tenure. Such actions would have bioresearch go in the wrong direction.

Several universities have avoided this disturbance by turning management decisions over to venture-capital partners. The group takes over when federal research funding is no longer available. Money is supplied after a determination is rendered that marketable products can be culled from the laboratory work in progress. "The university then has an option to buy a half interest in any spinoffs" [Dworkin, Gabor, 1988].

Despite the growing prospects for high profits, some universities shun entrepreneurship with corporations because it might produce a sideward view disfavorable to laboratory science. "Some universities are going too far" [Reimers, 1988]. At one university a planned multimillion dollars investment fund will operate to minimize potential conflict of interest. The schools rôle remains so sensitive that observers hold it up to ridicule. Professors in academia are not always adept at business as they are at home in the laboratory, and certainly not in a banker's office.

The AMA prohibits MDs from selling products at a profit. "The House of Delegates of the American Medical Association passed a provision on June 23, 1999 prohibiting doctors from selling health products to patients for a profit. The measure squeaked through by six votes and reverses the AMA's earlier stance. Selling products such as dietary supplements, vitamins, child car seats or skin creams 'present a financial conflict of interest,' according to a report by the AMA's Council on Ethical and Judicial Affairs [CEJA]. The AMA President noted that part of the purpose of the AMA's inception in 1847 was to put a stop to the 'snake oil' peddling that occurred in the 19th century. The AMA agreed, however, to permit doctors to distribute needed products free or at cost. However, critics allege such products may be otherwise unavailable. Other doctors claim product sales may make up for losses due to managed care and treatment of uninsured patients" [Nacmed, 1999].

Any commercial enterprise in medicine is in a clear and present danger for moral pollution. Medical money matters hoist with its flag of success its own destructive petard. An indepth overview with insight unfolds some new faces in business medicine and some face-lifted old ones looking new who are more business oriented than they should be as graduates of medical schools. When the idea of virtue is replaced by the concept of economic grandeur, intellectual and moral consensus is diluted.

Confluence of bioscience and industry comes at a particularly poor time for the medical profession. Many ethical implications have been made concerning the increasingly entrepreneurial nature of some physicians. "Never before have physicians seemed so intent on making money through means other than fees from patients they treat" [Relman, 1985]. Relatedly, never before have medical researchers pursued their financial interests in more diverse ways [Block, 1989].

"At the same time that physicians are being reviewed as greedy and motivated by self-interest, current methods of conducting clinical trials are being attacked on a number of fronts as unethical. Many believe that medical research currently has a not insignificant problem with out-and-out fraud in the form of altering data, omitting data, and fabricating data. Such fraud is often related to financial conflicts of interest. One concern is how conflicts of interest may shape investigators' decisions about the design and conduct of trials. An even more relevant consideration is simply unconscious bias created by conflicts of interest that may not be overcome by a researchers consciously honest motivations" [Prentice, 1999].

Certainly there are many bioscientists who defend to the utmost the right of medical researchers to gain financially from the companies whose products they are investigating and scrutinizing for imperfections, safety, and effectiveness. The concern should be with how conflicts of interest may lead investigators to make inappropriate decisions about the design and conduct of clinical trials. The issue is not primarily one of honesty but of unconscious bias which may be quite subtle and difficult to detect [Kassirer and Angell, 1993]. Many "economists conclude that one may gauge the effect of a conflict of interest by the strength and directness of the financial incentive it offers doctors" [Rodwin, 1993].

In the United States drug manufacturers try to influence physicians by offering gifts, payment for consultations, honoraria for presentations at meetings, and subsidies or hospitality for physicians attending conferences. Other pharmaceutical corporations sponsor continuing medical education, make direct payments to clinician-researchers, and personal detailing [Shimm et al, 1996].

The United Kingdom has similar tacticians in the pharmaceutical industry "whose largess has resulted in a position where the information given by doctors about medicine is not necessarily relevant, not necessarily clear and rarely complete, and where patients have their understanding artificially distorted by the intellectual atmosphere to which they are subjected. How has this come about? The position becomes clear when it is recognized that through its largesse the pharmaceutical industry determines the content and direction of the bulk of medical research and much postgraduate information and education, influences the publication and distribution of medical research data, the attitudes of the opinion formers, undermines critics, curries favor with patients/public, and finally has a special (favorable) relationship with government" [Collier, 1992].

"For many years, it has been argued by those concerned with the ethics of the medical profession that drug companies have so completely coopted clinical investigators with various forms of largesses that the reliability of the results of these investigations is questionable" [Shimm et al, 1996]. A study was reported in which 96 percent of the bioscientists who defended a controversial type of heart drug [calcium channel blockers] had financial ties to the drug's manufacturer [Stelfox et al, 1998]. Another example centered on a clinical trial to test a vitamin A-containing ointment. Optimistic reports indicated that it was efficacious for treating *keratoconjunctivitis sicca*. The researcher did not disclose that he owned stocks in the company that was to manufacture the ointment [Kuzma, 1993]. Further studies indicated the ointment was no more effective than a *placebo*. A state medical board ultimately dropped ethic charges against the researcher [King, 1992].

Senate hearings produced evidence that, in 1988, pharmaceutical manufacturers gave $165 million in gifts to physicians. Such gifts may undermine a physician's judgment and clearly give the appearance of being bribes [Wand, 1992]. That such gifts are allowed stands in stark contrast to the restrictions placed upon other fiduciaries. Unlike typical fiduciaries, who can not accept gifts that may influence their professional decisions, doctors frequently accept gifts from pharmaceutical firms and medical suppliers [Rodwin, 1993].

Because of the need for public confidence in the judgment of medical professionals and the attendant public responsibilities of the medical profession, attention must be paid to apparent and potential conflicts of interest as well as to actual conflicts of interest [Relman, 1980]. Questionable practices splotch bioethics that are easily generated by financial persuasion. The medical profession's code of ethics should prohibit explicitly medical-industrial unions that propagate deterioration of bioethics which is destructive of patient's confidence. Plus the harm done to the public's perception of the medical profession. Especially is this urgent at a time when physicians are accused, almost daily, of being greedy and when their integrity is questioned frequently. Many physicians have paid dearly for their errors. To preserve their probity they should not join forces with corporations in any enterprise that is questionable as to importuning the ethics of medicine.

Profit Motive Mission

When reliable physicians are brought into the environs of an invincible commercial empire, there is a probability that they can be jacketed in a solid, steel-like intellectual property incarceration. Business is armed with the hard-money driving force which can wear down even the ultra-ethical physician who is unprotected against the massive, financial onslaught. MDs and PhDs under the control of the pharmaceutical pachyderms find their research results are patented to prevent purloining. Most commercial institutions have a profit motive not a public service motive. Rarely do business executives display a blending of profit and genuine altruism.

An author wrote a book containing scathing words. The title is, *Prescription for Profits*. The theme centers on how the pharmaceutical industry financed an unethical union between science and the commercial world. It is a so-called insider's view of the rise of biotechnology. The commercialization of a new discipline exemplified in the establishment of technological science corporations is revealed. Included in the text is a reawakening of the alleged abuses, misuses, and misinformation at some laboratories at the National Institutes of Health [Marsa, 1997].

This author proclaims "the innocence and the financially disinterested character of biomedical research before the 1960s" [Marsa, 1997]. Then she derides the race to find the structure of DNA [deoxyribonucleic acid]. Under written attack are the selling out of academic biotechnology to industry and the funding of AIDS research. Allusions are made to the wheeling and dealing that launched the biotechnology industry, its cultivation of academic ties, and external and internal investigations at NIH [Marsa, 1997]. No mention is made of any irregularity in genomic projects, the study of genes, and their rôle in diseases.

Even without accurate documentation, what has been written is an unfavorable appraisal of the ethics in bioscientific research. It brands this sector of medicine with certain suspicions that are unbecoming a learned discipline. Ethical correction is required to eliminate any suggestion of impropriety to preserve the illuminating motto, *Scientia gratia scientiae* [Science for the sake of Science].

Business is not to be blamed entirely for the invasion into medical science. Researchers often took positive steps to recruit venture capitalists to support a project. An apparent simple endeavor such as the production of genetically engineered mice for research had a difficult beginning. "Men and mice have a lot in common—approximately the same number of genes" [Moukheiber, 1999]. This values specific mice as a great asset to the research community.

Inventors of medical devices have difficulty in securing a market for them without help from industry. Aggressive lobbying has to be resorted to at many levels sometimes for a worthwhile instrument to be used in hospitals and by physicians/surgeons [Alger, 1999]. Another example of initial difficulty for a beneficial discovery to succeed is in biotechnology. "The fruit fly which shares barely 15 percent of our genes . . . is turning a single snippet of DNA from a *Drosophila*, the geneticist's favorite fruit fly into a precious research tool" [Herrera, 1999]. From a troubled beginning this enterprise won a commitment from a well-endowed partner for up to $200 million [Herrera, 1999].

"The latest source of excitement in the biotech industry is pharmacogenomics, the study of genetic differences that affect . . . chances of getting sick or responding to a drug. Pharmacogenomics promises custom-made drugs" [Robbins-Roth, 1998]. The chief scientific officer of a large pharmaceutical firm "speaks of pharmacogenomics as the savior of the industry" [Poste, 1998]. This event is a contributing factor to "pharmaceutical stocks rise over the past five years claiming they were able to cure whatever ailed the average investor" [Leckey, 1999]. "Genomic research stock has had a good run on Wall Street. You could argue that this biotech subindustry is overpriced, but you can not deny that it is going to have an impact one way or another on 21st century medicine" [Robbins-Roth, 1998]. Who is aware of any ethical misdemeanors along the way?

"Ethical issues may prevent the gatekeepers of managed care from realizing the savings claimed for customized medicine. Patients may not want to hear that their genes make a seeming wonder drug non-cost-effective in their case. Many people may refuse to share their genetic information with a health maintenance organization's accountants. Genomic research, of course, may yet pay off in other ways than by making targeted drugs. For example, a genetic database created by Spectra Biomedical, a division of Glaxo Wellcome, found an unexpected correlation between migraine attacks, serious depression and variations in the dopamine D2 receptor (a molecule that sticks out of certain nerve cells). This receptor is a major target for drugs against psychotic disorders; now it may become a target for migraine drugs as well" [Robbins-Roth, 1998].

Medical suppliers have increased in number and are engaged in big business. Competition has corrupted some companies in the selling of bandages, syringes, and other medicosurgical equipment. To sell at a lower price used equipment is sold as new. "The pressure to cut costs is intense. We are looking to do it any way we can" [Pitta, 1999]. Hospitals and other medical outlets spend $23 billion a year just to process the purchases they make. The typical hospital buys $50 million in goods yearly from up to 2,000 suppliers, filing up to 70 purchase orders every day [Pitta, 1999]. No one knows what kick-back inducements and other unethical practices are hidden in these purchase transactions.

Nursing Home Business

Geriatric health care has become an industry in itself. It is not the same when the elderly were enrolled in a nursing home. Names have changed to assisted living, senior residence, and special cooperatives for the retired. A boost to which is medicare coverage. However the many threats to medicare leaves it open to manipulation. Hidden laws are passed which chip away at some medicare benefits which seem to twist ethical beliefs.

"A U.S. Court of Appeals has returned some patient freedoms to medical care for the elderly. Two years ago Congress, in a provision of the Balanced Budget Act known as Section 4507, in effect, prohibited doctors from treating Medicare-eligible patients outside the Medicare system. Any doctor who treated such a patient privately had to file a sworn statement with Washington that he would not treat any Medicare patients for two years. Even in Britain, the mother of socialized medicine, people are allowed to opt out of the national health care system.

"The Court of Appeals for the District of Columbia ruled in July 1999 that the elderly can indeed be treated outside of Medicare for procedures the government deems unreasonable—that is, procedures that the Medicare bureaucracy believes medically unnecessary, such as extra lab tests. The decision also permits the elderly to obtain, if they desire, nonreimbursed (by Medicare) services, such as plastic surgery, and to obtain experimental services or devices.

"For services covered by Medicare, alas, Congress' prohibition remains in place unless a patient says in writing that he does not want to fill out the myriad Medicare forms for reasons of privacy. If Medicare might not or will not pay for a service, a doctor and patient can fill out a form called the Advance Beneficiary Notice, which states that if Medicare does not reimburse the claim, the patient will pay for the service.

"Medicare's price control reimbursement regime also remains in place. The fees that Washington's Health Care Financing Administration, which oversees Medicare, has decreed providers may charge for many medical treatments that are unrealistically low, thus guaranteeing that the quality of health care for the elderly will suffer in the years to come" [Forbes, 1999]. Congress should repeal this poison pill and allow patients, if they so choose, to be treated outside of Medicare.

Placing monetary return over optimum health care may be slick business but it is bad ethics. Financial stringency pertinent to medicosurgical care automatically has bioethical considerations. Bad business ethics is like an express elevator that has no down button. Once the up-lift has started the elevator just goes higher and higher, appropriate propagable ethical standards do not permit tactical misrepresentation as a business stratagem. Ethics is not to be fissile. Always straightforward and unchangeable it has neither east nor west. The direction of its magnetic arrow is immutable, always pointed to the northern star without derogation.

Longevity increases with each passing year. The geriatric population marches on so that it is a recognized economic force with sociopolitical clout. However the inevitable day arrives when these worthy citizens need care as their physical strength declines. Then their mode of living changes. Often they must relinquish management of their own affairs and move from their long-time residence into a much different home. Ethical questions rise at this time which can be disturbing.

An analysis of many projects designated for senior care stress business as a major factor in managed care of the elderly. Conducting a business of this type lists as primary principles the debt-to-equity ratios and revenue yields divorced from the nursing/medical care of their client-patients. As business people who are executing well the task at hand and are producing positive economic results pleases the ownership. Even if this financial success is at the expense of low-salaried employees and the elderly under their surveillance.

Carping at senior citizen enterprises is necessary because too many ignore their ethical responsibility as they deflect constructive criticism dexterously. The issue should be medical/nursing care not one of financial return. It is ethically wrong not to assure the elderly that they will receive the health care services they paid for, need, and deserve. Attempting to satisfy these requisites there has come into being smaller residences for the elderly that are more home-like than most corporate— or church-run assisted living facilities. These residences for the elderly are expensive—nearly $3,500 per month. Such residence limit the number to six people which lessens the ambiance suggesting an institution. Yet with a sufficient number of people not to become forlorn [Booth, 1999].

The world of assisted living has a moral obligation to make homes away from home for the geriatric population that seeks such service. No excuse for ethical laxity in this regard is tolerable no matter the options chosen: home care, congregate housing [residential compound], assisted living, continuing care facilities or nursing home. This industry in overseeing those of advanced age should have a benevolent conscience.

Ethics Under Siege

American science has been a highly successful, disciplined enterprise in its graduate training, scholarship, the scope of its laboratory discoveries, and intellectual constructions. Over time, science has pierced through challenges to establish bioscientific paradigms. But many scientists in industry have neglected on occasions to participate satisfactorily in promulgating adequate ethical guidelines. Perhaps the urge to merge with success, riches, and fame were paramount.

Biotechnology firms can [and some do] offer surprising lucrative opportunities to succeed in a business setting. Once recognized they draw into the circle colleagues who seek similar remuneration and rewards. The flexibility of the opportunities are distributed widely and are independent of obstructing combinations of circumstances. This workplace culture has not eliminated ethical deficiencies as individual moral insufficiency continues to thrive. Unfortunately, bioscientific ingenuity has marched hand-in-hand with national, medical, pharmaceutical manufacturing corporations in the disregard for bioethics. The ethos of the separation of business from science with preservation of ennobled professional ideals have been excluded. Business movement into bioscience has matured into extensive financial empires. No economic coterie cares about past ethics as bioscientists shepherd their mental productions like sheep to be sacrificed on the altar of high finance.

Most taunts against the science-commerce union with predictions of tragic consequences are taken in stride by each component of the *entente cordiale*. No impertinence has occurred of sufficient magnitude to encourage either debate or contradiction. Defiance of ethical practices between science and industry has not been identified. Invariably, the harmony will continue unopposedly in a self-perpetuating representation of an artfully composed commercial reality. That is what counts in business.

Neither demonized nor blackened by the smoke from the fire of destructive criticism, the potential success of commercial medicine is predetermined. No reticence is discerned in the incessant monologue promotion of the scientific productions of manufacturing corporations. The outputs of science have been re-engineered to whirr the financial rate-return on the investment big business has made in bioscience. With the march onward is left behind many ethical postulates that are downgraded to jingling triviality.

Few bioethicists lambast commercial abuses of science in the professional journals, the media, and/or in proclaiming policy statements. It is inappropriate for business spokepersons to applaud the economic benefits derived from bioscience as it becomes subordinated to commercialism. No objections are forthcoming from the bioscientists who do not seem to have sufficient boldness to question the unquestioned, to think the unthinkable, and lack the spirited energy to do anything about them.

Bioscientists have become deluged with new criteria for measuring their success. Although they are the beneficiaries of this elaborate, appealing propensity, in the long perspective they may become its victims. No anodyne can make soporific the respectful conscience which effectively recalls the old-fashioned ethical codes which no longer have a viable audience. Which is not as it should be. Hence there is no visible moral tetchiness in those bioscientists enticed into business. They are oblivious to any ethical deviance in the transmission of scientific good-deeds into commercial money crops. This may be a preview of impeccable science's requiem.

Downloaded becomes the conscience that does not place importance on an upgrading ethical mind. Scientists can simulate robots who do not grow morally in any way and do not beget progeny steeped in high ethical principles. Bioscientists should not become machines racing across the landscape of technology ready to lock together materialism and science. This is no consolation for those who fear the day when moral imperatives are no longer persuasive. In high academic positions, there are scientists who believe they and their colleagues should accept this fate and forsake all ethics which are now fragile and frayed. By embracing commercialism's standards, there will be no ethical interference by a monitoring conscience. It is a shuddering thought at this happening. Because it may be an enslavement to the whims of tooled, inanimate commercialism whose only objective is to generate revenue.

Humanity is living at a period in modern history that is noted for moral stagnation, freedom of actions, non-restraint, and ethical immolation. Business advertisements are the profile makers, creators of demand, and molders of morality. Visibly they deliver incentives which they control. By their purchasing power, consumers exert strong pressure on what business offers for sale. In the shifting bioscientific marketplace the masses and corporations are in control. At the interface crossroad of the commercial world and science, the masters at demand fulfillment are not restrained by any ethical infringement. Like the doctor-made monster in Mary Shelley's *Frankenstein*, the tragic creature is not the manufactured anomaly but the scientist who made it.

Finally, when all that remains is reflection of self, who will explain what really matters? Called by any name, a good reputation is legendary. A current breed of replicants are trying to redefine what it means to be human. Among the failures to do this is the inability to distinguish the animate from the inanimate, the spiritual from the material, shadow from substance, and what is best from what may be good. Bioscientists should not become inhuman because they deal with other human beings and human creations. Each person is obliged to add his/her own hum to humanity.

Every painful dilemma is not solvable. For bioscientists their repetitious dilemma is either to adhere to old ethical rules or discard them. Does bioscience's forging with commerce require making new regulations that may change moral disaster? Nonconformity can be the progenitor of miserable risks that destroy faith and reason. "The best periods in history have been those when faith and reason were of equal weight . . . and when they eyed each other from a respectful distance . . . But such times of balance are always brief" [Karlgaard, 1999].

Eruptions in the future will include enormous ethical questions which can surpass in moral consequences those of the present that seem tremendous in science and technology. Instead of an industrial economy, bioscientists may find themselves cooperating with agriculturalists because of a formidable convergence on many complex mixtures of technology, culture, agriculture, and science. These developments will revolutionize the existing society, its economic structure, culture changes, new lifestyles, and new ways of thinking [Toffler, 1999]. With these new conversions from the past will arise new values. Resentment against previous norms may erupt to destroy moral traditions and ethical qualifications. This will be a challenge by the future reigning ideology. With a resurgence of religion and lessening of secularism moral issues will be discussed openly. New-millennium technology will foster differences on what is ethically permissible. Biotechnologies may converge with one another, but they may be in counterposition to civilized morality and monolithic, unshattered bioethical appropriateness.

Commerce's Only Code

Slatternly, leaders of industrial enterprises when questioned about unethical methods give meddled answers that are unsatisfactorily inappropriate. Unfittingly they judge their own coruscating activities. No warning has been sounded from an ethical horn against the impertinent arrogance of smug business executives. Unembarrassed, they continue to form their own codes of behavior in business. They dictate codes which often are unethical and whittle away at the common ideals.

Even non-Jeremiah stoics complain, after work-discovery efforts, that there is a continuous decline in the standards of most businesses. The fuliginous conclusion reached posits that today's corporations are caught in the dusty sweep-up of "smart" business. They regard honesty as an object for mockery, facts as inventable, and truth an irrelevance. Success at any cost is to be acquired even by misconduct without mischance. Sought after is assiduous avoidance of quarrels with ethicists. Undetected gross ethical misconduct and/or hidden ministerial negligence are not wrongdoings in the business world. This prevails even when proper safeguards are ignored that are hostile to human well-being. Executive idiologues drive businesses with financial policies that abound in zealotry not commonsense.

Ethical deficiency is pandemic. It is prevalent even among the lesser educated whom Karl Marx called the *lumpenproletariat* [underclass]: and concerning whom some British politicians speak of euphemistically as "the excluded." With this phrase, politicians palliate all offenders without accusing any social group of irresponsibility. Hence stretching situations, bumbling, floppy-fringed maneuvers are condoned as the norm. When pursued in business and the noble professions it becomes an egregious slur against them. Both are tainted when they worship the mighty dollar and accept all appended terms in the acquisition of wealth.

Abstaining from ethical patterns is protection of ill-deeds. Not requiring a choice between bad habits and moral sentiment fosters a complacent assumption which inevitably becomes a buttress against constructive and destructive criticism. Monstrously dishonest it is illustrative of the primacy of economics as an infatuation with treasury notes. The implication of this ethical descent to impotent emptiness is found in the words of scientific physics: "Nature abhors a vacuum." So too may it be said of an ethical vacuum. With this emptiness comes moral serfdom.

Sometimes the sociology of corporations includes the morals of the Mafia. Stubborn pride gives them the tenuous confidence that brazens them to stand while ethical propriety crumbles at their feet. A false epic quality is advertised in a non-existent sterile atmosphere which masks the truth of what goes on in the board rooms of corporations. Moments of elation at prosperity eliminates ethical requisites as lesser-to-no-grade factors to success. Dominance of greater income return is most influential in establishing business policy.

No article of faith has replaced this credo within the living memory of venture capitalism. In the world of finance ethicists have limited power, minimal influence, and are unemployed. Business does not choose to be confined within ethical boundaries. Like the Sistine Chapel metaphor, referring to Michelangelo's fresco of God and Man, their fingers are almost touching with a distinct, crucial space between which can never be bridged. So too business and ethics remain separated. Loyalty to the firm needs no exhortation. It will always transcend ethical objections with shameless defiance.

It is unnatural to commercialize intelligence even though under civil law it is accepted as intellectual property. Pursuit of riches has secluded more deeply bioethics as a non-integrated shadow of biological research, medical solutions, clinical practice, and scientific literary reporting. Once integrity is abandoned, the rest follows easily: like faking sincerity pleases the devil.

Sequestration of bioethics may sort of flatter the ego and bring prosperity. Without giving attention to ethics critical medicomoral problems are avoided. Announced boundaries of restricted actions are not enacted. Polemical confrontation is absent. Putative solutions to ambiguous, abstruse, recondite ethical contretemps remain *in limbo*. Bioethics becomes an imaginative study. Discarded thereby as a facile form of instrumental analysis of conscience all ethical norms and nuances remain socially unconstructed and culturally unbound. Commercialism is the ruler over bioscience and its moral matrix.

Because profit is the God of Commerce no moral impediment will alter its determined direction. It is similar to those economists who say that hurricanes boost business because of the need to rebuild homes, towns, and cities. No thought is given to the loss of human life and the physical suffering caused.

Corporations are the world's motivating economic force which are imitated by other companies of lesser skill, stature, and wealth. To all of them reputation is nothing more than a feeling. Business psyche capitalizes on advertising propaganda that is emotionally provocative. Many people resonate to simple exhortations like bargains and health benefits. Against this backdrop, bedrock business ethics fade as capitalism teaches that successful companies chase riches. Evaluation of a corporation's reputation dismisses any reference to ethical performance [Alsop, 1999].

"Reputation is much more than an abstract concept; it is a corporate asset that is a magnet to attract customers, employees, and investors. . . Reputations—good or bad—have real staying power" [Fombrun, 1999]. Other attributes that occupy attention in rating reputation are product quality, corporate leadership, and vision. Based on criteria established, the rankings are determined by each corporation's "reputation quotient", a calculation based on how the public rated twenty attributes asked in survey studies [Harris, 1999]. No question was raised as to the probity, ethics, and policies of the company under scrutiny. Quotation values of elevated ethical adroitness was not measured.

Perils of unethical deviation has no promise of legal remonstrance as long as nothing provocative leads to suspicion such as an employee on the *qui vive*[1] and someone who "blows the whistle" on an employee whose misconduct is one of cheating. Especially notorious is when the ethical misbehavior involves governmental agencies at the state or fed-

---

1. French sentinel's challenge: on the alert, vigilant, watchful. Literal translation is "who lives" in English: "who goes there."

eral levels. Known as the *Qui tam*[2] law it has been invoked frequently in the last several decades of the twentieth century. Brazenly, business places no restraints on what it does. Policing itself is a nonentity. Ethical irresponsibility is antithetical to moral values whose recognition is worthy of more than a Victorian comment. Unfortunately there is no sign of change for the better against ethical ineptitude. The pretentious, sometimes vulgar, display of commerce's dark glamour continues without slowing down because of the accompanied steady rise in profits.

Money fails to satisfy in an era of excesses marked by cultural relativism, rampant pleuralism, and adherence to the philosophy of getting rich and spending it. However it is dominant in putting ethics, morality, and religion out to pasture. Spendthrifts seem not to be using their money in ways that promote personal satisfaction [Frank, 1999]. The result is the formation of a lethargic morality event that does not even want to seek it. Preference is given to the abandonment of all things ethical whose decline mires business executives in commercial profligacy. That is why business plans are drawn up to make a corporation an equal competitor in its unstoppable drive to be on the Forbes 500 list.

Into this atmosphere of dowdy ethics bioscientists have found their way nibbling on hooked bait radiant with dollar signs. As alimentation for greed little thought is given to any violation of bioethics. Where does bioscience stand after entering the portals of commercialism? A climate of moral nihilism is too inclement to nurture bioethics. Contrarily the usual well-established designations of honesty, trust, fairness, accountability, and probity have disappeared like the mists of yesterday and the fog of today. Tempted bioscientists caught in the tangled web woven by business experts can easily make transparent fools of themselves. Ethical misconduct of whatever kind is social, civic, and moral irresponsibility.

Business and its publicity agents are deft at misspeaking, as they toy with non-binding guarantees. Value-free, when a failure occurs it is called an innocent mistake. Gauging sick people and those in need of preven-

---

2. *Qui tam* is précis for the phrase "*qui tam pro domino rege quam pro seipso.*" Translation is "he who as much for the king as for himself." Reference is to a private person as a *qui tam* relator is allowed to bring a civil action on behalf of the United States for alleged employee cheating. Explained with details in the "History and Development of *Qui tam* in Wash. Univ. Law Quarterly, Pgs 81-83, 1972. See also USC ¶3730, 1988.

tive disease medication and/or vitamins is unethical and morally reprehensible. Five pharmaceutical corporations were indicted for price-fixing which is unconscionable and is inexcusable. Business is adroit in acquiring profits. The methods employed are worth the risk for investors because the financial stakes are high. Lucrative returns ignore questionable business tactics. Ethics is not an ambiguity that serves profit. Business lives for financial increments and when necessary disregards any controlling ethical authority that can stifle it.

Science in almost all fields is becoming more and more fascinated by itself when corporations seek the fruits of their labor. With this acclaim, the darkest days of viable bioethics are before us. Monetary lures have overridden ethical fortitude decreasing it precipitously. There appears to be neither awareness nor appreciation of bioscientific accomplishments for their own sakes without reward of any kind. This was a research tradition that nourished bioscience with the preservation of robust bioethics as part of its insignia.

Now ethics is trashed to acquire social status, financial security, and gain a prize. Doubly appalling is the belief that the foundation for this downdrawing of bioethics is the quest for prosperity. No mention is made of giving back, no response is made to call to duty, no sacrifice is endured for the greater good that is made—unless paid for handsomely. Blame for this unsavory attitude is placed on the strong economy, cynicism over the usual moral standards exhibited by public officials in high places, decreased national pride, lack of patriotism, disbelief in God, and the strong materialism innate to modernity. All these seem to outweigh everything else in life. They have caused a well-founded worry that the old-fashioned behavior expected of bioscientists has been destroyed.

To some bioscientists the assumption is taken that to adhere to an ethical protocol is unduly burdensome, impractical, and contrary to the freedom of science. As part of the intellectual corps, bioscientists have enjoyed no restrictions, no statutorily defined parameters, and no established policies of restraint. Noncompliance to limitations is a tradition of long-term duration among bioscientists. No thought of inhibition was given to any act unless it was contrary to the bioethical standards all others accepted without constraint. No legal authority mandated imposed restrictions. To this day there is no surveillance over the alliance between science and commerce. Ethical concern for the results, employment relationship, and financial arrangements between bioscience and industry do not need the approval of an Ethics Committee at a university, research foundation, or institute with which the bioscientist has a primary association.

It is a dark night in the daylight when prestigious bioscientists tear down whimsically the ethical barriers that protect them from monstrous unethical falls. Such acceptance does not showcase the distinctive, aesthetic sensibility that, at one time, was the decoration of bioscience. With each moral demerit goes gravitatiously downward the intended upward mobile goodness that is not imitated but can be duplicated by a comparable action. Highly intelligent bioscientists may not survive in an ethical vacuum.

With biosciences' invasion into reproductive technology and the blindness to bioethics because of the financial return, some bioscientists are imitators of the Divine Creator. Thinking they are equal to Him, they do not adhere to His Commandments. Bioscience in all its formats has become so obsessed with its potential for fame, wealth, and commercialism, that it has acquired the false omniscience they believe is omnipotent. Self-mesmerism has overwhelmed the basic tendency for good instinct.

A land-mine confronts bioscience. Founded on its overconcern for financial gain, fame, the political aspects of medical care, and the need for influential power, bioscientists have lost their true purpose for existing. The appeal of the commercial direction does not add to their bioethical bibliography. When the judgment day arrives those participants should not whine plaintively when the verdict is rendered on their business activities.

That which is unethical can be termed anti-meritocratic against the masterful history of the biosciences. It is aimed at those given to popularizing the arguments of bioscientists in academia and elsewhere who have formed a lucrative link between bioscientific culture and economic enterprises. Most prominent among the standard-bearers of this seemingly unassailable position are those who seek to explain why this workshop attitude to research is neither unethical nor unprofessional. This appears to be an attitude upon which the academic-commercial relationship's advantage rests not only in manufacturing but in trade and finance.

Research prosperity is difficult to refuse by medicoscientists who receive the dollop of millions of dollars. Bioethically oriented conscience ought to spurn such monetary hyperactivity. However, those involved therein show no interest in doing it. A parody on an old dictum may be applicable: the business of bioscience is the science of business.[3] This is the *nouveau* research philosophy that leads to riches, but does not blend with the aristocratic grandeur of mental performances that have a touch of immortality.

Weathervanes of well-mannered, mass sentiment dislikes the energetic, business rowdiness in bioscience which follows the popular, pleasure, love of money and the excitement it brings. Medical journalism indicates, but is not sure that we are witnessing either a permanent fall or a temporary lull in the process of medicosurgical, bioscientific discovery over the last decade. Factually, discovery is down, inventions are up. Intricate cleverness has perfected inventions that produce inorganic anatomic parts literally. Discovery unproductivity is not a fable.

Dumbing-down of medical research discovery makes a public image completely at odds with what it is supposed to be. This sad situation notoriously exaggerates into a piacular outrage a negative verve that leaves dedicated colleagues aghast with humiliation. No compromise can be brokered between truly ethical bioscientists and the wall-street medical researchers engaged in laboratory production for profit.

Bioethics recognizes the dilemma and is cognizant of those who have chosen to follow the financial trail. Generous indulgence in this money-driven science tempts researchers to cut corners which stultifies the conscience into languorous morality. What is obvious and illuminating is that these commercial scientists have no zeal for humanitarianism and whose ethics are somnolent.

Sad to relate is that talented bioscientists have been taken into the fold of an auction-style medical marketplace that manufactures items that are biological merchandise. Money derived from assembly-line science can purchase prestige, influence, and power. But it does not give immortality to any name. Money is a piffle even if it manages to convey the appearance of something more than a person really is. None of these participants are so versed in ethics that they distinguish among acquiring money through human frailty, moral corruption, and honest intentions. *Mores* of the current generation is an array of ethical chaos, an immeasurable catastrophe without any visible sign of resuscitation.

---

3. Lord Lawson wrote "The business of government is not the government of business."

The functional node of ethical accountability is for the commonweal of humanity. Although there are physicians who believe it is easier to treat patients than to engage in bioscientific research, the burden of bioethics is not attenuated for either the clinician or the medical researcher. Bioethics is not easily fatigued when enthusiasm for good does not fade. Promotion of ethics leaves no question unanswered. Concerning not only what is done, but how, and why it is done. That is what counts.

Unadorned, fundamental bioethics is the quintessential liaison between the art of medicine and bioscientific research. This brings into being caring and compassionate health-care givers who are testimonials of exemplary bioscientists. As models to emulate they prevent bioethical dowdiness, making it difficult not to adapt to inflexible, concise bioethics.

There is a growing fear that with bioscience's embracing of material things, it is stepping away from what made it so great. No longer believing in the holiness of the Bible, much less its inerrancy, many self-styled scholars use mundane feelings to manipulate its narrations to suit their own ideas. Biblical deviation easily leads to unsubstantiated improvisations which may lack words of wisdom. The same may be written about bioethics when many changes are made to suit the contemporary culture. Hence a battle ensues between two warring codes: the code of decency and the code of the street [Anderson, 1999].

Reconstituted ethics on demand is ethics manufactured to suit the mood of commercial progress. It is fake on the make that does not champion the basic concepts of accountability and responsibility. It is a reflection of modern society with its own nigaab[4] that looks prosperly good on the outside but morally rotting on the inside. No one knows what is in someone else's heart. In this complex, dangerous world shouting down morals/ethics/religion by smears, insults, and name-calling is spiritual blindness. Too many forget that human beings were created good. Therefore, they are made for morality.

The perils of futurology may be dismaying to the disgruntled. But this should not dissuade anyone from thinking, concentrating, and encouraging better oral trends with high ethical goals. Energetic, positive efforts are imperative to bring hope for eventual change. Conscientious analysis is to encourage reshaping moral choices and amplify efforts to establish admirable, icon standards for bioethics. Contemporaneously

4. Nigaab is the veil on the face of Muslim women.

adverse, immoral consequences will be minimized. The apostolate for change is a good objective that should encourage trustworthiness. No misinterpretation should intimate that this wished-for hope is either a soothsayer prediction or the product of inventive insight.

Chapter 32

Bioethics And Legal Medicine

For too long attorneys-at-law and physicians have been accustomed to set one profession against the other. Physicians were prone to paint tort lawyers as invaders into the coffers of medicine's treasury. Sudden crises in bioethical necessities came through tumultuous brinkmanships nearing catastrophic clashes within the proud medical structure. The very historical culture was threatened. To assuage the grief, lawyers, judges, and the courts came to the rescue. With their own perspectives in legal fashion the bioethical storms were calmed. This gave a clearer perspective and newer significance to the physician-attorney cooperation. The frontiers that separated law from medicine were approximated.

The harmonious medicolegal relationship continues even when legal decisions are the last words in the settlement of many difficult bioethical questions. Amicable understanding did not falter when meeting of the legal and medical minds was hampered by either mental sluggishness or immobility and time was of the essence. On a practical level the law answered most bioethical queries with continual support for patients. Both doctors and lawyers learned that unethical deeds in medicosurgical care is akin to moral suicide.

Professional persons know or should know that morality inculcates into their practices the virtues of honesty, directness, and forthrightness that serve as the basis upon which ethical normal behavior is established. This is also the formula for medicolegal ethics which is the synthesis of bioethics and the canons of legal conduct formed by the American Bar Association and its constituted subsidiary state and county bar associations.

Medicine and law, each in their own inimitable fashion have a fascination. Medicine is acclaimed because the object of its study is the human body, its health, survival, and longevity. Law is captivating because it serves an essential purpose that regulates, controls, and preserves humanity's civilization. Thus personal, social, and business disputes are settled peaceably. Law is the vehicle through which conflicts are resolved. The medium of law through the courts avoid belligerent conflicts that could erupt into fatal incidents. Published case law is like the ancient *Gesta Romanorum*[1] which were serious, amusing, valuable, and non-historical literature.

Combination of law and medicine compose a formidable partnership. Both are involved in human destinies. Hence a linkage between the two was inevitable. Although sometimes loosely united and softly cooperative with a different goal in their sights, serious conflicts are solved. Massive commerce, health care, and biotechnology have pushed them closer due to their expansions which had to include the ethical credos from both disciplines. Disappointingly in the race to win and to be conspicuous in the modern scenario sometimes each profession ignores their own printed ethical laws and behavior codes.

Why have these educated professions spurned their own prescribed ethical code? By their own omissions and commissions each has given a hearse to ethical verse. When they do, sinfulness is downgraded to a schoolboy vice ending centuries of moral scaremongering. Without firm medicolegal ethical by-laws, entire nations can sink into moral indifference as apathy can lead to a total oblation of ethical safeguards. Suspicion persists that some lawyers and many doctors are reticent to join the anti-ethics cadre because they fear the loss of academic standing/tenure at religion run universities. The insouciance toward morality and its

---

1. *Gesta Romanorum* are the most curious and interesting of all collections of popular tales [by Aulus Gellius 2 AD]. Negatively, one thing they are not, that is, they are not *Deeds of the Romans*, the acts of the heirs of the Caesars. All such allusions are the purest fantasy. . . The entire background is, in truth, as unhistorical and imaginary as each tale itself. In the centuries before manuscript-writing filled up the long leisure hours of the monks, the *Gesta*, both in the Orient and Occidental World were brought forth. . . [T]hey are the form in which the men of ideas of those rude times approached and entertained, by accounts of human joy and woe of their brother men of action [Library of the World's Best Literature, Vol 16, Page 6261].

offspring ethics continues to grow. This is noted when moral and ethical statements are platitudes expressing an emotion. These are pseudonyms, non-verifiable sentences, hypothetical anecdotes that are as unwarranted as they are fruitless. Then the doctor-lawyer relationship becomes no more than theoretical propinquity.

Lawyers do not invade the cultural essence of physicians. The same is not to be said of business people. A great divide exists between medicine and industry which is tried to be bridged by commercial corporations and the pharmaceutical industry more particularly. Not always subtle the machinations are an ethical embarrassment by the frank and obvious pushing methods used to persuade and influence physicians according to predesigned plans, maneuvers, and strategies.

This is encouraged by the social mixture openly displayed at medical meetings where corporations sponsor parties, events, river excursions, and outings which are neither faintly nor immediately related to bioscience. No one feigns that these social amenities are even remotely contiguous to the advancement of science as they are so easily identified as product promotional. These inducements do not impinge upon anyone's conscience even those who suspect a deviation from ethical propriety. These social programs have made some physicians children of financial success, fools of fame, and unable to confront stern critics. This is an added imperfection in the crumbling moral pedestal that has kept aloft the marks of medicine's distinction as easily recognized as the caduceus, its inherited biblical, Mosaic logo.

Case Studies On Medical Ethics And The Law

Associated with medicosurgical practice is the constrictions placed upon it by insurance contracts purchased by patients. This situation raises ethical concerns that affect relations between physicians and their patients. Also implicated are legal issues involving potential informed consent and antitrust liability. "Gag clauses impede the flow of information from provider to patient thereby undermining the trust the law deems critical to therapeutic relationships . . . When an insurer restrains doctors from imparting certain kinds of information to those under their care, patients can suspect that their doctors really might not have their best interests at heart when recommending treatment" [Miller, 1996].

"The landmark case of Moore v. Board of Regents of California held squarely that a physician's financial conflicts of interest involving recommended clinical procedures are material to a patient's decision about whether to go forward with them. In that case, the defendants had patented a cell line derived from the patient's unique bodily tissues without ever informing him what they were doing, despite his explicit inquiries questioning the necessity of calling him back for so many follow-up tests. Although the California Supreme Court denied the patient's claim to a property interest in his cells, it decided that, in order to secure informed patient consent, a physician must disclose financial conflicts of interest that could bear on treatment. The Moore decision is not binding outside of California, but its underlying principle is persuasive to the judiciary elsewhere[2]" [Miller, 1996].

"A subtext to this discussion involves the chilling effect that some insurer contract termination provisions exert on provider behavior. Any contract that can be terminated by the insurer 'without cause' leaves providers dissatisfied with contract provisions—or the way the contract is administered—vulnerable to economic pressure. 'Without cause' termination provisions threaten to disrupt established provider-patient relationships, because a clinician who balks at insurance provisions impairing the quality of doctor-patient communication risks losing access to those insured patients altogether" [Miller, 1996].

"On October 27, 1997, Oregon legalized physician-assisted suicide. Although there have been many studies of physician-assisted suicide, there are no data on the experiences of patients and physicians when the practice is legal. Physician-assisted suicide is practiced in the Netherlands but is subject to criminal prosecution, even though such prosecutions are rare. The Oregon Death with Dignity Act allows terminally ill state residents to receive prescriptions for self-administered lethal medications from their physicians. It does not permit euthanasia, in which a physician or other person directly administers a medication to a patient in order to end his or her life. To obtain a prescription for a lethal

---

2. The AMA's Council on Ethical and Judicial Affairs has concluded that "physicians must disclose all relevant financial inducements and contractual restrictions that affect the delivery of health care to patients." Physicians subject to such clauses are thus theoretically caught between Scylla and Charybdis—their contracts purport to forbid them from doing both what the law and their ethical principles may require.

medication, the law requires that the patient be an adult resident of Oregon who is 'capable' (able to make and communicate decisions about his or her health care) and who has an illness that is expected to lead to death within six months. The patient must make one written and two oral requests to his or her physician. The two oral requests must be separated by at least 15 days. The patient's primary physician and a consultant are required to confirm the diagnosis of a terminal condition and the prognosis determine that the patient is capable, and refer the patient for counseling, if either believes that the patient's judgment is impaired by depression or some other psychiatric or psychological disorder. The primary physician must also inform the patient of all feasible alternatives, such as comfort care, hospice care, and pain-control options. To comply with the law, physicians must report all prescriptions that they write for lethal medications to the Oregon Health Division. Reporting is not required if patients begin the process of requesting a prescription but do not actually receive it. Physicians and patients who adhere to the requirements of the act are protected from criminal prosecution" [Chin et al, 1999].

"A federal court recently convicted a physician of submitting false Medicare claims. He was fined and expelled from the Medicare system. He then received a notice from the state board of medical examiners for him to show cause why his license should not be revoked. Can a license be revoked for an offense that has nothing to do with medical skills and ability? Yes. In most jurisdictions, conviction for violation of a criminal statute involving moral turpitude is considered unprofessional conduct. The medical board can then impose whatever penalties its state charters permit for unprofessional conduct. These usually consist of the right to suspend, revoke, or restrict the right to practice medicine" [Lessons, 1999].

Revocation of a physician's license is generally within the authority of a medical board. Conviction for violation of federal antifraud laws is certainly within the range of offenses that could merit such action. For example, the revocation of a physician's license was concluded by a New York appeals court to be not so disproportionate to the offense committed, namely Medicare insurance fraud, as to be considered "shocking to one's sense of fairness" [Bhatt, 1997].

"A physician whose patient suffered permanent injuries due to a prescribed theophylline-based medication successfully sued the drug manufacturer under the Washington State Consumer Protection and Product Liability Acts. He claimed damages for injury to his professional reputation and for his personal physical and emotional distress. Evidence showed that the drug company had engaged in deceptive trade practices by concealing from physicians information about the risks associated with use of theophylline. On appeal, the Washington Supreme Court affirmed the physician's claim under the Consumer Protection Act but reversed the award of damages under the Product Liability Act. The court decided that, although the Consumer Protection Act normally applies to the ultimate user of a product, physicians are appropriate parties under the act in the case of medication injuries due to the special relationship between physicians and drug manufacturers, in which manufacturers deal directly with the prescriber, not with the patient. The prescribing physician may be a 'private attorney general' under the act because the manufacturer caused harm to his professional reputation. The physician, however, could not recover damages for personal distress after injuries experienced by his patient because such damages are available only under the Product Liability Act, a law that applies to parties directly injured by a product, their relatives, and certain bystanders witnessing the injury" [Helminski, 1994].

"Sometimes, physicians feel like helpless victims of the legal system. Occasionally, however, physicians can use consumer protection laws against those whose actions cause injury to their patients. As is the case with all other professionals, physicians' livelihoods primarily depend on reputation and goodwill. Damage to reputation and goodwill because of the unlawful practices of others fully justifies the physician's transformation to private attorney general. As such, the physician acts as an advocate for the patient and for the public. The relationship is in the best tradition of medicine and in the best tradition of attorneys general" [Helminski, 1994].

The diverse medicolegal cases presented above are a few illustrations of the intertwining of law and ethics. At times law is at variance with a physician's personal bioethical beliefs. Nonetheless confrontations do occur with decisions that are not always compatible with standardized bioethics. The core of law is not concerned with morality. Its mission centers about upholding the written laws and to be guided by previous court decisions in deciding disputes. Medicine is primarily concerned with patient welfare. Sometimes this becomes a sentimental persuader that clouds moral judgments. But this human kindness must not control thinking correctly. Especially when misguidance tempts deviation from bioethics which must be protected.

Loss of Chance

Rising out of discussions on bioethics is the legal aspects of loss of chance. The category of loss is caused by the negligence of another. Specific to this contention reference is to physicians. This cause of action has been recognized since the early twentieth century [Chaplin, 1911]. The basis for the legal action is stated succinctly: "should liability be imposed for negligence which merely increases the probability of an already probable negative outcome? [I]n a present minority, but in a growing number of jurisdictions there is reflected courts' efforts to compensate plaintiffs whose prospects of recovery or survival were less than even. Under the majority theory, a plaintiff with less than a fifty-fifty chance can not be harmed to a compensable degree by negligent care" [Zimmerly, 1989].

Ethical considerations have not been considered on the loss of chance. Therefore few thoughts are expressed on the morality of implied negligence. Legal decisions are not voluminous on this subject. One of these memorable studies is known in court records as the Cooper case. It concerns a sixteen-year-old boy who was taken to a hospital emergency department by ambulance after being struck by a truck while riding his bicycle. His history emphasized a blow to the head, followed by headache, and low-back pain. While in the emergency area, he vomited. Xrays were taken of his skull and lumbar region. The boy was discharged, went home where he died. Autopsy demonstrated a basal skull fracture, subarachnoid plus epidural hemorrhages. The parents sued the hospital for medical negligence. The court denied recovery based on expert testimony that the patient had maybe a fifty percent chance to survive if surgery was performed [Cooper v. Sisters of Charity, 1971].

Much loss of chance litigation is hidden under the heading of medical malpractice. In Florida, the much quoted Gooding case held that while a hospital emergency department staff was negligent in treating a man, the evidence did not prove that the patient had a greater-than-even chance of survival. No liability was imposed on the hospital [Gooding, 1984].

Two cases from Arizona reflect the contemporary tendency of the courts toward relaxing the probability requirement for causation, and moving toward recognition of loss of chance as the compensable injury. Compensation for increased risk of harm is, in effect, a reduction of the probability burden, to a substantial factor test. The damages being an award for the actual outcome, not just the lost chance [Hizer v Randolph, Arizona 1980] [Thomas v Sun City Comm. Hosp, Arizona 1986].

"The concept of loss of a chance places a tremendous reliance on statistics. . . Unfortunately, accurate statistics do not always find their way into the courtroom. . . Reports of results are subject to inaccuracies . . . and laboratory studies may not be as helpful and as reliable an index—as we would like to think. . . Under the theory of loss of a chance—there [is] no attempt by plaintiff's attorney or by his physician expert to consider the natural history, the nature of complications, patient's compliance, and the autonomous decision-making of the patient, and others empowered to make the pertinent determination" [Razinski, 1989]. Loss of a chance requires that judgment be completely accurate. But there is no mention of bioethical infringement.

"The intrinsic unfairness of the loss of chance doctrine is its abrogation of traditional civil proof based on probabilities. . . Experts who evaluate the evidence in malpractice cases can usually find something wrong with what the defendant did and this is particularly true in emergency situations where potential defendants act often without the benefit of calm judgment. . . The fallacy of decisions favoring the doctrine is that they view the concept as one of causation rather than as one of injury, particularly when the chance of success, or chance of survival is less than probable" [Mills, 1989]. Most states do not favor the loss of a chance concept [Zimmerly, 1989]. Solution to the unfairness of loss of chance as the causation of the end result is to reconsider loss of a chance in terms of injury rather than causation [Herskovitz, 1983].

Shifting the focus away from legal involvement, no thought is given to the ethical concerns about the loss of a chance. Ethics is a moral obligation that is independent of the proper business of the law that evaluates evidence that will lead to successful prosecution or a victorious defense. There are ethicists who tend to believe that law has abandoned ethics—legal and otherwise. Nobody can propose as a truism that ethical judgment, widely shared, is embodied in the law. In terms of the loss of a chance it is unethical, suggesting irrationality, for a court of law to hold culpable a physician for a part of the complexities that caused harm to a patient.

When medical malpractice is alleged, the law ignores bioethics completely. Medicine does not. Even if the physician deviates from the established standard of care and causes no injury to the patient, the health-care provider is not answerable as to any bioethical digression. In a court of law when a comparative question is asked which weighs the law against bioethics: the law wins.

Good Samaritans

The interface of law and medicine discloses that the deterrent to the timidity of rendering emergency care at the roadside to accident victims has not been eradicated totally by State Good Samaritan Laws. The moral obligation to assist either an injured or ill person has not been effaced.

California in 1959 was the first state to legislate Good Samaritan immunity for civil liability alleged from emergency care. Since that year every state plus the District of Columbia have similar laws. The intention of the legislators was to encourage physicians to assist victims of accidents without fear of malpractice litigation. Amendments to state laws have expanded Good Samaritan immunity to cover emergency care in health care institutions.

"Although the latitude given to physicians by the courts occasionally has worked to the detriment of the malpractice victim, such deference is necessary if the statutes are to be effective in achieving their purpose of encouraging physicians to stop and assist" [Reuter, 1999]

Most physicians/surgeons have good intentions in their professional work whether it is in treating their private patients or strangers. By training and adherence to medical codes their disciplined manner does not change with the socioeconomic status of the patient. Thus bad intent[3] is not part of a doctor's personality.

Although Good Samaritan laws absolve physicians from civil liability, it does not offer ethical directions as to a choice in responding to a person in need of medicosurgical assistance. Some states are considering laws that would compel a physician to respond to emergencies. There are many physicians who will not stop to render emergency treatment at an accident scene. Many salve the refusal by stating they are not trained in emergency medicine which is not an essential requirement of their specialty board.

---

3. Scienter is a legal term for bad intent which is an element in many lawsuits. Ballentine's Law Dictionary 1143 [3rd edition 1969] defines scienter as knowledge, particularly that knowledge which is charged with guilt or liability.

For many years reliability of physicians to adhere to bioethical conduct was individualized. Nowadays courts of law have coopted this responsibility making it a duty to act in a certain way under specific circumstances. Dispassionate observers may see this as unnecessary, relying upon the good conscience of every doctor of medicine.

The general public accepts physicians as men/women in whom they have trust and confidence. Willingly they are pleased to accept assistance from any physician in time of need. They do not question the ethical conduct of physicians/surgeons. Therefore, they accept that any improvements in bioethical *milieu* should be generated internally within medical organizations. The medical professions' code of ethics should be clearly explicit with prohitions specified which do not breach the Hippocratic Oath. Medical surveillance of self is a laudable endeavor and should be given much thought by the medicosurgical and bioscientific communities.

Wrongful-birth Lawsuits

Difficult as it may seem to believe, physicians are in an ethical quandary because they can be sued for giving professional care. There is a remarkable increase in the number of lawsuits against doctors for wrongful birth the opposite to wrongful death which has been a long-time basis for legal actions. "A mounting number of obstetricians/gynecologists are being sued by patients who say they would have had abortions if prenatal tests had detected fetal abnormalities" [Rarey, 1999].

Advances in genetic testing can disclose abnormalities and deformities. Therefore it is the ethical obligation of physicians to disclose defects to future parents. When inadequate information is given or failure to test for defects can be proven a lawsuit is inevitable.[4] All states do not

4. Most of these lawsuits occur when a child is born with Down syndrome, a genetic defect that stunts a child's intellectual development whose IQ remains at the level of an 8-year-old. If an obstetrician fails to do an amniocentesis and a Down syndrome baby is delivered he/she can be sued for wrongful-birth. Amniocentesis is performed hardly ever after the 22nd week of pregnancy for fear of permanent fetal damage. Negligence is also founded on failure to recognize, appreciate, and discuss test results, especially ultrasound.

allow wrongful-birth lawsuits among them are Michigan and Georgia. Twenty-seven states permit such legal actions [Rarey, 1999].

Objections to wrongful-birth litigation are voiced by many individuals who look upon such lawsuits as a new, unexplored malpractice area. A group in Chicago has stated that: "This is directly contrary to our national and state policies promoting the lives and livelihoods of people with disabilities. . . What we are dealing with here is the promotion of eugenics as a birth policy whereby doctors are sued for not weeding out the unfit" [Forsythe, 1999].

Eager for litigation, there will be some lawyers who will make a specialty of this class of lawsuits. Undoubtedly this will broaden the field of "wrongful life" lawsuits. The doors of courtrooms will be opened to sick, deformed, and disabled children who will institute legal action on the basis that they would be better off never having been born.[5] Morally, this would give the courts the task of Solomon to determine the dollar value of human life. Then judges will need to calculate the financial damages that are to be paid for having allowed the person to exist. Physicians will be witnesses to help estimate these amounts. Will they be participants in unethical conduct if they do? Moreover who is to be sued? Is this a moral transgression to be born even with an imperfection. The beauty of life is found inside the person, not on the external appearance of the body.

---

5. Like the complaint of Job in the Old Testament story.

Chapter 33

Physicians As Witnesses

Natural law ethics supplies the logic for those scientific positions, performances, and conclusions that are admirable because of their indispensable moral merit. There should not be an apparent segregation of dogmatic morality and the vocation of science. This would separate spirituality into an indigenous discipline apart from systematic scientific endeavors as if there is neither intrinsic unity nor correlation between them. Restoration of this essential singleness of purpose can be most beneficial to scientists in their chosen, prescribed tasks when performed under the banner of a holy alliance between science and spiritual tenets.

A fabled enlightenment is to secularize ethics and medicalize morality to suit the scientific situation encountered. To disarrange the normal diminishes the image of laboratory bioscience and clinical medicine. An example is the nineteenth and twentieth century physicians, psychiatrists, and psychologists who legitimized "insanity" in the law-courts. Claiming scientific medical expertise which was beyond judicial ability to be authoritatively comprehensive of an inexact mental deviation. Persuasive, certified bioscientists are capable of influencing juries and judicial decisions. Morality and ethics are abandoned frequently in the eagerness to achieve a victory in the litigation drama.

Special notice in this regard is given to the voluntary action of humankind in conformity with the precepts of law which is called justice. Although the courts of law seek expert testimony and rely heavily upon the knowledge of the highly trained expert, nevertheless, the testimony of a family physician concerning alterations in the mental pattern of patients is evidence of extreme latitude given to physicians in a court of law.

Medical opinion stated in a criminal trial can mold the law under the *Stare decisis* doctrine.[1] It is realized that the authenticity of certain facts surrounding a medicolegal problem resides in the morality of the testifier. Therefore the moral weight of testimony given is only as good as the person giving it. Expert medicosurgical/psychiatric witnesses can be misled by an incentive coupled with financial interest which is not ethical. Legal restrictions regarding mental illness in alleged perpetrators of serious crimes and capital felonies are decided generally in favor of the accused when considered irresponsible because of insanity.[2]

Until 1800 the test of mental incapacity under Anglo-American criminal law was that the person involved was deprived totally of his understanding and memory and did not know what he was doing. In 1812 it was decided that the correct test was whether the criminal had the power to distinguish right from wrong. Since 1843 in England and largely in the United States the test has been that at the moment the crime was committed the accused had a sufficient degree of reason to know that he/she was doing an act which was wrong. In the United States, Maine took the lead in 1847 by enacting legislation that protected from severe punishment accused persons with mental deficiency. The Maine law provided a judge to commit the defendant to a mental institution for observation, evaluation, and determination that the plea of mental incapacity was valid. The medical profession contributed quantitatively to the changes in these laws. Hence they had a serious moral responsibility which was manifested to the ultimate [Ficarra, 1968].

---

1. *Stare decisis* is Latin translated to mean abide by, to adhere to decided cases. It refers to a policy of courts to stand by precedent and not to disturb a settled legal point. The doctrine is that, when a court has laid down a principle of law as applicable to a certain state of facts, it will adhere to that principle, and apply it to all future cases, where the facts are substantially the same (Black's Law Dictionary).

2. Insanity is a legal not a medical term. There is no medical disease called insanity. Insanity is a legal noun formerly used to designate a person who exhibits signs of mental illness. "A man is sane when he knows the nature and quality of his acts, and knows they are wrong" [10 Clark and F. 200 8 Canib.L.J.300]. Attorneys-at-law are familiar with the updated nomenclature of diagnosed mental illnesses as modernized by the American Psychiatric Association.

Continuing this munificence in legal medicine is demonstrated in England. The year was 1843. A man named McNaghten was acquitted of a murder charge because of mental incompetency. This verdict caused a furor among the English people. Fifteen judges were impounded to clarify the laws relative to criminal responsibility and mental illness. The judicial consensus after much consideration propounded the rule that the test should be "whether the accused at the time of doing the act knew the difference between right and wrong" [Snyder, 1959].

The first breakthrough of the ironclad McNaghten rule occurred in 1954 in the United States Court of Appeals for the District of Columbia. The accused was Monte Durham, who was charged with housebreaking. In this instance the court ruled "that the accused is not criminally responsible if the unlawful act was the product of mental disease or mental defect" [Snyder, 1959]. The conviction of Durham was reversed on appeal [Court of Appeals for the District of Columbia, Durham v. United States 1954].

The Durham decision ignited the fire of spirited discussion throughout the United States. Some psychiatrists hail it as solving the problem. Others disagree. The controversy stresses the vital part physician-psychiatrists have in the courtroom. This prominence argues for the necessity of high, unbiased ethical standards for those who testify. By their testimony expert witnesses mold the law and can add or detract from the administration of justice. This is a moral responsibility that demands the highest ethical requisite for honesty.

Errors by those who are experts can be detrimental to the innocent even as the guilty may be set free. Relying heavily on expert witnesses a judge stated: "It is argued that the relation of mental illness to criminal responsibility should be left to the determination of experts, the psychiatrists, psychologists, and the courts should be guided by their more enlightened diagnosis of the particular mental disease under consideration. But the problem then arises which experts shall we believe, for it is a matter of common observation that there are no certified psychiatrists or psychologists we are able to accept unconditionally" [Newsome v. Commonwealth of Kentucky, 366 SW 2d 174 Ky, Dec 15, 1962; dissenting opinion Jan 15, 1963; rehearing denied, April 19, 1963].

Conflicting views in a courtroom are common as part of the adversarial procedure of adjective law. Judges and juries realize that medical opinions are not infallible. Nonetheless much testimony given in litigation is vital to one side or the other. "A witness in a judicial proceeding is absolutely privileged to publish false and defamatory matter about another as a part of a judicial proceeding in which he/she is testifying if the defamatory matter is relevant to the subject or inquiry" [Dunbar v. Greenlaw, 128 A 2d 218 Maine 1956].

Serious burden is placed upon physicians as expert witnesses in a court of law. They must give honest opinions derived from personal knowledge with strict adherence to truth. Nothing should sway them from this moral obligation. To do otherwise is a violation of ethical integrity as an essential element in the pursuit of *pro maximo bono* [for the greatest good]. *Per contra* deviation from probity destroys the integrity of the expert witness. This can be damaging to professional reputation. Strong, upright character is the best defense against ethical misbehavior. Good intentions do not justify telling untruths, committing perjury, and being unethical. Beneath the attractive toga of intended social, altruistic benevolence may lurk an unethical, despotic, perfervid immorality.

When sued for malpractice a physician may find it necessary to be a witness in his/her own behalf. Under oath the testimony must be the truth, nothing but the truth: not truth as he/she believes it to be. Under the psychological trauma of being a defendant against allegations of negligence, a physician may try to improve his/her chance of defeating the plaintiff by bending the truth. It is unethical for a physician to speak untruthfully no matter the circumstances.

Hindsight might suggest that alterations to truth might bring victory. This does not give approval to any ethical transgression. The better part is to prevent malpractice by protecting whatever is done as a defense against what may suggest negligence. Especially is this applicable when obtaining consents of every category.

As a repetition for legal defense and security, when a physician obtains a written informed consent for surgery, human experimentation, administration of new drugs, and signing a contract of whatever kind, the patient should be asked to write in his/her own handwriting at the conclusion of the sentence the following. "I have read the above and I understand it." For the protection of both parties, incorporate in the body of the statement, consent or contract the words, "what is not included in this document is automatically excluded."

Chapter 34

Compliance With Government Medical Guidelines

Ethical obligations demand that physicians, surgeons, and every person in health care adhere to the rules, regulations, and requirements of federal, state, and county governments. An example is the Stark I and the later Stark II legislations. These were passed because of financial interests some physicians had in laboratories. The fear was that such affiliations would tempt them to order more laboratory procedures than were necessary. Aiming at cost-containment no mention was made of the ethical impropriety of these excesses. Stark II expands Stark I which was aimed at laboratory referrals [Physician's Guide, 1999].

Referring patients to companies, corporations, and any medical entity is not permitted if the physician has a financial interest therein. Billing medicare and medicaid for such claims is a violation of the law and considered an unethical practice. Filing false information would subject the perpetrator to criminal and civil penalties [Physician's Guide, 1999].

Managed care facilities and anesthesiologists are constantly suspected of wrongdoing in their billings to medicare, medicaid, Blue Cross/Blue Shield, and insurance carriers. Abuse is found frequently involving patients in nursing homes, especially those chronically ill who are unable to change the initial provider. As to anesthesiologists, suspicion arises when they supervise more than four operating rooms at one time. "Routinely some anesthesiologists are supervising seven rooms for concurrent one-hour surgeries" [Physician's Guide, 1999].

It is unethical and fraudulent for any health care provider to overbill, bill for services not performed, listing services rendered to a higher level for larger payment, falsifying claims, and altering medical records. Doctors, hospitals, and laboratories should make certain they are doing everything they can to comply with honest billing methods. Not to do so is not ethical business practice. Dishonesty is immoral for physicians from whom only the highest behavior is expected. Honesty establishes good faith just as making deliberate false claims destroy it.

Double payment is unethical. If an error causes this situation, it should be acknowledged and all overpayments should be returned to the sender. Sometimes hospitals and other health care providers bill medicare, medicaid, and insurers for services and medication given to patients as part of research grants, drug trials, and other experimental studies. Many such projects are funded by the National Institutes of Health, Public Health agencies, and private foundations like the Cooley's Anemia Foundation. It is a gross moral fault if claims for materials used in these projects are submitted for payment elsewhere. This would equate with duplicate billing which is contrary to medical and business ethics. Moreover mechanisms are in place and are "used by Federal and State Governments to detect, refer, investigate fraud, and abuse cases" [Physician's Guide, 1999].

Chapter 35

Physicians Union

Labor unions indicate a united workforce in manufacturing, industry, and commerce is necessary. Medicine is a profession which is not a primary business but a health care service. Contemporary medical doctors are not complainers by nature. However, the progressive intrusion of third parties into their loved discipline has alerted them to denounce this continually increasing interference. In their protesting conduct they must preserve equanimity in the presence of unethical tactics that threaten to misshapen their future destiny.

There is great dissatisfaction with the way physicians have been treated by managed care, the Medicare system, and Medicaid. Patients are dealt with the same way. Hope for improvement resides in protests from patients and their families. Physicians are not listened to as readily as when citizens speak out in the public interest.

In 1998, these changes forced physicians to organize to fight some of the changes imposed upon them by managed care. Among the restrictions disliked are limitations on treatments, curbs on fees, and procedural compensation decreases. In this situation the American Medical Association, State, and County Medical societies had to campaign to keep up a declining membership.

"In a setback to physicians' efforts to unionize, a regional director of the National Labor Relations Board (NLRB) turned away a request by more than 650 New Jersey physicians that they be allowed to form a union. Dismissing a petition filed by Local 56 of the United Food and Commercial Workers, it was said that the physicians are independent contractors of AmeriHealth HMO Inc. . . , not employees." The doctors argued that since AmeriHealth "controlled many of the details of their work, such as the maximum wait for patients, the size of their waiting room, and whether patients should undergo surgery," they should be considered employees of the HMO. However, a spokesperson said that the doctors are not employees since they run their own businesses, contract with other HMOs, and receive only about 4% of the practice business from AmeriHealth. It was said that the physicians "lack the close economic relations and integration with AmeriHealth that would support a finding of employee status" [Stechel, 1999].

"This case was widely viewed as an important test case, although some said the New Jersey doctors' particular arrangement represented an unfavorable set of circumstances for a test case because of the lack of integration with AmeriHealth and the relatively small amount the HMO contributes to the doctors' caseload. An attorney for the union said the group has until June 7, 1999 to petition the NLRB's main office in Washington. While the union has not yet decided whether to appeal the decision, it may turn its efforts toward federal legislation that would give physicians the right to unionize" [Stechel, 1999]. This was done.

There was a time in American medical history when it was considered unethical for physicians to unionize. This attitude has changed by dint of adverse circumstances generated by business agencies that have a strangle-hold on how physicians practice. To combat this ogre, physicians have to unite. Because in union there is strength. Past generations of physicians would not believe that this situation would occur. But it has and American physicians have been forced to become a fighting unit to battle a common enemy, known as big business in managed medical care.

The American Medical Association has shocked the managed health care industry. On June 23, 1999 its governing Board of Trustees voted to form an affiliated labor union for physicians who are salaried employees. But a union with an important caveat—no strikes. This national union will give physicians more leverage in outside-the-profession agencies that are attempting to mold medical practice. The cardinal issue is the undue influence of business administrators whose greatest concern is saving money on patient care, simultaneously increasing profit to be given to stockholders. This is the philosophy of successful business ventures which is now applied to health care and insurance carriers. Physician trust in outsiders is frayed because of the past performances of nonmedical administrations.

Unionization seems inevitable as physicians have no clout against dominating health insurance corporations, corporation ownership of hospitals, and giant HMOs. With group force doctors are in a position of strength to negotiate collectively for improved patient services rather than only money matters. Frustration with managed health care and ineffectiveness in discussions with insurers has prompted physicians to unionize. It is not unethical for professional people to form an alliance for mutual interest and benefit.

"Federal antitrust law prevents the A.M.A. union from representing self-employed doctors. But the association is strongly pushing for a bill in the House that would provide an antitrust exemption to allow independent doctors to band together to bargain collectively with health plans and insurers. The implications of such a change must be carefully examined by Congress. Some states are moving in this direction. Texas recently passed a law to give self-employed doctors more bargaining leverage. The rapid shift in the medical marketplace has been driven largely by employers and insurers eager to hold down high medical costs. For the most part, doctors have been bewildered observers of the upheaval" [Editorial, 1999]. The A.M.A.'s action shows that the profession is no longer willing to stay out of the discussions, disputes, and disagreements with all those non-professional executive leaders dictating how patients are to be treated. Joining together diminishes the feeling of helplessness each physician has when pressured by managed-care restrictions.

Most "physicians have some relief in the AMA union plan. Others call the move an inadequate solution" [Yellin, 1999]. All hope a union will help physicians provide better care to patients. With centuries of historical tradition as a stamp of approval, medicine has received endless accolades as an honorable profession practiced by selfless persons whose purpose is to serve the common good. Now it finds itself in a delicate situation in which it can no longer function individually to be effective. In the battle against managed care, may it never lose its heritage. Equally important, everyone involved in the management of health care must recognize that medical decision-making is best left to physicians, who are the sole persons trained and licensed to practice medicine and, therefore best able to determine what health services are necessary [Hirshfeld, 1999].

Chapter 36

Science And Religion

Researches and pharmaceutical corporations have pierced the human genetic secrets. Without adequate consideration of the implications, bioscientists have developed a talent to invade the code of life. This new scientific power has been a metamorphosis in many aspects of medicine. Among which are the advances in forensic medicine to assist in crime solving and eruption in the knowledge of pathology. Many scientific disclosures are frightening.

Involved with these developments tremendous ethical issues have arisen. In addition some scientists have assumed a superhuman propensity that makes them potential discoverers of life's secret. The biological laboratory often has gleaming equipment, automated machines, and robots that gives the appearance of a manufacturing enterprise. Organized like a factory the combined scientific efforts are the largest ever attempted. Perhaps the complexity is greater than the moon project for the sheer magnitude of the ambitious undertaking.

Bioscience's potential may come in conflict with religion. Because many sorting technologies carry with them thorny ethical situations that will give rise to questions that must be answered. They will come into being quickly as the rapidly acquired information is made known. The dreams of ancient scientists will be realized in the next millennium minus the separatistic propensity to alienate science from religion. In past centuries science and religion were blowing themselves apart. Perhaps the future scientists will return to a belief in religion.

With understanding there comes the unravelling of complexities. Therefrom orderliness is made easier. Then finally simplicity replaces what was a complexity. So it should be with religion that is not beyond resolution by scientists. To them religion is not confusing, illogical, and is not terrifying. Bioscientists especially should emulate Sir Isaac Newton [1642-1727].[1] He "ordered the universe to the glory of God, but forgot to build Him a throne to sit upon. . . Rational man became manipulated man, buffeted about by advertising, subliminal appeals, and spin" [Wolfe, 1999].

Building on a strong heritage science and religion should have mutual respect and understanding for one another. As parceners they could serve humanity in their own indigenous fashions. Thus the energy evaporated in persistently recurrent, mutual criticism could be utilized beneficially in altruistic service *pro re necesse* [as is needed]. This is a vision of the future that will make value-ladened knowledge of religion and science more accessible to both disciplines.

Protracted union of science and religion evinces a genuine, condigned love of virtuous behavior. Which is accompanied by sincere concern for the welfare of all persons encountered without either dissatisfaction or an unnecessary fastidiousness. In a very tangible way religion gives valued assistance to physicians in bioethical and medicolegal distresses. Especially "when professional testimony is required in cases of such peculiar malignity as to excite general horror and indignation [that] a virtuous mend, even though scrupulous and timid, is liable to be influenced by too violent impressions; and to transfer to the accused that dread and aversion, which before conviction, should be confined to the crime, and as much as possible withheld from the supposed offender" [Percival, 1803].

Thus religion is an aid to subsist a regular gradation from the slightest presumption to complete moral certainty without diminishing the probability of presented facts. Religion is of considerable importance in those circumstances that place all humanity in the great theatre of life's drama and does not weary mankind when involved with well-doing. The sphere of human duty in this regard has no limits in its extent. Every advance in charity widens its boundaries. Increase of which multiplies with diversification the objects to be reached, and the length of years of service evinces their unceasing succession. This is Christian warfare in the army

---

1. English mathematician, scientist, and philosopher whose major works included the theories of universal gravitation, terrestrial mechanics, color, and the invention of differential calculus.

of God which prompts humanity to carry on when the voice of wisdom is not heard.

Religion and biosciences should come together joining forces for the common good. Because moral and religious influence of sickness is favorable to the best interests of humankind and of espial society generally. This is regarded justly as an important, even an essential, constituent objective for the establishment of civic harmony. Blending of religion and medicine leads to the purest beneficence that enhances truth, probity, and ethics without any violation of professional liberality.

An *esprit de corps* between religion and bioscience is a principle of action that is founded upon human nature, and when duly acknowledged, is both rational and laudable. Discriminatory separation of science from religion is considered to be an intellectual inconvenience and impropriety. Equally afflictive if a dissociation persists is the languor of sorrow when religion is absent and therefore unable to exculpate misdeeds. Bereft of an aphoristic ethos of this type a preclusion occurs which leaves most remaining controversies unsolved. With an insufficient comprehension, even wisdom is unable to assist with determinate assurance and conformable rectitude to bring about rational solutions to grievous problems.

The necessity for friendliness between science and religion resides in the fact that both aim to serve humanity. This should be the dedicated purpose of political science as well. From the golden age of the Renaissance, a relationship has been recognized between science and the ruling political powerhouse. To this day science, its components, and subspecialties with its technical know-how have placed powerful instruments at the disposal of national leaders who are not exempt from ethical restrictions in their usages.

When bioscience is used politically, it may have added a new descriptive noun, biopolitics, to the world's vocabulary. What is more important is the proper use of such unprecedented mechanisms in governance. Biomedical resources available to politicians can be more deadly when used without beneficial intentions. Possession of bioscientific modalities give great power over humanity. Politicians can dominate bioscience for either good or for evil purposes. This influence is done through intermediary institutions and by direct authority. The final judgment as to the exercise of bioscientific products must be guided by ethical norms. Indifference to morality indicts biopolitics as unholy from the bioscientific, political, and ethical perspectives.

With the prominence of bioscientific technology plus the wide acclaim and its elitism, it has taken upon itself to dictate morality, ethics, and to form its own cultural standards. Changes have rarified the religious atmosphere that was attenuated previously. The new bioscientific illuminism is profoundly secular and is respected by many colleagues as either an alternate or replacement of religion. All things divine are repudiated as superstition, vulgar piety, as an importuner of intellectual freedom, and enemy of science.

Hence most bioscientists, bioengineers, and scientists in general are their own ultimate arbiters who decide what is good or evil, true or false. As secularistic interpreters of their own conduct a consensus decrees it is primarily agnostic. Thus secularism,[2] not religion, prevails as to correctness in what is affirmed and/or denied. Many ethical biomedical subjects are unresolved: claimed as being irresolvable. This is because those who are asked to unravel them lack moral stability. Plus an inability to recognize malice and the sense of sin. This deficiency detracts from the definition of bioscience and discounts any supernatural order in its integrity. It is similar to the "Commercially or politically inspired distortions of fact or of canonical texts or works of art that pose real and continuing challenges to the conscience and consciousness of civilization" [Dechert, 1999].

That bioethics derives from religion is not a surmise. Therefore scientists who have no religion do not appreciate the importance of this code. A neutrality on religion by some scientists is another excuse for neglecting bioethics. A certain ambiguity implicit in the religious connotation attached to ethics dismisses it. Religiosity in medicine is of long duration in many cultures.

Saints have been adopted in medical iconography, medical anthropology, and folklore. From the medical pluralism of the 12th century onward up to the industrial revolution educated physicians ceased to be monastic infirmarians. Monk-physicians were the vehicle by which Greco-Roman humoral medicine was embraced easily and readily by the Christians of the Middle Ages. With no affectionate embrace most modern, ontic physicians shun such provenience as intrusive monastic medicine.

---

2. Secularism pertains to temporal rather than to spiritual things. It is the view that the well-being of humanity should predominate over religious considerations in civil affairs, public education, government actions, and legislation.

This is a dichotomy dissimilar to ancient times when science and religion were regarded as the same side of the same coin. In those days religion brought beauty, sweetness, and light into the dullest life.

Relevance Of Religion To Science

A long-anticipated conference by an eclectic commixture of scientists discussed the interaction between science and religion. The multidisciplinary gathering was informed about the emerging new academic discipline of Theology and Science which is burgeoning on many American campuses [Wertheim, 1999].

The meaning of this resurgence is purely speculative since it has not been defined by its productivity. What is evident is the focus on Christianity and the absence of religious disparity. Although open to all religions, the major participants and authors on this subject had a Christocentric perspective. The influential views of many scientists of diverse specialties encapsulate religion and science without difficulty. Although each has his/her own views and explanations of the harmony that constitutes a support for "a triumphant new natural theology" [Polkinghorne, 1998].

Many writings demonstrate the powerful consonance that Christianity and science can exist side-by-side without confusion, controversy, and contradiction. Other writers "claim that some scientific laws or observations are the ultimate truth and are immune to revision or reinterpretation" [Keith Ward, 1998]. "That philosophical sophistication, however, comes at a price: it seriously complicates both author's goal [Ward and Van Huyssteen] of finding a synthesis of Christianity and science. That problem is further compounded by the relatively antifoundationist view both authors take of religion" [Wertheim, 1999].

Many great and wonderful accomplishments are attributed to scientists. Their marvelous deeds are due to their majestic intellects and the high caliber thereof. However when it comes to religion their intellects do not seem to be as astute as when they are in the laboratory. Their mind-set is one that does not allow going beyond the physical and that which is seen. To accept anything on faith is beyond their ken. It does not decrease intelligence if something is accepted either on faith alone or in conjunction with a physical manifestation.

Science and religion should heal their differences that has been termed an historical rift. The divide between science and religion may be due to the over-reaching by some branches of science and the uncanny suspicion on the part of church authorities. The latter looked askance upon scientists who had a certain rationalism that explained all things by scientific reasoning alone and maintained absolute truth did not exist. Scrutinizing God by rationalism alone made it seem devoid of meaning which led to a cautious and suspicious view of science as being tainted with atheism.

"Religion is often seen as an impediment to science. . . Some scientists have suggested a kind of necessary apartheid between the two. . . While it is true that science [with its emphasis on testing hypotheses to achieve proof] and religion [with its appeal to ritual and spirituality] represent quite different aspects of culture. There are benefits to seeing them as symbiotic. Going so far as to suggest that finding ways for science and religion to work together may be vital to our future . . . science needs religion because as Einstein put it, 'Religion without science is blind; science without religion is lame.' Second, over the long term, science needs religion to help persuade people that the scientific enterprise is a noble endeavor, worthy of their support. . . . Third, religion can inspire scientists with a vision of what is most valuable and worthwhile in the scientific enterprise" [Harper, 1999].

To mark the quincentary of the expulsion of the Jews from Spain in 1492, a symposium was held in Jerusalem to provide an interfaith comparative perspective on medical-ethical issues in medieval and early modern Spain. Fifteen papers were read by participants from Israel, Spain, Great Britain, and Canada [Amundsen, 1999]. Most of the lectures centered on ethical problems in the relationship between physicians and patients. Plus the attitudes of Christian and Jewish practitioners of medicine from the 14th century to the 20th century.

The variety of discussions included an adaptation of scholarly competence to the treatise of religion and medicine as "an extraordinary example of collaboration and mutual trust in Jewish and Christian Spain" [Kottek, García-Ballester, 1996]. Jewish physicians were a common feature, at times a majority, in Christian Spain during the high and late Middle-Ages. Hostility did arise from the church and civil authorities. They disliked "Jewish physicians practicing on Christian patients, but also halakhic[3] antagonism to Jews employing Christian physicians ex-

3. Halakah in Judaism is the legal part of Talmudic literature, an interpretation of the laws of the Scripture.

isted. . . . Religious tensions often appear to have been stronger than compatibilities" [Amundsen, 1999].

Islamic input asserts that "the majority opinion in Moslem law prohibits Moslems being treated by non-Moslem physicians [which] coincides with a natural tendency among Moslems" [Kottek, García-Ballester, 1996]. These authors conclude with the observation that in Israel "religious affiliation is thus very much a determining factor in the choice of doctors even today" [Kottek, García-Ballester, 1996]. With numerous themes forming a mélange there is discerned in this presentation contributions from ethics, theology, formal religion, philosophy, rationalism, and other disciplines. The collage amalgamates religion and science into a worthwhile, bioethical compote.

Convergence Of Theology And Science

As far as many scientists are concerned religion, theology, and its doctrinaires should be buried in the catacombs. These primitive sepulchres would assure silence. Here in epigrammatic monuments, immobile and inarticulate, no irritation is possible as science could be free of tribulations from the enemy of science as religion was and is thought to be. Science does not submit to examination of conscience to be unbiased in its criticism of theology. Science maintains it has demonstrated "that all of material existence can be traversed in an unbroken journey by the rational mind. The world turns out to be coherent, or more precisely, it is consilient"[4] [Wilson, 1999].

"Scientists are solving the problems that philosophers have fought to keep eternal. The origin of existence, the essence of life, the nature of mind, the meaning of human life, the wellsprings of ethics and religious faith—all these mysteries of mysteries are yielding to consilient explanation" [Wilson, 1999]. This statement with eloquent prejudice plus monumental arrogance reeks with hubris and does not have the tone of either scientific or philosophic clarion clarity.

"The borderland disciplines are inevitably triangulating on the ultimate question: Do religion and moral reasoning also have a biological

---

4. Consilient is the term philosophers use to describe the coming together of the disciplines by force of fact and maturing theory. Consilience is the intellectual glue of the world-wide technoscientific civilization [Wilson].

origin? Are they the products of evolution? So stated, the meaning of spiritual authority breaks into two possibilities, two competing hypotheses that now appear susceptible to empirical testing. Either humanity is guided by moral principles that were formulated outside human existence, in other words by divine will or natural law, or else humanity has evolved these principles on its own during its long genetic and cultural history. Many thoughtful writers have said, No, such an important issue can't be that simple. But the time has come to say, Yes, it can be that simple. Sometimes a seemingly impossible problem can be flanked, especially when it is composed mostly of metaphor. I believe that is what science is doing in the case of spiritual and moral authority" [Wilson, 1999].

"The naturalistic hypothesis arising from scientific knowledge holds that the powerful emotions of religious experience are entirely neurobiological, that they evolved as part of the programmed activity of the brain favoring survival of tribe and individual, and that the particular form they have taken was therefore shaped by the long and idiosyncratic genetic history of the human species. This hypothesis may be wrong, I will quickly grant. We will find out. If it fails, the opposing transcendental interpretation of morality and spirituality, favored by most traditional theology and ethical philosophy, will be strengthened. However, if the naturalistic hypothesis prevails, as I believe it will, a new, more secular mode will gain ascendancy. The great human dilemma will be recognized for what it is: We evolved biologically to accept one truth but then evolved intellectually to discover another. The transition from one foundation of thought to the other will be gradual and, because it is based on firm, testable knowledge universally shared, probably benign. In any case, it appears that this division wrought by science and the convergence of the disciplines will be the 21st-century version of the struggle for the soul" [Wilson, 1999].[5]

From the writings of research professors biotechnology will have a tremendous impact on theology. So they predict with more enthusiasm than positive, assimilable assuredness. No proof has been documented statistically to sustain the postulate that the available technology has in-

---

5. Edward O. Wilson is a two-time Pulitzer Prize winner and University Research Professor at Harvard University. His most recent book is Consilience: The Unity of Knowledge.

fluenced theology away from central religions. The inventing of the printing press was a technological achievement that enabled every literate person to read the Bible and thus with sufficient funds purchased one. This fact made people more religious and did not dilute their faith. When radio was popular and television was not invented, religious programs were attractive. In the early years of television lectures by clergymen had massive audiences. The internet has taken down all barriers which allows global communications, dialogue, and joint services among the world's great religions. Physics as a hard science has contributed to religious understanding. Perhaps in some way biotechnology will find in theology the solution to the hesitancy to adopt bioethical standards that will be acceptable to both disciplines as they find their final goal—ultimate criterion of truth.

This is an essential harmony because there is a prevalent indifference, even apathy, to a code of bioethics respected by all concerned. Without it, mounting uncertainties and labyrinthine confusion enters the life of the moral research scientist. Mental disquietude arises which brings with it an interference in creativity and productivity. Such internecine struggles gives energy to discord and birth to adversities that increase the dividing distance between science and theology.

In the forefront for reconciliation is The Catholic Academy of Sciences in the United States of America. This scholarly academy is dedicated to the resolution of the old conflict still raging between science and religion. As intellectual warriors whose only weapon is knowledge academicians are in combat against opponents who increase the dividing canyon between two former friends and allies.

Wherever religion and science converge The Catholic Academy of Sciences serves. It provides diverse, multi-professional, Christian support for medicolegal, bioethical issues arising in bioscientific research and socioeconomics. Recognized as a learned academy of scholars, its intellectual reservoir is *semper paratus* [always prepared] to assist the Christian Church in America. One of its aims is to amalgamate high ethical standards with upright scientific productivity. The Academy assists in the recognition of speculative, hypothetical possibility, and realistic conceptual probability. The moral mission of The Catholic Academy of Sciences is to invigorate certitude into the clinical setting of scientific practicality.

This Academy is a companionship whose harmony resounds in celestial songs of compatibility. Hence the intellectual laity who are religious and the devout religious who are *literati* are united as *periti* [senior advisers]. Combined into a scholarly gathering they are close to God and not distanced from their disciplines. By their professional accomplishments each one demonstrates a fungible theme that science and religion, faith and reason are miscible. At plenary, annual sessions, an interdisciplinary dialogue strengthens theology and science as complements of each other. Both are luminaries that dispel the darkness on the pathway leading to knowledge encased in truth. Although new as to time, The Catholic Academy is ancient in the conceptual adherence to Christian tradition, industriousness, altruism, and loyalty to God.

Catholic Academicians are stalwart in resistance to this world's mischief, disbelief, and non-belief. As men/women of exceptional scholarship, they are disciplined, innovative, and challenging. Dedicated to the mighty task of preventing discord between the visible world of materialism and invisible spirituality their efforts are ceaseless. With vivid thoughts nurtured by fermenting intellectual brilliance they envision a world in which truthfilled knowledge serves humanity in multiple, diverse dimensions of daily life.

Many scientist are lukewarm about religion. Others are either outright atheists or outspoken agnostics. "Einstein was not a conventionally religious man, but he spoke often of a deep reverence for nature, a cosmic religious feeling" [Davies, 1999]. In the later years of his life he acknowledged credence in the Judeo-Christian tradition. "Many other scientists share Einstein's deep sense of awe for nature's mathematical elegance and sheer breathtaking ingenuity. For some, their research takes on the form of a spiritual quest" [Davies, 1999].

A minority of well-known scientists in *academia* pronounce the word God but they call themselves atheists and are aligned with Darwinism. Lesser celebrities in science have religious beliefs. There are a few Anglican and Catholic clergymen who are theologians and outstanding scientists. They are in the forefront fostering dialogue between them. History records that science was an offspring of theology. This proof is substantiated by the publications of *L'Abbé Lazzaro Spallanzani* in the 18th century, and many more clerics who are outstanding physicists, geneticists, and bioscientists in the subsequent centuries.

Many scientists[6] believed their research was a means of discerning God's creations as they sought understanding of divinity. "The term natural theology was used by those who sought evidence for God in the processes of nature, in contrast to divine revelation" [Davies, 1999].

Theology and science became antipodal in the 19th century [1859] with the Darwinian uproar attended upon the publication of *The Origin Of Species*. Neither did Darwin nor the anthropological scientists of that century perceive the great antagonism religion would have against this theory until it eventuated. No matter the materialistic attitude perceived, scientists are unable to deny that the natural order of the universe has rational intelligibility even if they lack faith in God. Many scientists may not admit it but the convergence of science and religion may overcome this reticence.

The division between metaphysics and pure science is shortening although there is a great hesitancy to bring theology totally into the bosom of universal science. This is a reason why bioethical standards are not accepted with firmness, adherence, and without questioning. Ethics is neither arbitrary nor absurd. Validity is its strongest supporting structure which is amalgamated with the gift of faith in divinity.

Predicting science and religion will merge at some future date is not plausible. In general scientists are skeptics, challengers, doubters, and give little credence to what is unseen, neither identifiable nor tangible. Contrarily religionists are open-minded to accepting very much on faith. The closer science comes to religion the less will it ridicule spiritual longing for God and learn that faith is not negotiable.

An appropriate *caveat* is that many modern scientists whose writings and lectures sound religious but on close, meticulous examination are revealed to be no different from those of other scientists who are atheists. What they do is misuse language and redefine words as they compose a vocabulary of scientific and religious terms. "Goodenough happens to be a biologist, but this [her] kind of neo-Deistic pseudoreligion is

---

6. Galileo, Kepler, Newton and others. In his excellent book Professor James J. Walsh MD of Fordham university includes chapters on ecclesiastic scientists to be noted. Among them are Copernicus, Basil Valentine [a founder of chemistry, Linacre [physician and ordained priest], Father Kircher, Bishop Stensen [anatomist and father of geology], Abbé Hauy [father of crystallography, and Abbot Mendel [one of the founders of genetics]. Book listed in bibliography.

more often associated with physicists. In [Hawking's] case, I hasten to insist, the accusation is unjust. His much-quoted phrase, 'the mind of God', no more indicates belief in God than my saying, 'God knows!' as a way of indicating I don't. I suspect the same of Einstein invoking 'dear Lord' to personify the laws of physics. Paul Davies, however, adopted Stephen Hawking's phrase as the title of a book that went on to earn the Templeton Prize for Progress in Religion, the most lucrative prize in the world today" [Dawkins, 1999]. These are only a few samples of the search for God by scientists who try to mold religion to suit their own tastes because they are unable to accept the existing dogmas.

When moving beyond the realm of, and the comprehension of science, there are some ponderous questions about the cosmos that science does not answer. "The mistake is to think they are therefore beyond religion, too" [Dawkins, 1999]. Is this a secret confession that scientists believe in God? If it is so it is not equivalent to religion and science embracing each other. But it does mean that scientists no longer believe it is unthinkable and not permissible to speak openly of the integration of science with spirituality. Does this signify science will find God?—perhaps.

What is visible is that there is dialogue and communication between scientists and theologians. Many scientists in their research efforts and conclusions are not reticent to state their work does not deny theology but is "complimentary to the human religious quest. . . Both astronomy and biology are now being advanced by many scientists as religiously significant" [Clayton, 1999].

"Many scientists still see the crusade against religious belief as an obligation. Darwin made it possible to be an intellectually fulfilled atheist touts Oxford zoologist Richard Dawkins. . . Modern biology has been cleansed of divine purpose. . . But for every Dawkins, one finds a religious scientist who sees in the structure of the cell or the distribution of galaxies some evidence of the creative hand of God" [Clayton, 1999]. This is no indication that there will be an ultimate unification of science with theology. Contentment currently can be derived from the present flow of scientific knowledge that evokes a religious response to the astronomic discoveries of the magnitude, beauty, and orderliness of the universe.

At various junctures over the centuries, historians have written with askewed, personal input on the antagonism that has existed between science and theology. Intellectual allometric[7] development did not allow their drawing together with mutual understanding and reflexive appreciation. Comprehension of each was not totally conducive to annotated disrespect mutually shared with inequality. This was further accentuated by science's failure to recognize that it, like theology, seeks the ultimate truth. Of equal notice was the unwillingness of both to meet on the plethora of occasions propitiously available.

The furnaced fires that blaze upward with shady smoke engulfing science and religion are refueled by academic atheists in strategic, influential faculty positions at prestigious international universities. Prejudice does not permit the discernment that science and religion's common goal is truth. Harmony between them is difficult because of towering influential professors whose delight is to importune religion. Pleasure is derived for them in this iconoclasm which psychologically is noted as *schadenfreude*.[8]

Building of a sincere science-religion relationship is in the making as each is becoming more tolerant of the other. Each has a key objective to be an incentive for cooperation for which both are qualified. As high-styled, competent planners they can prompt themselves adequately to arrive at satisfactory solutions. No longer is science playing checkers and religion playing chess on the same *oui-ja*[9] board. Now their criticisms of each other have mellowed to wan, languid, gentle corrections. Random thought proposes that God, religion, ethics, morality, and science will eventually be a meshed network. Permanent, correct ethical conduct in science can be anticipated by this cooperative integration which will disallow every scientist to be his own Boswell.[10]

---

7. Allometry is the relative growth of a part in relation to an entire organism. Intimated here is that the intellect did not reach full maturity simultaneously as the body.

8. German noun for pleasure in the unhappiness of other people.

9. *Oui-ja* is a trademark for a board with the alphabet and other symbols on it, and a planchette [small triangular moving board] that is thought, when touched with the finders, to move in such a way as to spell out spiritualistic and telepathic messages on the board. Derived from the French *oui*, yes plus the German *ja*, yes.

10. Boswell means an assiduous and devoted admirer, scholar, and recorder of another's words and deeds. After James Boswell [1740-1795], Scottish lawyer, writer, and biographer of Samuel Johnson.

The performance philosophy of morally correct, determined, honorable, respected bioethicists is rooted in the spiritual understanding of human persons. Those who reserve their hearts entirely for spirituality renounce firm attachment to temporal things. This is a witness to the acceptance that only God can satisfy the human heart with lasting, genuine, joyous contentment with fulfillment. With this recognition the realization is attained that demonstrates fidelity to humanity's true vocation.

Applicable to bioscientists this same fidelity is pertinent. With its proper place assumed there will be attained that dimension of bioscience which illustrates its true purpose toward the acquisition of natural perfection. Then bioethics will receive its own merited acknowledgement and not be looked upon as a deuteragonist to bioscience.

When bioscientists try to muzzle the suggestions, requirements, and demands of bioethics, bioscientific educational norms are plunged toward decadence. Once fallen, not even moral justice, social docility, and scientific apology will be powerful enough to return it to where it belongs. Because the concrete, collaborating unity of faith and fidelity has been demortarized into pulverization.

Religion, Science, And Population Control

Bioethics is placed in a rear compartment when discussions arise on population control at the World Health Organization, the United Nations, other international, and national benevolent organizations. In China there is the most horrific population control program in the world. No historic period has recorded such denial of human rights with its brutality, wickedness, and draconian immorality. Officials of the Chinese government take pregnant women from their homes and families as if they are criminals. Locked up like prisoners they are forcibly aborted and sterilized even when they are in the final month of pregnancy.

Outbursts against such atrocities are infinitesimal in the United States and no contrary voice is heard arising in other countries in the western and occidental world. This indifference is compounded when overpopulation propaganda has persuaded many high-ranking government officials that limiting every woman to one child is a good idea. Sad to relate, United States tax dollars are used to fund population control programs. Slaughter of the innocent not only is an ethical violation, it is contrary to God's Commandment, Thou shalt not kill. Government population controllers are not exempt from this divine law in China, Latin America, Africa, Asia, and elsewhere.

Anti-natal policies in the United States are wicked just as they are in foreign lands where human rights abuses are committed in the name of population control. The justifying excuses are both myths and mistaken theories which emphasize that economic prosperity is impossible with population growth. Basically a control of population is a war against helpless people under the deception that prolific people are the poorest producing a threat to the well-being, advancement, and peace in their own nations.

Accentuating the evil is that economic assistance is conditioned on the acceptance of the anti-birth policy. Unjustly the poor are the targets of population control. "More and more, the United States and other countries inform the poor all over the world not to feed their hungry children, but to keep from having children who might one day be hungry [Mosher, 1999]. A review and analysis of worldwide population control activity labels it as unethical, immoral, contrary to religious teaching, and nature.

"Credible statistics show that the world is better able now than ever before to feed and clothe today's populations, and many more to come. In fact, the statistics also show that the real problem facing the world today is not overpopulation, but underpopulation. At the present time, 61 countries around the world are having too few children to maintain their current populations. Yet the mainstream media and pro-population control groups like Planned Parenthood have bilked millions of Americans into believing that limiting families to one or two children—or even no children—is necessary, even virtuous. We are surfeit with hearing that the world is overpopulated, that there's not enough food to go around, or that a massive world famine is just around the corner. The doomsayers who spread these lies would rather abort, sterilize, and contracept people than respect them for what they are: our greatest resource. People are an asset, not a burden" [Mosher, 1999].

The foundation of the United States of America is a covenant, the Declaration of Independence. It commits its citizens of every generation to work for, not against, the right to life, liberty, and the pursuit of happiness. Charged with these responsibilities, we are remiss in this duty if no effort is made to object strenuously against population control aimed at the "least of our brethren."

Specific, special authority for the solution of human ethical questions regarding biotechnologic, demographic, and other medicolegal impasses is not the indispensable right of attorneys, politicians, the clergy, and biological scientists. The obligation belongs to all disciplines plus many other learned persons. These include philosophers, ethicists, and the educated laity. As a universal, communal duty dispersed among them, with an especial responsibility placed on attending physicians, it begets a shared mutual obligation to decide the multifaceted bioethical conundrums which are foreseeable in this twenty-first century that has arrived and is moving onward rapidly.

Chapter 37

Bioethics And Moral Theology

Engraved in stone is the validation of bioethics by Greco-Roman, Hebraic, and Christian theology. This moral code may be amended, added to, improved but never discarded. The strength of bioethics is that it does not accommodate to alternatives, images, impressions, near-truths, hyperbole, and embellishment. Within its immobility no duplicity and dissimulation can survive. Bioethics is stupendous in its overtness, overwhelming in its directness, superb in straightforwardness, and is stated with positive conviction. Uncompromising in its rejection of mundane materialism bioethics is a reflection of active Christianity.

The truth of Christianity needs no public relation advertisement. "It is an amazing fact that we celebrate 2,000 years of a faith now shared by more than two billion people, which was founded by an unknown man of poor family who came from a much despised part of what was a backward province of the Roman Empire" [Johnson, 1999].

"Jesus of Nazareth could read and write and he knew the scriptures. But he had no special training in evangelism. No resources whatever, and the men he called to follow him were illiterate fishermen or, like Matthew, from unpopular trades such as tax-gathering. The ablest of them, Saint Paul, was a tent-maker. . . Yet within a few decades it [Christianity] had set the world of antiquity ablaze, and its flames continue to flicker in the hearts of men and women across the world" [Johnson, 1999]. Christianity with its teachings of moral goodness, ethical virtue, honesty, and love is the greatest long-distance runner of history whose efforts are winning the race and the eternal prize.

Adherence to Christian principles does not allow deviation from bioethical standards founded on its basic rules. In bioscience there is a population segment whose ideology tolerates deceit, guile, and worships greed. Concealed ineptitude idealizes untruth. Hideous in essence it is hidden by silent acquiescence. Christian bioethics abhors all this as it is bound to moral theology. Therefore there can be no bowing simpering to the evil mundane, monster of materialism.

But it remains difficult to think of bioethical dogmatists encountering contrarians who disagree with the concept that moral battles are fought best by theologians. Public discourses on bioethics sometimes utter ethical positions that are bent to serve the speaker even if it alters truth. Purposefully any synchronism between moral theology and bioethics is avoided assiduously. Rarely is it popular to listen to the voice of religion in discourses on bioethics. Theologians and religious scholars are considered fanatic, non-scientific, and theologically one-sided. Often embarrassed theologians shrink from these assignments. Much is lost when bioethics is deprived of a religious input on delicate topics.

Extreme uses of bioscience threatens rationality and objectivity when progress is the *via vitae medicinae*.[1] In the name of progression immorality can be discounted easily. "There is readily apparent evidence that religion provides bioethics a missing ingredient. . . Consistently despite the ubiquitous faith in secularity, pleasure, and science, there is a persistent yearning to see a moral, meaningful trajectory in one's private life, in one's workplace, and in the social goals of the state. Religion persists in asking about goals, ultimate meanings, and long-term consequences—religion insists on the question of moral meaning in the way that science insists on the question of replicable physical data. . . The systemic theology of science is quite powerful; tantalizing not only to the clinician, but also to the ethicist. It takes a serious regard for religious faith to remind us that our faith in science and philosophy alone may leave us unfulfilled" [Zoloth, 1999].

In its final interpretative purpose bioethics is expository of the final teachings of Judeo-Christian-Muslim moral codes. With many mainstream debates anticipated over central moral issues in medicosurgical research, clinical care of patients, not-fully-explained, and undisclosed proposed scientific intentions, these teachings are not to be dismissed.

The fundamental, common-ground, overarching carapace of all three religions is an admonition to preserve the moral integrity that is consis-

1. Medicine's way of life.

tent with the *dicta* found in the Bible and the Koran. As is contemporary civil life, the world of bioscience has become very complicated. With the complexity is confusion wherein may be lost totally the already weakened sense of bioethics. Busy with an intricate bioscientific *prospectus*, sensitivity to morality as an essential component to the project may be ignored. Threatened is disrepair of responsible bioethics. Under this circumstance some bioscientists may not "fulfill the true purpose of their vocation—glorifying God in service to others" [Rae and Wong, 1996].

Uncomfortable as it may seem to some bioethicists to think moral theologians are trespassing on their territory, they are not to be ignored if the most treasured concepts of bioethics are to be preserved. Christian moral theologians are always advocates for strangers, prodigal children, the powerless, and the abandoned. Bioscience has thoughts on euthanasia, physician-assisted suicide, medicalized death, and pre-birth abortion. God's Commandments of love and justice can never allow these grievous actions. Historical tradition scorns the society that abandons these Sinaitic, Mosaic laws. Bioethics is the voice of these commandments in the bioscientific communities. By dint of distributive justice moral medicine must be active, vociferous, and credible in a world that needs humility, charity, understanding, and good-will.

By their works are they known. Bioethicists by their good deeds can bridge theory with theology and bring morality where it was not and enter those scientific disciplines primarily atheistic.[2] This will lessen the tension that is fomented by those scientists who believe and teach that Christianity opposes science with the additional concept that ethics and science are incompatible. From a pensive viewpoint bioethics is a coming together of scientific inquiry, morality, and theology. Ethics also is a source for ecclesiastics to be informed of progress in the biosciences, technology, ecology, and other scientific endeavors. Bioethicists are in the forefront of organizers of centres for the study of science and religion on many university campuses.

---

2. "Many, if not most, in the 4.9 million-member scientific community tend to be atheists." Statement by Robert Royal, a Catholic scholar author of "The Virgin and the Dynamo" [quoted by Larry Williams listed in bibliography]. He states "Members of the National Academy of Sciences are almost all disbelievers, while only 40 percent of those listed American Men and Women of Science believe in God and an afterlife."

Moral teaching in bioscience must be ongoing even when facing dissent. Intellectual currents of dissent can be made attractive as they undermine traditional ethical values. Theories are advanced to justify, excuse, and/or bolster scientific acts that are contrary to natural law. Traditional moral doctrine is turned aside by anthropological presuppositions and ethical presumptions. Even degrading situations that are intrinsically evil [abortion, euthanasia, assisted-suicide] find defenders even though they are disgraceful and are a blotch on civilization. Responsibility is denied for unethical conduct under the subjective approach to morality sustained by behavioral scientists.

Doubts and objections to moral bioethics is a way to an elimination of theology in its structure which will make it less absolute and authoritative. Thus immoral acts may be justified if the consequences are good [consequentialism] or if the acts bring about a "greater good" through a lesser evil [proportionalism]. [Pope John Paul II's encyclical, "Veritatis Splendor."] Moral theology and bioethics are not derived from a democratic policy. Its laws are not determined by consensus, and ethical teachings are not according to human practices.

Divine natural law and the Ten Commandments are inchoate to bioethics. The universality and permanent validity of its precepts are for all people, at all times, and in all places. Bioethics in conjunction with moral theology forbids certain kinds of behavior. Whatever is offensive to human dignity is not permissible under the moral code of bioethics which is the subordination of bioscientific actions, procedures, and research to the preservation of the harmony between God and humanity.

Epilogue

Leave axes, books, and picks,
    Instruments of woe,
The scythe[1] of time, with deadlier tricks,
    To line the borders of the Styx[2]
Too soon will bring them low.

John De La Fontaine [1621-1695]
in his appeal to the woodman.

On occasion dramatic literature vividly portrays the lavish, picturesque scene of victorious Julius Caesar [100-44 BC] poised as the general who conquered the known world. Nearly bursting with pride he rides in a filigreed, elegant, resplendent chariot pulled by two virile, caparisoned, white steeds. With verdant laurel-wreath on his regal head, he listens to the excited, cheering, boisterous populace. *Ave Rex, Imperator Maximus*[3] rang in his ears incessantly. His ornamental toga ruffles in the breeze touching his smiling face. More exhilarating than the roar of the multitude is his alertness to the dynamic, tingling joy of the occasion that runs engagedly throughout his responsive, erect, military body.

Behind the monumental warrior standing like a statue is an oracular servant-scrivener whispering discretely into the master's attuned left ear: Remember Caesar, thou art mortal. Applicable to all humanity, this is often forgotten by persons in high social strata, political positions, and

---

1. Symbol for old-man father-time
2. In Greek mythology, the Styx is one of the rivers of Hades across which Charon, the boatsman, ferried the souls of the dead.
3. Translation is Hail King, Greatest Emperor.

the noble professions. *Forsan et haec olim meminisse invabit*[4] [Perhaps at some time it will aid you to remember these things].

Modern bioengineering has eliminated the need of the human uterus for the origin of conception. Every human being still grows in the womb. Bioscience may be contemplating an artificial incubator to supplant the anatomic structure. With this success the grandiose next step will be to strive for physical immortality. Then there will be no need to be mindful of mortality. The scientific world believes there is no limit to its ability. "The reverential attitude toward the womb, however, has changed in recent years. New reproductive technologies have been an important factor in bringing about this change. As the incubator replaces the womb, the vice of alienation replaces the virtue of compassion" [De Marco, 1999]. And so goes the decline and fall of bioethics as the personal touch falls into oblivion during the onward march of technology that replaces God.

There are many advocates of artificiality in bioscience who believe it is superior to nature. An argument is presented "that an embryo developing outside the body can be more easily monitored for birth defects and, eventually, for desirable gene patterns. He [Asimov] also endorses this type of gestation because it would help women gain an important measure of equality with men. If a woman could, as he puts it, "extrude the fertilized ovum for development outside the body, she would then be no more the victim of pregnancy than a man is'" [De Marco, 1999]. "Grossman predicts that the time will come when natural pregnancy will become an anachronism and the womb will shrink to appendix-like proportions" [De Marco, 1999].

With these thoughts floating in the minds of scientists, will there be a time when girls, teenagers, and women can choose to be superovulated? Their eggs can be collected, frozen, and thawed out later. Whenever they decide upon the time, the process of artificial fertilization and incubation can begin. Such progeny will have a newly established category which to some equates with pathophysiological distortion and the psychological grotesque.

Ongoing changes in bioscientific thought has approached a critical juncture with bioethics. This leads to a continuation of the intensive

---

4. Spoken by Dido, a Tyrian princess founder of Carthage, to Aeneas, hero of Trojan War in the Latin, classical, epic poem 'Aeneid' by Publius Vergilius Maro [70-19 BC].

debate on what is permissible, what is questionable, and what is impermissible. Just because a biological procedure is feasible technically, does not *ipso facto* mean it is sanctioned ethically and morally. Having had many current challenges, the future augurs for more serious, profound, sensitive, and ethically critical decisions to be made.

At this time poignant debates are anticipated since the accelerated technological advances are outdistancing ethical vigilance. The separating distance will increase as the expanding, contemplated bioscientific research has no commitment to bioethics. This is proven by the geometric rise in assisted reproductive technology. In 1999 there were about 50,000 embryos in various cryobanks distributed over the various geographical states. These are in storage for distribution for use within 5-6 years which is the limitation on preservation. There is no doubt they will be utilized before the expiration date when one considers that in 1997 there were 24,000 babies born by *in vitro* fertilization [Nathanson, 2000]. Geneticists are running wild in their quiet laboratories.

In this new millennium effort must be energized to prepare new ways and means to sustain moral and ethical principles as a necessary element in the framework of science. No reason can be given for an escape from this responsibility. Bioscientists of moral reputation do not disengage ethical duties from their work if it is to resonate with admirable acceptance. Reconceptualization of the relationship between bioscience and bioethics may be necessary to verify that moral concerns are of the highest priority.

A mentally healthy bioscientific society finds its roots in vigorous moral dicta that originate in religious faith. Upon which the good life patterns are formed into a culture that gives meaning, dignity, and purity to it. Bioethics has within its core religious traditions. Many of the laws adopted by civilized nations stem from religious teachings. Such laws are constitutional and acceptable as serving secular needs and purposes. Discussions on bioethical issues from a variety of perspectives do not endorse a particular religion. The religious infusion disallows watered-down ethical concepts which are worse than none at all. Because the latter may sanction that which is prohibited by all religions—a lamentable, improvised evil.

Sociologists whose specialty is not religion distinguish between belief and knowledge in their discussions on morality. "Some things I know, and some things I believe . . . Generally speaking I do not have to believe what I know . . . statements express strong convictions but not indisputable evidence" [Berger, 1999]. Left unsaid was the result of this concept. Does it give an excuse for ethical divergences and dismiss both faith and belief which are human acceptances in morality, ethics, and character-building. Granted faith and belief are not identical and not strictly synonymous. Faith is more subjective than objective. Belief is arrived at intellectually whereas some aspects of faith are a divine gift beyond ordinary comprehension. Most supernatural tenets are not within the grasp of the human intellect. It is not always easy for human beings to possess true faith and honest belief in God because the world has forceful methods that foster disbelief and make it easy to deny faith.

Living a life of good reputation, admirable character, true value, and unbending morality is difficult in the modern world of excitement, desire, ambition, and self-gratification. Hence few are receptive to the return of traditional ethical conduct whose repetition is a deference to precise rectitude. Bioethics has its own resonance, absoluteness with a philosophic relativeness to medicine that is historical and uncomplicated. There is no ancient past associated record that links medicine to economic gain, therefore it is tenuous bioethically.

Noted in recent decades is the change in bioscientific thinking that has been influenced by financial persuasion. Physicians have been distracted by the dominating attention given to commercialism in their professional activities. Unfortunately many bioscientists are blinded to the adverse consequences that are inclusive with commercialism as it carries with it another dimension to medicine. Biotechnology is a contributor to money-matters in this profession unskilled in finance. Highly touted, meagerly understood it has not added either to medicine's respectability or pristine image.

The bioethicist has another burden to bear in regard to business matters in the biosciences. At all times and under all circumstances bioethicists must be trusted advisors to patients, colleagues, and every person who seeks their counsel. As goodwill distributors of moral decisions they contribute to the establishment of a firm ethical code without easing of verisimilitude standards which would be an innate folly.

How much and to what degree finance influences science is not determinable with extreme accuracy. However certain policies seem to suggest there is some persuasion from this source. An example is the bioengineering of foods. At Food and Drug Administration hearings scientific and biotechnology industry officials staunchly support genetically engineered crops. Alliances for biotechnology groups support genetically altered foods. Persistence remains even when opposition claims that "genetically engineered organisms released into the environment pose risks that are potentially irreversible, untraceable, and uncontrollable" [Barboza, 1999]. Science is no longer an autonomous entity. Instead it is a stressed interplayer in the economic, social, ethical forces in modern culture. At the same time, particularly in studies of biotechnology there is an emphasis on economics at the expense of bioethics.

The influence of economics, the social sciences, and politics have had a greater persuasion on bioethics, medical thinking, and practice than is realized. The consequences of the interaction between biomedicine and these influences have major significance for the moral, ethical, and healthful future of modern society. Because it is feared that highly technical biomedicine is becoming less humanistic without understanding the social relations of health to morality.

An interrogatory is the formidable assault society has made on healthcare. Socialization of which is an aim of sociologists who are not trained in medicine and have no experience in its practice. They attack the present medicosurgical system in all its components including its knowledge, its teachings, scholastic methods of education, organization, political power, and lobbying influence. The friendliness between the sociologic-scientific relationship has become estranged. This may be illustrative of the perspective potentiality of biomedicine and the current socioeconomic culture to be at odds in determining professional behavior toward social transition which at present is an unresolved paradox [Porter, 1997]. From a morality viewpoint it has been written: "As political and economic freedom diminishes, sexual freedom can compensatorily be increased" [Aldous Huxley, 1932].

The notion of compassion has adulterated bioethics. A great deception has inveigled itself into morality under the cloak of sympathetic empathy that has diluted ethical structures to a weakness that is inexcusable. This has given rise to a falsehood that compassion is a moral principle itself with primacy over all others. In its proper place compassion is a virtue but it is not an ethical mandate. Compassion becomes a persuading force when difficult moral problems are to be resolved by lukewarm bioethicists. Reference is made to those bioscientists who follow policies that lead to popularity, acclaim, and awards *via* political correctness. Thus abortion is legal, euthanasia is practiced in some geographical locations, and unmonitored bioengineering continues. Compassionate excuses are given to justify the alienation of ethics from bioscience. To undermine motherhood by abortion that converts the womb into a tomb is to turn off the fountainhead of compassion. Killing of innocent babies is not an act of compassion for the mother's feelings, social situation, and/or economic status. Compassion is an expression of love motivated by wishing good to another.

Loss of moral sense in research science, biomedicine, law, diplomacy, politics, commercial enterprises, personal lifestyle, and intimate relationships is pervasive. Having their origins in curiosity and skepticism, some new research enterprises have brought forth the question: Is it as desirable a development as some bioscientists seem to think it is? Moreover when some animal experiments are applied to human beings they challenge grossly the asseverated morality and ethical high-values of a proper society. Both simple and complex bioscientific undertakings require much circumspection when probability does not justify their accomplishment.

Accompanying this is the waning of religion, impedimented judgment, and multiple variations on the theme of inquisitiveness. Indubitably all contribute to ethical decadence. Simultaneously there is a recognizable rise in superstition and heterodox cultism. Attached to which is no common-sense concept of aesthetic spirituality so reminiscent of the alchemy and magic of the 16th and 17th centuries.

Science and technology give such instant results that human beings have been spelunking themselves when immediate and visible outcomes are not expected. Long-term benefits of ethical behavior and moral stability are not always immediate but result after more than one episode of spiritual goodness. To many this is through religion. The Dalai Lama [Tenzin Gyatso] believes it is easier to put ancient wisdom into modern ethics within the structure and rituals of a religion. Although he stresses that religion is not a necessary prerequisite for leading a good life. But "His ethical promulgations do not allow us to do without the basic spiritual qualities" [Anderson, 1999].

Threateningly the constant emerging technology is redefining bioethics. Changing is the quality of moral standards as technology harnesses the new resources of burgeoning learning and by utilizing its productivity to alter fundamental, natural biology. The new bioengineering supposedly was to simplify. But in fact it made many complexities. Some newly designed perfervid permissibles are the springboard for injustice that rambles undetectedly, as it destroys old-time ethics. The old standards are indicted as chastened legislature that subverted bioscience.

Sciences merited redemption from restrictions contained in an environment of religious paranoia mixed with stringent puritanical, turbulent Christianity is applauded by most scientists.

Encouraged by agnosticism, the jiggling of bioethics is from the well-upholstered clique who benefit from the change in some substantial way. They do not put people before a personal ideology that commands the publicity limelight with patent signs of its undeterminate continuance. This is so, even though their ethics is neither faithful to natural law nor has meticulous adherence to the dicta of Hippocrates and suggest a forced awkwardness in composition. Medical history verifies that original bioethics died two world wars ago when enthusiasm for change overawed the pleasantry of respect that chanted "off with the old, on with the new." Official bioethics as an honorable symbol is not always worth caring about to some bioscientists. Therefore it is easily eliminated as an unnecessary moral venture.

Those who have been educated into scholastic respectability as bioscientists have the moral duty as well as the responsibility of intellectuals to seek, sustain, and be engrossed in truthfully oriented bioethics. In truth is found the splendor of wisdom. Because of its radiance, medicine like philosophy has the unavoidable obligation to form honest thoughts and create marvelous ideas that guide the world's direction into right channels as part of its vocation in accordance with its innateness.

Most scientists are adept at compartmentalization in their professional activity. They enjoy each new challenge, every new result, each new device presented, and every new theory under review. Rarely do they think beyond. This is a probable explanation, not a reason, how in the name of science, they can launch immoral experiments. It is disturbing ethically "when scientists lose touch with their humanity in the single-minded pursuit of scientific advancement . . . brilliant minds miss the ethical markers along the way—sometimes even to their own detriment . . . [a] scientist, so caught up in the thrill of science that he treated atomic physics like a parlor game. . . While much scientific research today may be carried out ethically, the exceptions can still fly below the radar" [Welsome, 1999 and reviewer of the author's book, Deborah Nelson].

Pioneering perserverances of biomedicine are not to be minimized as progress and substantial achievements. But it has aroused some discordance between biological research and bioethics. At the top of the divergence is scholarship and vocationalism versus religion and morality. Future medical historians may wonder why research bioscientists risked the warm relationship formerly enjoyed between biomedicine and professional ethical conduct. The varied attitudes toward religion by the general public has found a *nidus* in the sciences. The *nexus* has become attenuated in a relaxation of previously promulgated codes which are seen as either decadent or outdated. Hence science has no crucial rôle in promoting bioethics as an awareness against the dangers of its loss. A considerable proportion of the bioscientific population is not concerned with bioethics as they are addicted to the profits from research and the revenues it generates [Lock, Reynolds, Tansey, 1998].

Colleagues are often subjected to vituperation because of the immoral acts and palter of other bioscientists. The strange disjunction between ethical propriety and personal dislike is not a great distance. Factually, not incidentally is the opprobrium heaped upon the bioscientific profession as illustrated by the many liability lawsuits of the past, present, and future. Under the eagle-eye scrutiny of lawyers bioscientists are interrogated for verification of records, certification of ability, and not for sanctification. These notable changes have taken place in response to present day social contextual pressures that underscore the thinking on health care. Questioning the authority of biomedicine as a policy-maker in its own discipline has demoralized the people who serve in it [Mooij, 1998].

Moral disorder in biomedicine arises in the biosciences ranging from simple blood transfusion to bioengineering. Technology is to support biological functions, not change them. It appears technology dictates ethical conduct as it seems to have overcome sociobiology. Important is knowing when to do something and when to retreat from doing it. The feasibility of which is not the ultimate indication for its performance. Bioscientists have an ethical obligation to refrain from doing things simply because they have the knowledge to do them if they are immoral.

For the biosciences ethics is their guiding light to reach the apogee of perfection. Bioethics separates good science from bad science. It reenforces traditional dogma as promulgated by past bioscientists of excellent moral merit. Thus goodness in the laboratory is separated from evil. Within the meridian of bioethics is preserved the sphere of patterns that are real, reliable, regulatory, and righteous.

In its moral movements bioethics defends the good as its mission by adherence to its principles and abhorrence of what is not good. The existence of misconduct is not discerned easily as it is disclosed in other non-scientific professions. Furthermore it is not expected from physician, surgeons, and bioresearchers. By inheritance they are the pacesetters for establishing moral codes of professional behavior which taught respect for duties, obligations, and responsibilities. Perhaps it was because they believed with Albert Einstein [1879-1955] his memorable aphorism:

> Science without religion is lame;
> religion without science is blind.

The whirlwind developments in medical technology and surgical technique have made it most impracticable for ordinary people to understand that physicians and surgeons are not miracle workers. In turn some medical scientists do not discourage this misbelief. Failing in the application of metaphysical norms to the mandatory standards of their profession they encourage the falsity. A world spellbound by fame, notoriety, glamor, mechanization, and money easily subordinates human dignity to these alluring enticements.

Deceptive trickery is rampant in those persons motivated for the wrong purpose. Shallow arguments of pseudo-science and pseudo-sociology are used to sustain actions that are intrinsically and philosophically not genuine. Hypocritical munificence can be a device to accommodate those who lack even a minuscule of the anthropic component. An integral element in bioscience is adherence to impeccable conduct which is its luminous beauty worthy of emulation.

Misbehavior by any subterfuge wears down slowly, but resolutely, the glorious reputations and illuminating character of the scientific professions. Honorable scientists of every genre renounce unconditionally anything that brazenly distorts morality, ethics, and the time-honored laws that have guided them since the Hippocratic era.

Spectacular research in genetics, reproductive medicine, cloning, and organ transplantation has acclaimed bioscientists with stunning recognition. Such medical advances have triggered diffuse, mixed reactions concerning probable risks inherent to these remarkable endeavors. Appended to which is the threat of bioethical transgressions. Thus has arisen hidden complexities that question the unrestrained usage of this gained knowledge.

Among the thought-provoking topics that ruffle the tranquil biomedical scene are the following for ethical evaluation.

1. Manipulation of the genetic makeup of children that could be passed on to future generations;
2. Cloning of human beings; and
3. Bioengineering.

Powerful probabilities in these research areas can place bioscientists on a slippery slope downward. Many bioethical issues confront them which are not to be ignored categorically.

Of necessity this state of bioscientific recognition has given bioethics a resurgence as a reaction to erratic biological experimentation and excessive medical technology. These research endeavors have questioned the motivation of bioscientists which in turn raises character questions of the participants. Defects in moral character are reflected in the propulsive force that is ponderous in ethical choices.

Decades ago British opinion poll ranked the medical profession first in trustworthiness with a 75 percent rating. Other trust ratings were 55 percent for judges, 23 percent for lawyers, 7 percent for civil servants, six percent for cabinet ministers [including all politicians and parliamentarians]. Journalists and those in electronic media were given 4 percent for trustworthiness and dependability as to factual truth. Present-day health-care providers of every genre should try to recoup and strengthen this confidence so that once again the biomedical profession may enjoy and regain the privilege of service to humanity with acknowledged, faithful reliability.

Thus the bioethical decisions made by bioscientists will be virtuous ones that are habitual dispositions to perform actions that are in accord with fidelity to trust, justice, integrity, and self-effacement. This demands courage and the probability of severe destructive criticism. Adherence to these virtues beget principles that are a phronesis.[5]

Health care is and must be a social good rendered to fulfill a human need. Because of this requisite it is not to be manipulated to reap profits. Legally and morally any misuse of medical ability is degradation of this

---

5. "Phronesis is the capacity to discern what moral choice or course of action is most conducive to the good in a given set of circumstances. It embodies prudence, the link between the intellectual, moral, and supernatural virtues. Fortitude-courage is said to be the hardest to practice in today's environment. Justice is the only concept that is both virtue and principle" [Pellegrino and Thomasma, 1993]

aptitude. Bioscientists have the obligation to be aware of the distinction between what is a moral requirement [the preservation of life] and what is a moral option [to select ordinary over extraordinary health care].

Cloning of human beings has stirred the commercial entrepreneurs who are expressing the financial gain to be gathered by this Dolly imitation. They do not indicate any choice in selecting who is to be cloned. If this process continued for many generations most human beings would look alike. Diversity of beautiful people would vanish. Life would lose its charm in the monotony of similarity. If clones became the majority population, would the rest become slaves?

Other advocates of cloning propel the plan that would concentrate on cloning a person's organs in test tubes. Keeping a set of spare organs cryophysiologically for future use in the event they are needed. This is a craving for those who cherish immortality. "In our desperate search for immortality we have come to see life as an obstacle to overcome. We have used every means at our disposal to fight the prospect of our own demise" [Nathanson, 2000]. Use and abuse of the magic of cloning is not without future hazards and ethical impurities.

Of all the majestic progresses in medicosurgical procedures, kidney transplantations are in greatest demand. Associated with this sought after urgency are many covert activities which are illegal, immoral, and horrendous. In far away India homeless people are murdered. Their kidneys are removed to be sold. The bodies are cremated and the ashes thrown into the Ganges River. Other people emigrate from their countries to go elsewhere to sell one of their kidneys. Eventually most of them become illegal immigrants. In an Asiatic country executed criminals have their kidneys removed which are sold to the highest bidder.

The United States of America is no exception to nefarious deeds in organ transplantations. In the 1980s a pathologist at a DC hospital was arrested for removing kidneys from cadavers soon after death. More recently federal agents searched the home of a Los Angeles man who allegedly advertised that he would arrange organ transplants for fees of \$125,000 to \$225,000. In the USA it is estimated that there are available 10,000 cadaveric kidneys for the more than 200,000 patients requiring transplants. All have end-stage renal disease awaiting to be recipients of a donor kidney.

Limited supply of cadaveric kidneys is far below the demand for these transplantable organs. The eagerness to acquire these renal organs has given rise to a hidden system of international commerce in various nations of the world. An example occurred in 1989. A Turkish peasant was flown to London to donate a kidney for $4,400 [Kinsley, 1989].

When any aspect of organ transplantation becomes a business for profit the altruism diminishes and the procedure is tainted with moral decay. Professionalism is erased quickly by commercialism. "The sale of human organs by donors living or dead is indefensible under any circumstances" [Merrell, 1971]. For this reason the USA, the UK, and other nations have outlawed the sale of human organs.

Crass, banal, and opportunistic commercialism encourages sinister practices that take advantage of death as a prologue in the grand cyclic stage of pseudo-beneficence. Subjecting bioscience to a futile, sectarian frenzy to sell human organs for financial profit is an egregious offense against humanity. Discomforting morally this is unethical deportment that degrades the once high-caliber practice of classical medicine.

Scholars are not impressed by strident calls from some scientific cabals who sanction with encouragement salvage of organs from executed criminals [Lu, 1998]. Overtures are heard by those bioscientists who abhor the reaping of organ harvests for financial gain.

With the adherence to modern relativism which pervades every stratum of modern society, it is not shocking to the flabby conscience that stealth of human organs flourishes. Little thought seems to be given that such practice is disordered and incompatible with accepted bioethical standards. Conventional thinking does not arouse fulgent opposition to this venture. To be vociferous against this practice does not appear to be a moral obligation of bioscientists. This is a reflection of current laxity that looks upon such criticism as an old-fashion and antediluvian. Because the moral climate is inundated with uncertainty, it has become sluggish with no noticeable shift toward any betterment.

Seriously grave ethical issues are faced by managerial bioscientists and bioengineers. They must possess innately prescribed core valued guidelines. These should be crystallized in written formats that are the basis for ethical decision-making. Embodied therein, as a supplementary, is needed a preorganized process that settles the conflict between scientific reality and ethical utility. In this hopefulness the critical imperative of arriving at honorable ethical conclusions is facilitated by scientists in this contemporary world of education that supposedly gives intellectual enlightenment.

Everyone engaged in mental pursuits could benefit from the reputation of the 1998 winner of the Nobel Prize in Medicine. Doctor Robert

Furchgott, 82, worthily he is characterized briefly in the New York Academy of Sciences Member Newsletter [Winter 1998-1999]. The last sentence of this written accolade is: In football, as in science, Furchgott is ever gracious, ever honest, and plays his heart out.

Legendary bravery, as recognized in this Nobel laureate, is an exigency in present day biomedical engineering and biomechanics. Even a person with the strongest resolve can be overcome under the forceful pressure of external, destructive, unethical forces. When internal morality is weak it is easily abandoned. Divinely-given strength must remain vibrant if one is not to succumb to ethical illiteracy.

Victory of goodness over addled evil is not universally customary. When it eventuates, difficulty arises as to which is paramount the unrehearsed admiration or the spontaneous astonishment. Eminently firm for principles of probity in barking against public sentiment, without even the slightest cavil, is a rarity. Where fortitude is strong, integrity is not weak. This conventional epithet applied to scientific heroes of yesteryear is like the Jurassic age. They are primitive.

Sartorily metaphoric, rueless evil is unpostured, shabbily dressed in a dark suit, furtively made odiferous by clouds of cheap cigar smoke that hides the face. Even so evil is still magnetic because it has the temptation promise of a sybaritic reward. Without this ephemeral superficial attraction wickedness is repulsive.

Goodness dressed in white robes stands erect regally as wafted incense rises upwardly from a bronze thymiaterion upon which it rests solidly. Goodness possesses the tremendous power of quality-giving which brings joy wherever it pervades.

In many instances some human beings have selected the abdication of reason to satisfy their desires. Hence they adopt utilitarianism and a theory of morality that is governance by selfishness. The modern world does not yearn for the old view of character which is a refutation of modernism, relativism, and free-expression. Exemplary influence that stimulates morally helpful ideas is found in a minority of people including bioscientists. The vanity and madness of foolish people are the majority.

Few are they who are inflexible in principle, zealous in humility, exacting in parochial, and distant good works that vibrate with divine appreciation. The world is on the brink of being lost. Too many people are living immorally. This causes the mental misery behind many shows of violence. Spiritual carelessness is expressed in a 19th century poem written by Richard Harris Barham [1788-1845].

> Oh! grief and despair
> I vow and declare
> What words can express
> The dismay and distress
> With many a moan
> and many a groan
> When incurring the fate
> Of the Master's hate.

Human systems that degrade morals, deal in sensitivity instead of sense, in caprice instead of reason, in darkness instead of light which lead to inferiority, naiveté, and disingenuousness. While in action human beings so afflicted think they know well all aspects of practical life. Hence they do not feel the shock of incongruity, and fail to recognize their duties and liabilities.

Medical History United With Bioethics

Since World War II's aftermath Germany has been striving to regain its 19th century prestige as a scientific community with high ethical excellence. Accompanying this anticipation the assertion is made that the disciplines of bioethics and medical history are to be intertwined. German medical historians have had a long-standing mutual admiration with engagements in the constructive debate on bioethics. Historians recall the great respect the western world had for German bioscientists in past generations. Hence teutonic medical historians have included bioethics in their research projects and teaching programs at universities.

In response to the question of relevance of one to the other, the answer is found in reference to seeking past experience which could contribute to the answering of current medicomoral problems. Bioethics in turn can profit from medical history that records how our medical ancestors solved with professional dignity and purity, the same or similar medical and ethical intricacies. From past medical history can be learned the criteria that permit the differentiation between appropriate and inappropriate decisions. Additionally it assists in the establishment of structural paradigms for bioethics as landmarks in medical history.

With such aid given right decision-making is facilitated. Concurrently the physician-patient relationship is enhanced which gives a favorable perspective to medico-social history [Toellner and Wiesing, 1997].

Medical History United With Bioethics in the curricula of German medical schools shows a promise of ethical revival in Europe. The North American continent does not demonstrate a similar enthusiastic rejuvenation. It is recognized that in the United States of America there are many excellent institutes of bioethics. Some are part of university post-graduate courses leading to a terminal degree. Others are not serving as centres for advanced studies in philosophy. Outstanding faculties teach the best moral principles. Unfortunately their voices are not heard by those who should listen. Whatever the American epitaph for the 20th century may be, it will not include fidelity to morality, a model for a way-of-life, adherence to gladdening, apodictic truth, and the infusion of the theological virtues of faith, hope, and charity into daily life.

Absent on the tombstone will be prudence. One author has called prudence the virtue of the golden mean. "Virtue stands in the middle between extremes. Prudence is the virtue active in the practical reason that facilitates finding a happy middle path. Prudence seeks to determine the moral truth of a proposed action. It answers [with immediacy] the question: is this action good or bad?" [Miller, 1990].

Prudence is elsewhere when notice is given to the shrill attacks launched against morality. Bioethical standards are ignored, altered, and discarded when prudence is absent. For neither morality nor bioethics has an obituary been written. A short time remains. The hurrier it passes, the behinder we get to see a renewal of morality and all its subdivisions. In this regard hours have become precious as they evaporate hastily. Not even updated, sophisticated technology is able to produce a time-saving apparatus. With the new century, perhaps, there will be an improvement in morality and desiderative, salubrious bioethical principles will flourish brilliantly.

The new millennium is the momentous time to design programs for indepth analysis of the most seriously important bioethical and medicolegal issues that must be settled. This is an historical era of medicosurgical changes, advanced bioscientific engineering, newer technology, and pharmaceutical productions. The range of controversial topics to be formalized into a salutary composite are broad but not too numerous that they are not countable. They are poignantly momentous because they will determine answers to life and death issues.

An apparent need is for the establishment of detailed, consistent bioethical standards that ensure with assurance that known issues have rational moral solutions. Among the requisites is adherence to the highest quality of moral terms for rendering medicosurgical service. As an exemplary strategic partnership among physicians, patients, and health care facilities, conclusions agreed to will provide an accessible, searchable archive for all concerned with doing what is right. These available, adopted criteria will diminish the frequency to revamp decisions on future bioethical questions.

Profiled subjects in the archival reservoir of answers would be the majority of medicosurgical challenges that experience has placed in the forefront. Accountability for decisions would be established. From these reformatted codes the authority for decisions will be derived. This reservoir of intelligence centralization would not permit picking and choosing answers that are not in accordance with the established dicta. Legal sanction would be a protective prevention against any disgruntled person who would seek to challenge what has been formulated, sanctioned, and accepted. That which has been endorsed will sustain the distinction between good ethics and the opposites. It is from such principles that medical excellence radiates. No mystery is there to know that unity of good medicosurgical research/practice and upright bioethics sustain each other. Both united are a dynamic force for good deeds subordinated only to God.

Bioethical responses to command moral decisions are not to be arrived at cursorily and should bear the *imprimatur* of justice and kindness. With these assets the highest quality of bioethics will possess confidently the verve to be the cultural icon of the biosciences throughout the third millennium.

Bioethics was born in the clinical practice of medicine and surgery—not in the laboratory. It arose from the interactivity of the physician-patient relationship. An ethical framework was developed which more specifically was clinical ethics. Now bioethicists require a much broader agenda that includes bioscientific research, genetic engineering, resource allocation, and prioritization. Also this involves the justice of healthcare systems, the distribution of health care, and the economics thereunto pertaining.

Ethical theorizing may survive when applied in the abstract to the right to health care. When prioritization and distribution of limited medicosurgical resources are to be decided, moral truth makes decision-making an ethical complexity. Danger lurks in the shadow of social determinating factors rather than bioscientific verity in selecting patients for therapy. Access to restricted healthcare demands serious bioethical considerations. Without bias conclusions are to be reached according to the highest moral criteria. Political correctness, manufactured philosophy, and empirical, unexplored theories are not to broaden to weakness the bioethical credo that experience proves to be sane, sound, and scientific.

Required is the fortifying of moral, ethical, social, and civic reawakening to this necessity. No consideration in this regard is to be given to any personal, political, and social gain. When ethics and morality are lost the world is troubled by chauvinism, jingoism, jihads, and ethnic cleansing. Loss of morality and ethics in physicians, bioscientists, and researchers will expose them to analogous perils from which there is no extrication.

Updated bioethics must stand firm against what is wrong. It is to be the clear, clean mirror that reflects the best in bioscience. Bioethics is the vehicle that carries the best assets of medical science. It is the master disciplinarian guarding the determination to pursue only goodness. At the same time it is the refuge from threats that when succumbed to, bring desolation to an elevated, high-level, unstinted, altruistic vocation.

Bioethics A Necessity

There is nothing more tragic in diminishing human dignity than to glorify unethical behavior as the accepted norm in an alert, educated society. Immoral deportment can neither be excused nor elevated to the plane of normalcy. Acceptance of these deviations erodes the higher faculties of the mind. Contemporaneously they disengage the supernatural matrix that sustains these intellectual traits which distinguish humankind from irrational, savage beasts.

No corporeal autogenous immunity exists against temptations that seduce into evil conduct. However the berm against immoral actions is discerned in the human spiritual defense system that is fortified by a discerning, discriminating conscience. In the specialized subjects of bioscience, it is incumbent upon medically trained persons to be in the forefront as advocates of proper ethical conduct. The perfection of an ethical code must emanate from the talents of bioscientists. Ethical guidance, practical training plus clinical/research experience lead to a firm scientific basis for the conclusions discerned.

Formulation of honorable bioethical parameters can not be the exclusive, self-acclaimed acquired domain of theorists of whatever origin. Physicians must have a vital rôle in guiding medical morality. In this way physicians will not be considered merely as providers of healthcare and patients will not be categorized as consumers.

The advancement of biological sciences in all phases depends upon serious research, imaginative inventions, astute observation, reliable documentation, and precise authentication of programmed preclinical studies. All these educational endeavors must have certain philosophical base lines as their leading spirit. These are moral stability, reliability, and untarnished adherence to truthfulness. Such sentimental refinements promulgate a strong commitment to the full score of an elevating medical *ethos*[6] from defined norms to professional attitudes. The aim of progressive, developmental advancement in medicine is not to obtain glamorous publicity. A more laudable goal is to do good with all those graces that goodness implies.

All bioscientists must not abandon the fundamental concept of monitoring themselves. With this self-appointed ombudsman the primary medical moral truths will prevail. Unworthy as it may be one recalls that it is an unpopular cause to teach etiquette, proper behavior, morality, and the need for ethical manners. A quatrain written by Don Marquis[7] explains this travesty very well.

For him who fain would teach the world,
The world holds hate in fee—
For Socrates, the hemlock cup;
For Christ, Gethsemane.

---

6. In Greek usage to indicate character to specific people, groups, and/or culture that sustain fundamental values and mores.

7. Donald Robert Perry Marquis [1878-1937] an American journalist and writer of prose and poetry; author of *Archy and Mehitabel* published in 1927.

Predictions

Moral intrangencies from ethical issues arise in everyday medicosurgical inhospital and outpatient practice. Multiple questions are thrust upon the physicians and surgeons who have no alternative but to decide (often with much haste) what to do in order to solve the bioethical problem at hand. Future medical practice will demand the ethical and legal obligation to warn patients against complications associated with their physical activities, contemplated biological engineering procedures, therapeutic expectations, and their rights of informed refusal or consent. Among these new imperative categories mandating a physician's obligated duty to inform patients are the following:

1. Strenuous physical exercise alters the integrity of various neuroendocrine systems. In women an exercise-induced deficiency of the hypothalamic secretion of the gonadotropin releasing hormone results in the syndrome of "hypothalamic amenorrhea" [Jacobs, 1982].
2. Long-distance running in men can cause a deficiency in hypothalamic gonadotropin-releasing hormone (similar to women) resulting in suppression of testosterone production decreasing spermatogenesis [Reame et al, 1985; Ayers et al, 1985; McConnie et al, 1986].
3. In underweight patients with *anorexia nervosa* the pituitary responds to corticotropin-releasing hormone being restrained in its response by the elevated levels of cortisol suggesting that hypercortisolism in anorexic patients reflects a defect at or above the hypothalamus, a return to eucortisolism after correction of the weight loss indicates resolution of this central defect despite persistence of abnormalities in adrenal function [McConnie, 1986].
4. Studies in pulmonary fibrosis indicate that alveolar inflammation occurs in about half the clinically unaffected family members at risk of inheriting autosomal dominant idiopathic pulmonary fibrosis, evidence that pulmonary inflammation without fibrosis will proceed to clinically evident pulmonary fibrosis is not known [Bitterman et al, 1986].
5. A survey of ballet dancers (mean age 24.3 years) suggests that hypoestrogenism occurs in them causing amenorrheic

intervals, further data indicates that a delay in menarche, prolonged intervals of amenorrhea (reflecting prolonged hypoestrogenism) may predispose ballet dancers to scoliosis, stress fractures or both [Warren et al, 1986].

6. Sexually transmitted organisms have been infective during artificial insemination by a donor, such transmission can cause local, disseminated, or fatal disease in the recipient or harm the fetus, screening of the donor plus the donated semen is necessary to avoid infectious complications, semen samples are not able to be evaluated completely on the day of donation, the usage of fresh semen for artificial insemination should be discouraged, until accurate rapid diagnostic tests are available, only fresh semen that has been screened should be used which is an additional argument against this procedure [Mascola et al, 1986].
7. Enthusiasm in the pursuit of a diagnosis often deceives the physician either into minimizing or neglecting to warn patients against the evil effects of ionizing radiation to those administering radiotherapy or those in the area of ionizing radiation. Known dangers are cancer induction, genetic damage or both [Mattler et al, 1985].
8. Withholding or withdrawing life-prolonging medical treatment demands a standardized conclusion which the American Medical Association attempts to promulgate in this advisory: "Even if death is not imminent but a patient's coma is beyond doubt irreversible and there are adequate safeguards to confirm the accuracy of the diagnosis and with the concurrence of those who have responsibility for the care of the patient, it is not unethical to discontinue all means of life-prolonging medical treatment. Life-prolonging medical treatment includes medication and artificially or technologically supplied respiration, nutrition or hydration. In treating a terminally ill or irreversibly comatose patient, the physician should determine whether the benefits of treatment outweigh its burdens. At all times, the dignity of the patient should be maintained.

The litany of the above eight awarenesses are not the complete list of areas of necessary knowledge to the physician which must be imparted to patients to whom these facts pertain. Basically any medical demerit should be standard information freely given by medical practitioners. Lack of this information with remissiveness to give such knowledge to the patient entitled to these safeguards is improper, unethical medical practice. This indicates that bioethical determinations may be formulated in social solitude but their promulgation must be universal.

The preludium to this epitome's ending is not a prophesy. But all misbehavior that is shameful, fosters hypocrisy, is ethically thoughtless, and has lost moral essence will be destroyed from the fatigue of sheer exhaustion due to its own iniquity. Even momentous, unrestrained, strong driving force is depletable. All evil reaches its denouement with the passage of time. Never is destroyed the powerful, indestructible finery of goodness by contrasting evil.

Envoi

Originally this book was intended to accentuate the substantial need for bioethics in medicosurgical practice and bioscientific research. With progression in writing it, there came into being an advocacy for the preservation of the historical dignity of medicine and its allied disciplines. To preserve and continue the historical tradition and scholastic heritage of this learned profession civilized faith, civility, and civic consciousness could not be ignored. Bioethics' progress will include history and law as *aides-de-camp*.[1] Out of this union will come firm efforts to solve the many future delicate intrangiences. Bioethical impasses will be solved intellectually, morally, and scientifically. Thus

> When strife of life is over.
> Each day's battle is finally done.
> In death the victor's triumph's won.
> Let the elegy of praise be sung
> With echoes of alleluia.

---

1. French for "camp assistant" of military origin, i.e., a confidential assistant to an officer of high rank.

Bibliography

ACOG [Am College Obstetrics and Gynecologists Committee on Ethics]. Multi-fetal pregnancy reduction and selective fetal termination, Opinion 94,38. International Jour Gyn and Obs, Vol 140, No6, Pgs 140-42, 1992

Aitkinhead, New Lease Of Life—The struggle for life: Fresh dilemmas have boosted the anti-abortion lobby, but the basic issue is unchanged. The Independent of London, Pg 17, Aug 11, 1996

Akron vs Akron Centre for Reproductive Health, Sup Ct USA, Dissenting Minority Opinion of the three Justices O'Connor, White, and Rehnquist, 1983

Albanese AA. Iatrogenic cataracts. NY Jour Med, Vol 63, No 2, P 514, 1963

Alger A. Surgical strike. Forbes Magazine, P 92, Sept 20, 1999

Allman WF. Drowning in a sea of knowledge. U.S. News & World Report, Pg. 59, Sept 12, 1988

Alsop R. Reputation's nothing more than a feeling. The Wall Street Jour [International Business], P B15, Thurs Sept 23, 1999

Altman LK. Promise found in alternative to vaccine barred for babies. NY Times [National], P A13, Friday, July 23, 1999

American Institute for Cancer Research. Annual Research Conference, Wash, DC, Thursday morning, Sept 2, 1999

Amundsen [Darrel W] of Western Washington University. Review of Book edited by Samuel S. Kottek and Luis García-Ballester. Bulletin of the History of Medicine, Vol 73, No 3, Pgs 494-95, 1999

Anderson E. *Code of the Street*. New York: WW Norton, 1999

Anderson S. Accentuating the positive. Book review of Tenzin Gyatso, the Dalai Lama in The Spectator, P 39, June 5, 1999

Anderson WF. Human gene therapy: Why draw a line? Jour Medical Philosophy? No Vol, No 14, Pgs 681-693, 1989

Angell M. New ways to get pregnant. N Eng Jour Medicine, P 1200-1, Oct 25, 1990

Angell M and Kassirer JP. Clinical research—what should the public believe? Editorial, N Eng Jour Med, Vol 331, No 2, Pgs 189-190, 1994

Annas GJ. Death with dignity. Health Care Choices For Today's Consumer [MS Miller editor]. Pgs 297-308, 1995

Annas GJ. Why should we ban human cloning? New Eng Jour Med, Vol 339, No 122, Pgs 122-25, 1998

Annas GJ. The Shadowlands—secrets, life, and assisted reproduction. N.Eng Jour Med, Vol 339, No 935, Pgs 935-39, 1998

Annas GJ [School of Health Boston U]. Quoted by John Leo q v infra

Anonymous. FBI Searches L.A. Home In Transplant Fraud Case. The Wash Post, National News, Sunday, P A16, Nov 8, 1998

Armstrong J. *On The Injurious Conduct And Defective State Of That Corporation*. London: Baldwin, Craddock, and Joy, 1825

Asimov Issac. Quoted by Donald De Marco q v infra

Associated Press. Clinton's advisers propose limited embryo research. Reported in Wash Times, P A3,Monday, May 24, 1999

Associated Press Report. The Wash Times, P B11, Thursday, July 29, 1999

Atchley WA. The patient and public policy. The Pharos, Vol 62, No 2, P 39, Spring 1999

Aunger R. Culture Vultures. The Sciences, Pgs 36-39, Sept/Oct 1999

Auzepy P, Durocher A, Gay R et al. *Accidents médicamenteaux graves chez l'adulte*: *Incidence actuelle dans le recrutement des unitiés de réanimation. Nouveau Presse Medicale* Vol 8, No 2, Pgs 1315-1318, 1979

Ayers JW, Komesu Y, Romani T, Ansbacher R. Anthropomorphic, hormonal, and psychological correlates if semen quality in endurance-trained male athletes. Fertility and Sterility, Vol 43, No 7, Pgs 917-921, 1985

Baird Patricia quoted by Naomi A. Schaefér q v infra

Baker D. Finn says Virginia should pay more. The Wash Post [Metro Section], Pgs B1 and B8, Thurs, July 22, 1999

Baker RB, Caplan AL, Emanuel, Latham SR [editors]. *Am Med Ethics Revolution: How AMA's Code of Ethics Transformed Physicians' Relationships to Patients, Professionals, and Society*. Baltimore: Johns Hopkins U Press, 1999

Barboza D. 2 sides square off on genetically altered food. The NY Times [National], P A25, Friday, Nov 19, 1999

Bean WB [Editor]. Guest Editorial comment, Page 1221. Current Medical Digest, Dec 1972

Benacerraf Baruj. Harvard Magazine interview. Quoted by Daniel Greenberg in US News and World Report, Pgs 72-73, June 8, 1987 q v infra

Benzenhöfer U. *Der Gute Tod? Euthanasie und Sterbehilfe in Geschichte und Gegenwart*. Munich: CH Beck, 1999

Beresford D. Dolly is old before her time. National Catholic Register, Vol 75, No 25, P 15, June 20-26, 1999

Berger P. A Far Glory: The Quest for Faith in an Age of Ceredulity. Quoted by E.J. Dionne Jr. q v infra

Bernard C. *Introduction to Experimental Medicine*. New York: Dover, 1957

Berwick DM. From Measuring to Managing the Improvement of Prevention. Am Jour Prev Med. Vol 11, No 6, Pgs 385-387, 1995

Bhatt v Defuono, 661 NYS 2d 66 App Div 1997

Billups A. Forbes backs Princeton protest against hiring 'Professor Death'. The Washington Times, Page 1, Thurs May 20, 1999 also in Washington Times, Page A3, Triday July 23, 1999

Bioethics Law of July 29, 1994, J.O., July 30, 1994, 11056-68. Royal Commission on New Reproductive Technologies, Canada

Bitterman PB, Rennard SI, Keogh BA, Weavers MD, Adelberg S, Crystal RG. Familial idiopathic pulmonary fibrosis: evidence of lung inflammation in unaffected family members. New England Journal Medicine, Vol 314, No 6, Pgs 1343-1347, May 22, 1986

Blakeslee S. New medical research tool: Human tissues in lab mice, NY Times, P A1, Tuesday, Oct 30, 1990

Bloch E. Statement of Dir Nat Sc Foundation Intergovernmental Relations Subcommittee of House Comm on Gov't Operations, 101st Cong 1st Session 179, 1989

Bloomberg News. Warnings issued about Viagra, report in NY Times, P C5, Friday, May 22, 1998

Booth C. Taking care of our aging parents. Time Magazine, Pgs 48-51, Aug 30, 1999

Bobbio N [Norberto]. *In Praise of Meekness: Essays on Ethics and Politics*. London: Polity, 2000 [Translated by Teresa Chataway]

Borg [Susan] and Lasker [Judith]. *When Pregnancy Fails*. Boston: Beacon Press, 1985

Bosk CL. *Forgive And Remember: Managing Medical Failure*. Chicago: University of Chicago Press, 1979

Boston [Associated Press]. Eminent medical journal's editor quits. The Wash Times, P A13, Tuesday, July 27, 1999

Brandt AM. Bioethics: then and now. Medical Ethics, Spring 2000, Pgs 1,2. Publication of Lahey Clinic, Burlington, Mass

Brody H. *Ethical Decisions in Medicine*. Boston: Little, Brown and Co, 1976

Brown D [Book reviewer]. History of Sciences. The Uses and Misuses of Medicine. Book review of 'The Nazi War On Cancer' in The Wash Post, P 7, July 25, 1999

Buchanan AE, Brock DW. *Deciding for Others: The Ethics of Surrogate Decision Making*. Cambridge: Cambridge U Press, 1989

Buckner F. Cedars-Sinai Med Centre vs Sup Ct and the Tort of Spoliation of Evidence. Legal Med Perspective. [Pub Am Coll Legal Med], Vol 6, No 1, Pgs 1-2, Jan/Feb 1999

Bud R. *The Uses of Life: A History of Biotechnology*. NY: Barnes and Noble, 1993

Buesseler JA [Texas Tech] Un Health Science Center, Lubbock Texas. From managed care to managed neglect? The Pharos, Letters to the editor, P 40, Winter, 1999

Bunge RG. Fertilizing capacity of frozen human spermatozoa. Nature, Vol 172, Pgs 767-769, 1953

Caffarra C [Msgr]. Consultor for the doctrinal congregation and director of the John Paul II Institute for Studies on Marriage and the Family at the Pontifical Lateran University, Rome. Taken from his Terrence Cardinal Cooke Lecture given in New York, Oct 7, 1998

Cahill L. National Bioethics Advisory Commission. Report on cloning by the US Bioethics Advisory Commission: Ethical considerations. Human Reproduction Update. Vol 1, No3, Pgs 629-41, 1997

Cameron N [Presbyterian theologian at Trinity International University, Deerfield, Illinois. Quoted by Nicholas Wade, q v infra

Canby TY. Reshaping our lives. National Geographic Magazine, Pgs 746-760, Dec 1989

Caplan AL. *Bioethics From Womb To Tomb*. Gary: Indiana Un Press, 1997

Caplan AL. *Am I My Brother's Keeper? The Ethical Frontiers of Biomedicine*. Bloomington: Indiana Univ Press, 1998

Casey K [Reporter for Charlottesville Daily Progress]. UVA studies turning vegetables into vaccines. The Wash Times, Aug 15, 1999

Castiglioni A. *History of Medicine*. New York: Alfred A. Knopf, 1941

Catholic Un of the Sacred Heart, Milan Italy. Can human cloning be therapeutic? Document from the Centre for Bioethics. Reported in L'Osservatore Romano, N 7, Pgs 6-7, Feb 17, 1999

Cedars-Sinai Med Centre v Sup. Ct Los Angeles, 74 Cal Rptr 2d 248 Cal 1998

Chaplin v Hicks, Kings Bench, UK, 1911

Charen M. Another kind of adoption. The Washington Times, P A 17, Thursday, March 1, 2001

Chavez L. Faculty furor at Princeton. The Washington Times, Page A16, Thurs May 6, 1999

Chicago Tribune. Briton's decry plan to abort healthy twin fetus: Single mother says she can afford to raise only one child. Chi. Trib., P 6, Aug 6, 1996

Chin AE, Hedberg K, Higginson GK. Legalized physician assisted suicide in Oregon—The first year's experience. New Eng Jour Med, Vol 340, No 7, Pgs 577-78, Feb 18, 1999

Clagett OT. This time is a very good one, if. Archives of Surgery, Vol 96, No 4, Pgs 485-492, April 1968

In the matter of Claire Conroy. NJ Court of Appeals 1983. Quoted by Mark Rust q v infra

Clayton P. The Ultimate Hypothesis. Forbes ASAP, Pgs 241-242, Oct 4, 1999

Cleaveland C. Beauty In Unlikely Places. Philadelphia: Am College of Physicians, 1998

Code of Medical Ethics: Current Opinions with Annotations. Chicago, Ill: American Medical Association; 1996

Cohen T. Jokes: *Philosophical Thoughts on Joking Matters*. Chicago: Un Chicago Press, 1999

Colber A. Conflicts between pharmaceutical company largess and patient's rights. Medico-Legal Jour, Pgs 243-44, 1992

Colburn D. Redefining Death. Washington Post, Health Section, Medical Ethics Page 7, Nov 20, 1985

Colliton WP Jr. M.D. Medical affairs Director for Am Life League, Inc. Stafford, VA 22554 in *All About Issues*, Vol 35, March-April 1992

Concetti G [Rev]. An offensive horror story. L'Osservatore Romano, N 44 [1314], P 10, Nov 3, 1993

Cooper v Sisters of Charity of Cincinnati, 27 Ohio 2d, 242, 272 NE 2d 97, 1971

Corson V [Genetic counselor, Johns Hopkins U]. Getting Counseling: A personal decision. Wash. Post, Health Section, P 15, Nov 15, 1986

Cousins N. A layman looks at truth telling in medicine. JAMA, Vol 244, No 17, Pages 1929-1930, Oct 24/31, 1980

Cover Story. Medical Electronic Products, Issue 177, P 2. Published in Pittsburg, Pa, June 1999

Cowell FR. *Cicero and the Roman Republic*. London: Isaac Pitman and Sons, 1948

Crichton [Sir Alexander]. *An Account Of Some Experiments Made With The Vapor Of Boiling Tar*. Printed by James Ballantyne and Co. For Manners and Miller, Edinburgh; and T. and G. Underwook, 32 Fleet Street, London 1817

Cronquist T [Thomas A]. Personal communication from the Institute for the Psychological Sciences, Arlington, Virginia, March 20, 2001

Crossley, Choice, Conscience, and Context, 47 Hastings L J 1223, 1996

Culver CM. Ask the ethicist: Would you tell the patients? Medical Ethics, Spring, 2000, P3. Publication of Lahey Clinic, Burlington, Mass

Curran WJ, Hall MA, Bobinski MA, Orentlicher D. Health Care Law and Ethics. New York: Aspen Law and Business, 1998

Cushing H. *The Life of Sir William Osler*, Vol 1. London: Oxford-Clarendon Press, 1925

Dalton Vs Legg. 441 P2d 28 Oregon 1968

Davidson RA. Source of funding and outcome of clinical trials. Jour Genl Int Med, No 1, Pgs 155-158, 1986

Davies P. At the Crossroads. Forbes ASAP, Pg 231, Oct 4, 1999

Davis BD. Lecture: Future trends in biomedical research. Tenth annual National Institutes of Health Research Safety Symposium, Bethesda, Md, Dec 3, 1987; Bernard D. Davis, MD is professor of bacterial physiology at Harvard Medical School

Dawkins R. Snake Oil and Holy Water. Forbes ASAP, Pgs 235-37, Oct 4, 1999

Dawkins R. *The Selfish Gene*. London: Oxford U Press, 1976

Dawkins R. The Blind Watchmaker. Quoted by Philip Clayton q v supra

Deam J. Infertile couples shop on line for cyber-donors' eggs, sperm. The Wash Times, P A2, Thurs, Jan 13, 2000

Dechert CR [Prof. of Politics, Catholic U. of America]. Personal communication, March 15, 1999

Dechert CR. Truth Values and Cultural Pluralism. Am Maritain Assoc News, Wash DC, Pgs 259-271, 1999

Declaration on Euthanasia, Sacred Congregation for the Doctrine of the Faith, Vatican City, Rome, Italy, June 26, 1980

Delay Tom [House Majority Whip]. Quoted in Psychology group regrets publishing pedophilia report by Julia Duin q v infra

Delicate Balance: Scientific Communications vs. National Security. Issues in Science and Technology, 1989

De Marco D. The Virtue Corner: Compassion. Social Justice Review, P 153, Sept/Oct 1999

Dennison BA, Rockwell HI, Baker SL. Excess fruit juice consumption by preschool-aged children is associated with short stature and obesity. Pediatrics, No 99, Pgs 15-22, 1997

Dennison BA, Rockwell HL, Nichols MJ, Jenkins P. Children's Growth Parameters Vary by Type of Fruit Juice Consumed. Jour American College of Nutrition, Vol 18, No 4, Pgs 346-352, Aug 1999

DeWachter MAM. "Euthanasia in The Netherlands." Hastings Centre Report, 22[2]:23, 1992

Dictionary of Philosophy, edited by Dagobert D. Runes. New York: Philosophical Library, undated

Dillon WP et al. Life support and maternal brain death during pregnancy. Jour AMA, Vol 248, Pgs 1089-91, 1982

Dionne EJ. Take it on faith. The Wash Post Magazine, Pg 7, Dec 12, 1999

Doughty O [Oswald]. *Dante Gabriel Rossetti.* A Victorian Romantic P 96. New Haven: Yale U Press, 1949

D'Souza, Dinesh. *The Virtue of Prosperity*: *Finding Values in an Age of Techno-Affluence*. New York: Free Press, 2000

Duin J. Psychology group regrets publishing pedophilia report, The Wash Times, P A10, Thursday, June 10, 1999

Dworkin P, Gabor A. From ivory tower, US News and World Report, P 51, May 2, 1988

Dyer AR and Brazil P. Should doctors cut costs at the bedside? Hastings Center Report 16[1]:5-8, 1986

Edinburgh. Laws Of The Medical Society Of Edinburgh, Instituted 1737, Incorporated by Royal Charter 1778. Edinburgh: Printed by C. Stewart Printer to the University, 1803

Editorial. Surgical team's professional poll [on cheating]. The Surgical Team, Pages 8-11, Jan/Feb 1977

Editorial. Unionized Medicine, The NY Times Editorials/Letters, P A26, Friday, June 25, 1999

Elkeles B. Der Moralische Diskurs über das medizinische Menschenexperiment im 19. Jahrhundert Medizin-Ethik, no.7. Stuttgart: Gustav Fischer, 1996

Elliott C, Lantos J [editors]. *The Last Physician: Walker Percy and the Moral Life of Medicine*. Durham, NC: Duke U Press, 1999

Ericsson RJ. Don't worry about sex balance. USA Today, P 14A, Monday, Oct 19, 1987

Ethical and Religious Directives for Catholic Health Facilities No 28E, 1991

Ethics Committee of the Am Soc For Reproduction Medicine, Ethical consideration of assisted reproductive technologies, Pub. No 67, 1997

Etzioni A [Sociologist at Columbia University]. On problem of cheating. [Study done at University of Illinois]. Science 192: 325, Nov 1976

Evers JC and Byrne PA. Brain death—still a controversy. The Pharos of Alpha Omega Alpha, Vol 53, No 4, Pgs 10-12, Fall Issue 1981

Farr M. Holy Grail, sliding scale, and refusal as symptom: Competency determinations for medical and psychiatric patients. The Pharos, Vol 62, No 2, Pgs 2-9, Spring 1999

Federal Policies for the Protection of Human Subjects: Notes and Rules. 56 Fed Reg 28002-28032. June 18, 1991

Fenigsen R. "A Case Against Dutch Euthanasia." Hastings Centre Report, 19[1]: 22-24, 1989

Feverherd P. Medical ethics dilemma: facing the limits of technology. The Long Island Catholic, P 5, Nov 6, 1991

Ficarra BJ. *Newer Ethical Problems in Medicine and Surgery*. Westminster, Md: Newman Press, 1950

Ficarra BJ. *Surgical And Allied Malpractice*. Springfield, Illinois: Charles C. Thomas Publisher, 1969

Ficarra BJ. A Physician's Bioethics. Jour of Med, Vol 29, Nos 5 and 6, Pgs 241-258, 1998

Field DR et al. Maternal brain death during pregnancy. Jour AMA, Vol 260, Pgs 812-22, 1988

Fisher M. The Chosen. Wash Post Magazine, P 6, June 20, 1999

Fishman S. Inconceivable. Vogue Magazine, P 306, Dec 1994

Fletcher J. *Morals And Medicine*. Princeton, New Jersey: Princeton University Press, 1954

Fletcher J, STD. The moral dimension in clinical decision making. *The Pharos*, Pgs 2,4, Spring Issue, 1987

Fletcher J. Quoted by Gina Kolata in NY Times, Pgs 1 and 22, Sunday Oct 24, 1993 q v infra

Fletcher JC. Testing for sex choice is bad for society. USA Today, P 14A, Monday, Oct 19, 1987

Florman SC. Engineer's pursuit of honor. Forum Section, Issues in Science and Technology, Vol IV, No 2, Pages 11-12, Winter 1989. Published quarterly by National Academy of Sciences, Washington, DC

Fombrun Charles, Management Professor at NYU and Executive Director of the Reputation Instituted in New York. Quoted by Ronald Alsop q v supra 1999

Forbes Magazine. Going native, P 70, Aug 9, 1999

Forbes S. Fact and comment. Forbes Magazine, p 32, Oct 4, 1999

Forsythe C. President of Chicago-based Americans United for Life. Quoted by Matthew A. Rarey q v infra

Frank RH. *Luxury Fever: Why Money Fails to Satisfy in an Era of Excess*. New York: Free Press 1999

Frankl VE. *Man's Search For Meaning*. Vienna: University Press, 1946

Franklin S. Embodied Progress: *A Cultural Account of Assisted Conception*. London: Routledge Ltd, 1997

Frazier L. Seeking a safe path toward fatherhood. Wash Post, Pgs A1 and A16, April 18, 1999

Freedman B. Competency, marginal and otherwise. Int Journ Law Psychiatry, Vol 4, No 53, P 72, 1981

French R. *Doctors and Ethics: The Earlier Historical Setting of Professional Ethics*. Pgs 72-97 [Editors: Andrew Wear, Johanna Geyer-Kordesch, and Roger French]. Amsterdam: Rodopi Press, 1993

Fridolf K. Medicine as a Liberal Art and the Question of the Physician's Income. J Hist Med and Allied Sc, Vol XXXI, Pgs 448-459, 1976

Friedman Orrie M. The ethics of genetic screening. Issues in Science and Technology. Page 13, 1989

Frommeyer WB [JR] [Prof Med Univ Alabama Med Centre, Birmingham]. A Physicians Prayer. The Distinguished Faculty Lecture for 1971. Reprinted in part from the Bulletin of the American College of Physicians, Vol 13, No 2, Pgs 100-102, Feb 1972. Also in The Alabama Jour Med Sciences, Vol 8, Pgs 145-148, Apr 1971. Quoted in editorial by William B Bean, MD q v supra

Fukuyama [Francis] writing on 'The Great Disruption' in the May issue of the Atlantic Monthly. Quoted in The Washington Times, Page A2, Thursday, April 29, 1999

Galewitz, P. Arthritis drug's sale gives makers cause to Celebrex, The Wash Times, Pgs B6-B7, Tues, Aug 3, 1999

Galewitz, P. Similarity of names causes drug mix-ups. The Wash Times, P B12, Thurs, Aug 26, 1999

Gaylin WM. The problem of psychosurgery. In. Gaylin WM, Meister JS, Neville RC, editors. *Operating on the Mind*: *The Psychosurgery Conflict*, p 13. New York: Basic Books; 1975. Cited in Freedman, Competency, marginal and otherwise, p 55

Gaylin WM, Meister JS, Neville RC [Editors]. *Operating on the Mind*: *The Psychosurgery Conflict*, P 13. New York: Basic Books, 1975

Geertz C. Common Knowledge [1997]. Quoted in Wilson Quarterly, P 135, Autumn 1997

Gibbs, RF. The "ubiquitous" medical expert. Legal Aspects of Medical Practice, Official Publication of the American College of Legal Medicine, Vol 14, No 8, Pg 2-3, August 1986

Gilbert S. Fatherhood from the grave: an analysis of postmortem insemination. Hofstra Law Review, 22, Pgs 521-549, 1993

Gladwell M. Scientist retracts paper amid allegations of fraud. The Wash Post, Pgs A1 and A6, Thursday, March 21, 1991

Goldrich S. RU-486 or against it. The Wash Times, P B8, Thurs, Sept 3, 1998

Goldstein A. Clearing the air about a rare disease. The Wash Post, Pgs C1 and C9, Sunday, April 4, 1999

Gonzalez T [Bishop]. Catholic World News communication from Santiago, Chile, August 1, 1998

Goodenough U. The Sacred Depths of Nature. Quoted by Richard Dawkins, professor at Oxford Un, q v supra

Gooding V University Hosp Bldg, 445 SO 2d 1015 Florida 1984

Gosden RG. Transplantation of fetal germ cells, Jour Assisted Reproductive Genetics, Vol 118, No 2, Pgs 118-23, 1992

Gosden R [Edinburgh University]. Quoted by Gina Kolata q v infra, 1994

Grady D. Trek in remote Pakistan leads to hair-loss gene. NY Times, P A8, Friday, Jan 30, 1998

Greenberg D. Publish or perish—or fake it. US News and World Report, Pgs 72-73, June 8, 1987

Gregory DR. Current status of No-Code Orders. Read at annual meeting of Am College of Legal Medicine, May 9, 1985

Griese Msgr Orville, director of research for the Pope John XXIII Medical-Moral Research and Educational Center. Quoted in The Long Island Catholic, Page 6, Thursday, April 21, 1988

Grimsby Vs Samson 530 P 2d 291 Wash 1975

Grossman Ed. Quoted by Donald De Marco q v supra

Guilford Handbook. Psychological Evaluations for the Courts: A Handbook for Mental Health Professionals and Lawyers. Guilford, Conn: Guilford Press, 1996. Quoted in Washington Post, Sunday, Pg C2, June 27, 1997

Gyatso, Tenzin, *His Holiness the Dalai Lama. Ancient Wisdom, Modern World: Ethics For A New Millennium.* Boston: Little, Brown, 1999

Haakonssen L[isbeth]. *Medicine and Morals in the Enlightenment: John Gregory, Thomas Percival, and Benjamin Rush.* Atlanta: Amsterdam Press, 1997

Hamilton, DS. Extraordinary means to preserve life. Long Island Catholic, Sept 1, 1983

Hansen B. *Perlman's Ordeal.* New York: Farrar Strauss Geroux, 1999

Harper C. When great minds think alike. The Wash Post [Sunday Section on Outlook-Science and Religion], P B3, June 13, 1999

Harris Barbara. [Anaheim, Calif.] Founder of CRACK [Children Requiring a Caring Kommunity. Quoted by Irvine q v infra

Harris Interactive Inc, a New York research group. Quoted by Ronald Alsop q v supra 1999

Harris J. "Goodbye Dolly?" The ethics of human cloning. J Med Ethics, No 23, Pgs 353-60, 1997

Harvard Medical School report. Ad Hoc Committee to Examine the Definition of Brain Death. JAMA 205, 337-40, 1968

Harvard Law Review. "Physician Assisted Suicide: The Right to Die With Assistance." 105, 2021, 1992

Hausen, JDL, and Smith, CA: Effects of withholding fluid in the immediate postnatal period. Pediatrics 12:99-113, 1953

Heilleron JL. The Sun in The Church [page 29]. Quoted by Peter G. Brown, Editor, in Initial Conditions, Editor's Notebook under title, Beware of Greeks Bearing Science. The Sciences, Vol 39, No 5, P2, Sept/Oct 1999

Helminski F. The physician as private attorney general. Mayo Clinic Proc, Vol 69, No 6, Pgs 393-94, 1994

Hentoff N. Columnist for *The Village Voice*, syndicated columnist for the Washington Post in 'Jewish atheist' writes for life. The Long Island Catholic, Page 7, Thursday, Oct. 22, 1987. Published by Diocese of Rockville Centre, Hempstead, L.I., New York

Herald [Glasgow]. Minister expresses "Deep personal concern" over case inquiry call over abortion of twin. The Herald of Glasgow, P2, Aug 8, 1996

Herrera S. Lord of the flies. Forbes Magazine, P 164, Sept 6, 1999

Herskovitz V Group Health Cooperative of Puget Sound 664 P2d 474 Wash State 1983

Hillebrecht JM. Regulating the clinical uses of fetal tissue. A proposal for legislation. Jour Legal Med, Vol 10, No2, Pgs 269-322, June 1989

Hilts PJ. Fetus-to-fetus transplant blocks deadly genetic defect, researchers say. New York Times, P B14, Thursday, Nov 21, 1994

Hilts PJ, Stolberg SG. Duke University's research unethical. The Globe And Mail [Canada], P A13, Friday, May 14, 1999 [From NY Times Service, Durham, NC]

Hirsh H. Medical Malpractice predicated on the tort of "outrage." South Med Journ, Vol 71, No 2, Pgs 818-820, 1978

Hirsh H. That's outrageous, another legal curb on your behavior, Med. Dimensions, P29, May 1978

Hirschfeld AH, Behan RC. The Accident Process. I etiological considerations of industrial injuries. Jour AMA, Vol 186, No6, P 163, Oct 10, 1963

Hirshfeld EB, Nino K, Jameson H. Structuring Provider-Sponsored Organizations. The Legal and Regulatory Hurdles. Jour Legal Med, Vol 20, No3, Pgs 297-363, Sept 1999

Hister A. "Kevorkian Offers Cold Comfort on Euthanasia Debate." *The Globe and Mail* [Toronto], P C8, Sept 14, 1991

Hizer V Randolph 126 Arizona 608, 617 P2d 774 Court of App 1980

Horizons. The new rules of reproduction. US News and World Report, Page 66-69, April 18, 1988

Hunckeler D, Prokop A, Cherrington AD, Rajotte R, Sefton M. Bioartificial Organs II: Technology, Medicine, and Materials. Proceedings of a conference, July 18-22, 1998. New York Academy of Sciences

Hunt M. *The Story of Psychology*. New York: Doubleday, 1993

Huxley, Aldous. *Brave New World*. New York: Harper and Row, First Perennial Library Edition, 1969

Huxley A. Brave New World. London: McMillan, 1932

Ibrahim YM. Ethical furor erupts in Britain: should embryos be destroyed? NY Times, P A1, Aug 1, 1996

Ibrahim YM. Planned abortion of one twin stirs furor in Britain. NY Times, P A3, Aug 6, 1996

Ingelfinger F. Editorial. N Eng Jour Medicine, Vol 294, P 334, 1976. Quoted by Irvine H. Page q v infra

Innaurato A. Hairy-chested sopranos. Forbes Magazine, Pg 154, Aug 9, 1999

Irvine M. Addicts paid to not have children. Washington Times, P A2, Tuesday, July 27, 1999

Italian Olympic Committee. No prosecution of Pantani over blood test. The Wash Post, Planet Sports, P D8, Sunday, July 25, 1999

Jacobs HS. Amenorrhea in athletes. British Journal of Obstetrics & Gynecology, Vol 89, No 3, Pgs 498 to 500, 1982

James KC. Use the law to ban test for sex selection. USA Today, P 14A, Monday, Oct 19, 1987

Jick H. The discovery of drug-induced illness. New Eng Jour Med, Vol 296, No3, Pgs 481-85, 1977

Johnson vs Women's Hosp 527 SW 2d 133 Tenn Ct Appeals 1975

Johnson P. Whited sepulchres, spin-serpents, the world, the flesh, and the devil. The Spectator, P 37, Oct 30, 1999

Jones P. Ancient and Modern, The Spectator, P 17, Oct 17, 1998

Jonsen AR, Siegler M, and Winslade W. *Clinical Ethics: A Practical Approach to Ethical Decisions in Clinical Medicine*. New York: Macmillan Publishing Co., 1982

Jonsen AR. What does life support support? *The Pharos of Alpha Omega Alpha*, Vol 50, No 1, Pgs 4,7, Winter 1987

Jonsen AR. *The Birth Of Bioethics*. New York: Oxford U Press, 1999

Juengst ET [Centre for Biomedical Ethics, Case Western Reserve University Cleveland, Ohio]. Can enhancement be distinguished from prevention in genetic medicine? Jour Medical Philosophy, No Vol, No 22, Pgs 125-142, 1997

Juengst ET. Genetic enhancement: A conceptual and ethical challenge for gene therapy regulation. Medical Ethics Journal, Pgs 1-2, Lahey Clinic Medical Centre, Burlington, Mass, Spring 1999

Karch FE, Lasagna L. Adverse drug reactions: A critical review. JAMA, Vol 234, No12, Pgs 1236-41, 1975

Karlgaard R. Three cheers for nonconformity. Forbes ASAP Magazine, P 147-48, Oct 4, 1999

Kass LR. The wisdom of repugnance. New Republic, No 216, Pgs 17-26, June 2, 1997

Kaufman IR [Judge]. Life-and-death decisions. NY Times, OP-Ed, Oct 6, 1985

Keller EF. *The Century of the Gene*. Cambridge: Harvard U. Press, 2000

Kellner T. Resurrection insurance. Forbes Magazine, P 45, Aug 24, 1998

Kennedy Institute of Ethics Journal [Advertisement Brochure]. Johns Hopkins U. Press, Baltimore, Md, Feb. 2001

King. Charges against 2 dropped: Eye researchers had been accused of ethical violations. Boston Globe, at 50, Apr. 13, 1992

Kinsley M. Take my kidney, please. Time, Mar 13, 1989

Kolata G. Scientist clones human embryos and creates an ethical challenge. New York Times, Pgs 1 and 22, Sunday Oct 24, 1993

Kolata G. Fetal ovary transplant is envisioned. New York Times, National Section, P A16, Thursday, Jan 6, 1994

Kolata G. Medicine's troubling bonus: surplus of human embryos. NY Times, P A1, Mar 16, 1997

Koren G. *Textbook Of Ethics In Pediatric Research*. Melbourne, Florida: Kreiger Pub. Co, 1993

Kottek SS and García-Ballestar L [Editors]. *Medicine and Medical Ethics in Medieval and Early Modern Spain: An Intercultural Approach*. Jerusalem: Magnes Press, 1996

Kuhn T. The Structure of Scientific Revolutions [1962]. Quoted in Wilson Quarterly, P 135, Autumn 1997

Kuhn CG. Claudü Galeni *Omnia Opera* [20 volumes, citation from volume 14, P 602]. Leipzig, 1821-33

Kuzma. Criminal liability for misconduct in scientific research. Un. Michigan Jour Law, Ref 25, N 53, Pgs 357-73, 1993

Lahey Clinic Medical Centre Magazine. Interventional Cardiology: The heart of the Matter, Pgs 10-11, 1999

Larson R. Report concedes pot has medical benefits. The Wash Times, P A3, Thurs, March 18, 1999

Law E. Deformed clones greatly outnumber normal creations. The Wash Times, P A3, Thurs, Aug 19, 1999

Lawson-Tancred H. The start of an intellectual battle. [Book review of consilience by Edward O. Wilson published by Little, Brown, Boston, 1998] in The Spectator, P39, 10 October 1998, London

Leckey A. Drug stocks no cure as holdings anymore. Wash Times, P B8, Tues, July 27, 1999

Legal Lessons, Publication of Am College Legal Medicine. Revocation of license for Medicare fraud. Vol 7, No 3, P3, June 1999

Lejune J. Geneticist opposes use of fetal tissue. Quoted by Pete Sheehan q v infra, 1993

Leo J. Genetic advances, ethical risks, US News and World Report, P 59, Sept 25, 1989

Leopold A. *A Sand County Almanac and Sketches Here and There*. New York: Oxford University Press, 1949

Levine R [Ethicist at Yale U Med School] quoted by Kolata q v supra, 1994

Levran D, Dor J, Rudak E, Nebel L, Ben-Shlomo I, Ben-Rafael Z, Mashiach S. Pregnancy potential of human oacytes—The effect of cryopreservation. N Eng Jour Med, Vol 323, No 17, Pgs 1153-56, Oct 25, 1990

Lewis A. Physician, heal thyself. NY Times, P A15, April 4,

Lind LR. Studies in Pre-Vesalian Anatomy: Biography, Translations, Documents. Memoirs of the American Philosophical Society, Vol 104, Pgs 141-156, 1975

Linden DEJ. Gabriele Zerbi's *De cautelis medicorum* [On rules of caution for physicians]. Bulletin of the History of Medicine, Vol 73, No 1, Pgs 20-21, Spring 1999

Linenthal AJ. Past and present—Dealing with uncertainty. The Pharos, P 51, Spring, 1995

Lipsey JH. Cautions raised on deciding who should be treated. Am Med News Letters page 5 [Nov 18, 1983]

Lock S, Reynolds L, Tansey EM. *Ashes to Ashes*. Atlanta: Amsterdam Press, 1998

Lu L. Commerce in organ transplantation. The Pharos, Pgs 2-5, Spring 1998

Lynch NT, Clay RL, Hegmann KT, Greaves WW, Gold JA. Advocagenic Illness: A New Name For an Old Phenomenon. Legal Medicine Perspective S, Vol 5, No 4, Pgs 1-2, July/Aug 1998

Lynn J: A guiding hand needed for guardianship programs. *Medical Ethics*, Vol 2, No 1, Pg 3, 10, Feb 1987

MacConnie SE, Barkan A, Lampman RM, Schorek, MA and Inese BZ. Decreased hypothalmic gonadotropin-releasing hormone secretion in male marathon runners. New Eng J Medicine, Vol 315, No 7, Pgs 411 to 416, Aug 14, 1986

Makulowich JS. Genetic Engineering grows safer, Potomac Gazette, Science Section, P B-28, Wed Dec 9, 1987

Marsa L. *Prescription for Profits: How the Pharmaceutical Industry Bankrolled the Unholy Marriage between Science and Business*. New York: Scribner, 1997

Mascola L, Guinan ME. Screening to reduce transmission of sexually transmitted diseases in semen used for artificial insemination. New England Journal Medicine, Vol 314, No 7, Pgs 1354-59, May 22, 1986

Matthews M. The pharmatech industry in the new economy. National Review, P 11, Dec 18, 2000

Mayers KS. When attorneys contribute to emotional and behavioral problems in their mentally ill clients. Am Jour Forensic Psych, Vol 12, No 1, Pgs 55-65, 1994

Mayo Clinic Proceedings, Rochester, Minnesota, Vol 68, No6, June, 1993

McFarland-Icke BR. *Nurses in Nazi Germany: Moral Choices in History*. Princeton: Princeton U Press, 1999

McFarling UL. Experts Skeptical Cloning of humans could be prevented as ethical questions about it are being pondered scientists are racing ahead unrestricted. Phila Inquirer, P A3, Nov 18, 1998

McGee EM, Maguire Jr GQ. Implantable brain chips: ethical and policy issues. Medical Ethics, Lahey Clinic Newsletter, Pgs 1-2, 8, Winter 2001

McTeer M. Putting a price on life. Comment Section, The Glove And Mail [Ottawa, Canada], P A13, Friday, Oct 29, 1999

Mehlman MJ and Botkin JR. *Access to the Genome: The Challenge to Equality*. Wash DC: Georgetown U Press, 1998

Meilaender G. Dialogue: Feminist approaches to bioethics. Page 6. Publication of Lahey Clinic Medical Centre, Burlington, Mass, Spring 1999

Melani D. Insurers urged to cover the costs of contraceptives: Number of unplanned pregnancies cited. Washington Times, P A2, Tuesday, July 27, 1999

Merrill JP. Statement of the Committee on Morals and Ethics of the Transplantation Society. Annals Internal Med, 73: 631-633, 1971

Mettler, FA Jr and Moseley RD Jr. *Medical Effects of Ionizing Radiation*. Grune and Stratton, Orlando, Florida 1985

Milbauer B. *Drug Abuse and Addiction*. Winnepeg: New American Company of Canada [Signet Books], 1970

Miller F. Gag clauses, medical ethics and the law, Medical Ethics Newsletter, Pgs 2,8, Lahey Clinic publication, June 1996

Miller JH [Rev]. *Love Responds*. St Louis: Catholic Central Union Press, 1990

Mills DH. Loss of a Chance. In Health Care Law and Ethics by Southby and Hirsh q v infra

Mooij A. Out of Otherness. *Characters and Narrators in the Dutch Venereal Disease Debates 1850-1990*. Atlanta: Amsterdam Press, 1998

Moore v Board of Regents of California, 793 P 2d 479 Cal 1990

Moore V Regents of Un of Calif, 271 Cal Reptr 146, 1990

Moreno JD. Ethical considerations of industry-sponsored research: the use of human subjects, Jour Am College Nutrition, Vol 15, No5, Pgs 35S-40S, 1996

Moseley R. Quoted by Debbie Salamone q v infra

Mosher S [President]. Population Research Institute Review, Summer 1999, Special Edition 1999

Moukheiber Z. Crossbreed. Forbes Magazine, P 116, Sept 20, 1999

Mudge J. *A Radical And Expeditious Cure For A Recent Catarrhous Cough*. London: Printed by E. Allen, Fleet Street, 1978

Mulligan JJ [Monsignor]. Frozen Embryos. Catholic Standard, Vol 41, No 49, P2, Dec 5, 1991

Mulligan JJ [Msgr]. Pandora's Box. Catholic Standard, P9, Nov 14, 1991

Mulligan JJ [Msgr]. Real Persons. Catholic Standard, Vol 20, No 42, P 20, Oct 18, 1990

Mumford E. *Interns—From Students to Physicians*. Cambridge: Harvard U Press, 1970

Muniz vs United Hosp Med Centre, Presbyterian Hosp 379 A 2d 57 1977

Myer JS. *Life and Letters of Dr. William Beaumont* [Third Edition]. St. Louis: Mosby, 1981

Nacmed News publication of Nassau County Medical Society on Long Island, NY, No 217, P2, July-Aug, 1999

Nangia S. Perception of harm and hidden benefits from human cloning by somatic cell nuclear transfer. The Pharos, Vol 64, No 1, Pgs 11-14, Winter 2001

Nathanson B. Ex-NARAL leader now argues against abortion culture. The Wash Times, P A2, Thursday, Feb 10, 2000

National Bioethics Advisory Commission, May 1999. Quoted by Nicholas Wade in NY Times, July 2, 1999, q v infra

National Centre for Education in Maternal and Child Health, Wash DC 20057

National Commission for the Protection of Human Subjects of Biomedical and Behavioral Research: "The Belmont Report: Ethical Guidelines for the Protection of Human Subjects of Research." DHEW Publication No [OS] 78-0012, 1978

Nelson HL. The architect and the bee: some reflections of postmortem pregnancy. Bioethics, No 247, P8, 1994

Nelson D. Review of Eileen Welsome's book, the Plutonium Files in Book World, The Wash Post, P4, Nov 21, 1999 q v infra

News Briefs. L'Osservatore Romano, N44, P12, Nov 3, 1993

New York State Task Force, Assisted Reproductive Technologies 295, Pgs 295-98, 1998

Obituary. Sidney Gottlieb, 80, CIA scientist, Wash Times, P C4, Friday, March 12, 1999

O'Brien NF. Conference explores ethical aspect of fetal tissue use. Catholic Standard, Page 24, Dec 10, 1992

O'Donnell, E [Bishop]. Time to stay vigilant. The Catholic Standard, P7, Nov 21, 1991

Origins [NC documentary Service]. Instructions on respect for human life in its origin and on the dignity of procreation. Replies to certain questions of the day, by the Congregation for the Doctrine of the Faith, page 697, on file page 698, Datebook page 698. Memorandum from US Bishop's Liturgy Secretariat, page 712. From Origins Vol 16, No 40, Pgs 698-711, March 19, 1987

Owen MJ. Fear fuels fetal tissue research. Catholic Standard. Special feature: News of The District of Columbia, Pgs 16,17, April 30, 1992. The essay reflects testimony offered at a U.S. congressional briefing on human fetal tissue transplant research. Debate on lifting restrictions on federal funding of such experimentaton was scheduled for the week of May 23, 1992 as the National Institute of Health reauthorization bill (HR 2507) was considered.

Page A. [Middlesex, NJ]. Why teach child to be good? Parade Magazine, Pg 6, Ask Marilyn column, June 27, 1999

Page IH [editor]. Profession of faith: faith in the profession. Modern Medicine, Pgs 8-10, Aug 15, 1977

Palumbo PJ. Editorial. Transition: A new editor. Mayo Clinic Proceedings, Vol 62, No3, P 230, March 1987

Parens E. Is better always good: Hastings Centre Report, 28[1]: S1-S17, 1998

Pauker SG, Kassirer JP. Therapeutic dicision-making: A cost benefit analysis. New Eng Jour Med, Vol 293, No 20, Pgs 229-234, 1975

PDF [Parkinson's Disease Foundation] Newsletter, Page 4, Winter 1993-94. Publication of Medical Research Centre [William Black Building], Columbia-Presbyterian Medical Centre, NY 10632-9982

PDF News. Published quarterly by the Parkinson's Disease Foundation, 710 W 168 St, NY, NY, 10032 Spring/Summer 1999

Pellegrino ED, Thomasma DC. *The Virtues of Medical Practice*. New York: Oxford U Press, 1993

Percival T [MD]. Medical Ethics or a code of Institutes and Precepts adapted to the Professional Conduct of

Physicians and Surgeons. Printed by S. Russell, for J. Johnson, St Paul's Church Yard, and R Bickerstaff, Strand London 1803

Perkins J. Payoffs for junk science, The Wash Times, Commentary, P A17, Tuesday, August 3, 1999

Physician's Guide To Medicare Compliance Issues. Published by Am College of Gastroenterology, Arlington, Virginia. Under license from UCG/Physicians Compliance Alert, Rockville MD, 1999

Pierce G. Inside Politics, 'Slipshod science.' The Wash Times, P A8, Thursday, July 29, 1999

Pitta L. Rx for $$ [dollars]. Forbes Magazine, Pgs 224-25, Sept 6, 1999

Polkinghorne J. *Belief in God In An Age Of Science*. New Haven: Yale U Press, 1998

Pollack A. Drug used against advanced breast cancer is also effective in early treatment, study finds, NY Times, P A14, Friday, May 22, 1998

Pollard J et al. *Drugs and Phantasy: The effects of LSD, Psilocybin, and Sernyl on College Students*. Boston: Little, Brown, 1965

Pollner F. Penultimate will deals in advance with question of life prolongation. Medical Tribune, Wed, Oct 1, 1930

Pope Pius XII. Encyclical *Humani Generis*: AAS 42, 575, 1950

Pope Paul II. Man is alive and free only if he observes Gods commandments. L'Osservatore Romano, N 44 (1314), P1, Nov 3, 1993

Pope John Paul II. Consciences must be formed to discern the objective moral law. L'Osservatore Romano, N.26, Pgs 3-4, July 1, 1998

Pope John Paul II. Address to pilgrims in Pope Paul VI Auditorium, Vatican City State, July 28, 1999

Porter D. *Social Medicine And Medical Sociology In The Twentieth Century*. Atlanta: Amsterdam Press, 1997

Porter, Kurt and Roy. *From Physico-Theology To Bio-Technology: A Festschrift For Mikulas Teich*. Atlanta: Amsterdam Press, 1998

Pouillet T [Theodor]. *Essai médico-philosophique sur les formes, les causes, les signes, les conséquences et le traitment de l'onanisme chez la femme*. Paris: Adrian Delalahaye, 1876

Prentice RA. Clinical trial results, physicians, and insider trading. Jour Legal Medicine, Vol 20, No2, Pgs 195-222, June 1999

Proctor RN. *The Nazi War On Cancer*. Princeton, NJ: Princeton U Press, 1999

Prosser W. *Handbook on the Law of Torts*. Paragraph 56, Pgs 348-350. St Paul: West Pub Co, 1966

Rae SB and Wong KL. *Beyond Integrity: A Judeo-Christian Approach to Business Ethics*. Grand Rapids: Zondervan, 1996

Rapp R. *Testing Women, Testing the Fetus: The Social Impact of Amniocentesis in America*. New York: Routledge Ltd, 1999

Rarey MA. Wrongful-birth lawsuits put doctors in ethical dilemma. Wash Times, P A2, Thurs, Aug 5, 1999

Razinski DC. Less of Chance—Less Emotion and More Science. In Health Care Law and Ethics by Southbey and Hirsh q v infra

Reimers Niels, Director of Technology Licensing at Stanford University. Quoted by Peter Dworkin and Andrea Gabor q v supra 1988

Reame, NE, Saunder, SE, Case, GD, Kelch, RP, Marshall, JG. Pulsatile gonadotropia secretion in women with hypothalamic amenorrhea: evidence that reduced frequency of gonadotropia-releasing hormone secretion is the mechanism of persistent anovulation. Journal Clinical Endocrinology Metabolism, Vol 61, No6, Pgs 851-858, 1985

Reinisch K. Spokeswoman for Planned Parenthood of the Rocky Mountains. Quoted by Debra Melani q v supra

Relman. The new medical-industrial complex. N Eng Jour Med, 303, Pgs 963-68, 1980

Relman J. Dealing with conflicts of interest. New Eng Jour Med, 749,313, Sept 19, 1985

Reuter SR. Physicians as Good Samaritans. Jour Legal Med, Vol 20, No2, Pgs 157-193, June 1999

Reuters Dispatch. The Boston Globe, P11, Thurs, Oct 25, 1990

Reuters, NY from UK. Reported in NY Times, International Section, World Briefing, Europe, Friday, June 25, 1999

Rigter H. "Euthanasia in the Netherlands: distinguishing Facts from Fiction." Hastings Centre Report, 19[1] Special Supp 31, 1989

Robbins-Roth C. Tailor-made drugs. Forbes Magazine, P 172, July 6, 1998

Roberge LF. Aborted fetal cell use in rubella vaccines: a medical and ethical conflict. Bulletin of Scientists and Engineers, April/May 1999

Robertson JA. *Children of Choice*: *Freedom and the New Reproductive Technologies*. Princeton: Princeton University Press, 1994

Robertson JA. Posthumous Reproduction. Indiana Law Journal, 69, 1027, 1994

Robertson JA. Human cloning and the challenge of regulation. N Eng J Med, No 339, Pgs 119-21, 1998

Robinson V. *Story of Medicine*. New York: New Home Library, 1943

Rockhill vs Pollard 485 P 2d 28 Oregon 1971

Röder T, Kubillus V, Burwell A. *Psychiatrists, The Men Behind Hitler, The Architects of Horror*. Los Angeles: Freedom Publishing, 1995

Rodriguez KF. Suing Health Care Providers For Saving Lives. Liability For Providing Unwanted Life-Sustaining Treatment. J. Legal Med, Vol 20, No 1, Pgs 1-66, March 1999

Rodwin MA. *Medicine, Money, and Morals*: *Physicians' Conflict of Interests*. New York: Oxford University Press, 1993

Rodwin M. Medicine, Money, and Morals: Physicians' Conflict of Interests. 97-111 [1993]. Quoted by Prentice q v supra

Rorty and Pinkerton. Elective Fetal Reduction: The Ultimate Elective Surgery, 13 Jour Contemp Health Law and Policy, 53, 53, 1996

Ross PE. Nine mistakes doctors make Forbes Magazine, Pgs 116-117, Aug 9, 1999

Rothman BK [Baruch Un. NY]. Quoted by Sally Squires in Wash Post, Nov 25, 1989, q v infra

Rothman [Barbara Katz]. *The Tentative Pregnancy*. New York: Viking Press, 1985

Rust, M.: Court vacates murder charges against MDs, Am Med News page 1,15, Oct 28, 1983

Salamone D [staff writer, Orlando Sentinel]. Medical Ethics Section of Health Magazine, Washington Post, Pg 13, Nov 11, 1986

Sanders A. Doctors and dollars. Forbes Magazine, Pgs 128-130, April 5, 1999

Sandquist MA. Do not go gently. The Pharos, Pgs 14-16, Fall 1996

Sass H-M. Reichsrundschreiben 1931: Pre-Nuremberg German Regulations Concerning New Therapy and Human Experimentation. Jour Med and Philosophy, No8, Pgs 99-111, 1983 Quoted by Moreno q v supra

Sauer MV, Paulson RJ, Lobo RA. A preliminary report on oocyte donation extending reproductive potential to women over 40. N Eng Jour Med, Vol 323, No 17, Pgs 1157-60, Oct 25, 1990

Schaefer NA. Eggs for sale. The Weekly Standard, Pgs 19-20, Nov 15, 1999

Scheer, RL. Decisions of life and death require our judges' guidance, letter to the editor, NY Times, pg 26, Oct 19, 1985

Schlozman SC. Book Review [Fits and Starts] Review of Books on Tourette Syndrome. The Sciences, Pgs 38-42. Nov/Dec 1999

Schlotzhauer A and Liang BA. The Ethics of selective termination cases. Opening the door to abortion extortion. Jour Legal Med, Vol 20, No4, Pgs 44-456, 1999

Schneider CE. *The Practice of Autonomy*: *Patients, Doctors, and Medical Decisions*. New York: Oxford U Press, 1998

Schuster E. A child at all costs: posthumous reproduction and the meaning of parenthood. Human Reprod, Pgs 2182-85, Nov 1994

Schuster E. The Posthumous Gift of Life: The World According to Kane. Jour Contemporary Health Law And Policy, Vol 15, Issue 2, Spring 1999

Schwartz H. Make sure doctors charge big fees. USA Today, P 14A, Monday, Oct 19, 1987

Selye Hans. *The Stress of Life*. NY: McGraw-Hill, 1960

Seper J. Black cocaine able to avoid detection. The Wash Times, P A6, Wed, April 28, 1999

Sexual or Romantic Relations Between Physicians and Key Third Parties. Report of The Council on Ethical and Judicial Affairs of the American Medical Association, Chicago, Ill: American Medical Association; June 1998. No. 92.

Sgreccia, E [Bishop]. Right to life begins at conception. L'Osservatore Romano, N45, P5, Nov 10, 1993

Shattuck Lecture—The Politics of Medicine in Britain and the United States of America. Presented as the Shattuck Lecture before the Annual Meeting of the Massachusetts Medical Society on May 10, 1986. Published in the New England Journal of Medicine, Vol 315, No3, Pgs 168 to 173, July 17, 1986

Shea WR, Spadafora A [Editors]. From the Twilight of Probability: Ethics and Politics. Pgs 91-105 Canton, Mass: Science History Publications, 1992. Reference to chapter, "Messages from Three Contemporary Images of Medicine: Failed Medicine, Miracle Medicine, and Science Fiction Medicine by Margaret A. Somerville, Director, McGill Centre for Medicine, Ethics, and Law in Quebec, Canada

Sheehan P. Geneticist Opposes use of fetal tissue. Long Island Catholic, P 9, April 21, 1993

Sheehan P. Moral experts concerned about reported cloning. Long Island Catholic, P9, Nov 3, 1993

Shepard Vs Superior Ct 76 Cal App 3d 16 142 Cal Rptr 612, 1977

Sherman E and Annas GJ. Reproductive Genetics And The Law 234, 1987. Quoted by Schuster 1999, q v supra

Shiffmar, Melvin. *Ethics in Forensic Science and Medicine*. Springfield: Charles C Thomas Ltd, 2000

Shimm DS, Spece RG. Ethical issues and clinical trials. Drugs, No 46, Pgs 579-584, 1993

Shimm, Spece, and Di Gregorio. Conflicts of interests in relationships Between Physicians and the pharmaceutical industry. Quoted by Moore q v supra 1996

Shoshone A. Jour Fertility and Stability, Pgs 449-51, 1992 Quoted by Schuster q v supra

Shulman S. Patent Absurdities. The Sciences, Pgs 30-33, Jan/Feb 1999
Silver LM. Quoted by David Beresford q v supra
Siraisi NG. *Medieval and Early Renaissance Medicine: An Introduction to Knowledge and Practice.* Chicago: Un Chicago Press, 1990
Slotnick RN and Zanjani E [University of Cal at Davis]. Reported by Philip J Hilts q v supra on experiments performed in 1993
Smith GP. Australia's frozen 'Orphan Embryos': a medical, legal, and ethical dilemma. Jour Family Law, Vol 24, Pgs 27-28, 1995
Smith MM, Sifshitz F. Excess fruit juice consumption as a contributing factor in nonorganic failure to thrive. Pediatrics, No 93, Pgs 438-443, 1994
Smith RE [Rev]. Hastings Centre Report. Pope John XXIII Centre, Boston, March 15, 1988
Smith V Superior Ct 198 Cal Rptr 829, 1984
Smith WJ. *Culture of Death: The Assault on Medical Ethics.* New York: Encounter Books, 2001
Snyder L. Unlawful acts and mental disease. JAMA, Vol 171, No 6, Oct 10, 1959
Snyder L. Murder: The most overlooked cause of death. Medical Economics, New Jersey, Aug 31, 1959
Somerville MA. The Song of Death: The Lyrics Of Euthanasia. Jour Contemporary Health Law And Policy, Vol 9, Pgs 1-76, 1993
Southby R McK F and Hirsh HL [Editor]. Health Care Law And Ethics. George Washington U Health Policy Series—Vol 3. Wash DC, 1989
Spaemann R. Even the best of intentions does not justify the use of evil means. L'Osservatore Romano, N50, P11, Dec 15, 1993
Spicker SF. *The Healthcare Ethics Committee Experience: Selected Readings from HEC Forum.* Melbourne, Florida: Kreiger Publishing Co, 1998
Spratt JS. The death of Socrates. Letter to the editor. The Pharos, P 42, Spring 1998
Squires S. The ethics of genetic counseling. Wash Post, Health Section, Pgs 12-13, Nov 25, 1986
Stechel RP. Presidents Message. NACMED News, Publication of Nassau County Med Society, NY, No 216, P1, June 1999
Stedman's *Medical Dictionary* [23rd Edition]. Baltimore: Williams and Wilkins, 1976 Also 26th edition 1995
Steinbock B. Sperm as property. In, Harris J, Holm S [eds]: *The Future of Human Reproduction: Ethics, Choice, and Regulation.* Pgs 150-61, Oxford: Clarendon Press, 1998

Stelfox, Chua, O'Rourke, and Detsky. Conflict of interest in the debate over calcium-channel antagonists, N Eng J Med, 101, 338, 1998

Stockhammer, M. Thomas Aquinas Dictionary. Philosophical Library, New York [16] NY, 1965

Sumner DE [Ball State University journalism professor] in a letter to the editor in the May issue of the Christian Challenge. Quoted in the Washington Times page A2, July 27, 1999

Tallarida RJ, Murray RB, Eiben C. A scale for assessing the severity of diseases and adverse drug reactions: Application to drug benefit and risk. Clinical Pharmacol Ther, Vol 25, No7, Pgs 381-390, 1979

Terry J. *An American Obsession: Science, Medicine, and Homosexuality in Modern Society*. Chicago: U of Chicago Press, 1999

Thomas C. Lying in the rights vineyards. Wash. Times, Page F3, Thursday, June 2, 1988

Thompson DF. Understanding financial conflicts of interest. N Eng J Med, Vol 329, No6, Pgs 573-576, 1993

Thomson V Sun City Community Hosp, Sup Ct Arizona 1986

Toellner R and Wiesing U [editors]. *Geschichte und Ethik in der Medizin: Von den Schwierigheiten einer Kooperation. Medizin-Ethik, No.10.* Stuttgart: Gustav Fischer, 1997

Toffler A and Toffler H. Eruptions from the future: The next 50 years will raise enormous ethical questions, Forbes ASAP Magazine, Pgs 185-86, Oct 4, 1999

Tong R. Feminist approaches to bioethics. Med Ethics Newsletter. Publication of Lahey Clinic Medical Centre, Burlington, Mass, Winter 1999

Trombley S. President of Planned Parenthood in Chicago. Quoted by Martha Irvine q v supra

Trunet P, Le Gall JR, Lhoste F, Regnier B, Saillard Y, Carlet J, Rapin M. The Rôle of iatrogenic disease in admissions to intensive care. JAMA, Vol 244, No23, Pgs 2617-2620, Dec 12, 1980

Uniform Determination of Death Act 12 ULA Civil Proc and Rem Laws, 1, Pages 320-23, 1990

United States vs Karl Brandt. Trials of War Criminals Before the Nuremberg Military Tribunals under Control Council Law No 10, Vols 1 and 2. "The Medical Case" [Military Tribunal 1, 1947; Wash DC, US Govt Printing Office, 1948-1949]

Vanderhoef KD. Collision Course: technology may prove to be the nemesis of abortion advocates. The Long Island Catholic, Page 4, Thurs Oct 8, 1987

Van Huyssteen JW. *Duet Or Dual? Theology and Science In A Postmodern World.* Hartford: Trinity Press International, 1998

Von Balthasar HU. *Tragedy Under Grace: Reinhold Schneider on the Expience of the West.* San Francisco: Ignatius Press, 1997

Von Kraft-Ebing R. Quoted by Röder et al p 23, q v supra

Wade N. With no other Dollys, cloning report draws critics. The NY Times, National Report, P A8 NE, Friday, Jan 30, 1998

Wade N. Animal's genetic program decoded. NY Times P1 and A26, Friday, Dec 11, 1998

Wade N. Embryo cell research: a clash of values. NY Times National, P A11, Friday, July 2, 1999

Wade W., Esq. Treatment decision breaks legal ground. Quoted in Am Med News page 15 [Oct 28, 1983].

Waldholz M. Technology and Health. Synergen finds protein that may offer path to new treatment for Parkinson's. The Wall Street Journal, P B8, Friday, May 21, 1993

Walsh JJ. *Catholic Churchmen in Science. Sketches of the lives of Catholic Ecclesiastics who were among the Great founders of Science.* Philadelphia: The Dolphin Press, 1906

Ward K. *God, Faith And The New Millennium: Christian Belief In An Age Of Science.* New York: Oneworld Publications, 1998

Warren MP, Brooks-Gunn J, Hamilton LH, Warren LF, Hamilton WG. Scoliosis and fractures in young ballet dancers: relation to delayed menarche and secondary amenorrhea. New England Journal Medicine, Vol 314, No 11, Pgs 1348 to 1353, May 22, 1986

Washington Times. Culture, et cetera. P A2, Tuesday, July 27, 1999

Waters R. Some epistemological questions concerning the non-medical use of drugs. Revue de l'Université d'Ottawa, Vol 45, No 4, Pgs 518-540, Octobre-Dècembre 1975

Wattenberg B. To sir with love. The Washington Times, P A18, Thursday, June 24, 1999

Watts A [Lan]. *The Joyous Cosmology. Adventures in the Chemistry of Consciousness.* NY: Random House [Vantage Books], 1962

Watts WD. *The Psychdelic Experience: A Sociological Study.* Beverly Hills: Sage Publications, 1971

Wawd. Pharmaceutical promotions—A free lunch. N Eng Jour Med, 327, P 351, 1992

Weinberg N. Blood money. Forbes Magazine, Pgs 123-126, April 5, 1999

Weinberg R [Whitehead Institute for Biomedical Research, MIT]. Nature, July 29, 1999, Associated Press release. Quoted in Wash Times, P A11, Thurs, July 29, 1999

Welsome E. *The Plutonium Files: America's Secret Medical Experiments In The Cold War*. New York: Dial Press, 1999

Wertheim M. The Odd Couple. The Sciences, Pgs 38-43, Mar/April 1999

Weston JK. The present status of adverse drug reaction reporting JAMA, Vol 232, No6, Pgs 203-235, 1968

Wigmore [3d edition] Paragraph 278, p120, 1940 Quoted by Buckner q v supra

Wilson EO. Hardwired for God. Forbes ASAP, Pgs 132-134, Oct 4, 1999

Wisconsin Rules of Professional Conduct for Attorneys, SCR 20:8.4[c], 1998

Wise BC, Vicini S, Carmingnoto G. Neuronal plasticity and neurotrophins. Georgetown Medicine [Inquiry, Discovery, and Opinion]. Publication of Georgetown University School of Medicine, Vol 2, No2, Pgs 13-20, Fall 1993

Witham L. Catholic scientists look to bridge theory, theology. The Wash Times, P7, Monday, May 24, 1999

Wolf SM. "Final Exit: The End of Argument." Hastings Centre Report, 22[1]:30-33, 1992

Wolfe T. Disciplines. Forbes ASAP, P 205, Oct 4, 1999

Yardley J. Book review of Perlman's Ordeal by Brooks Hansen q v supra, 1999

Yellin E. Some doctors see relief in plan for AMA union. The NY Times National, P A18, Friday, June 25, 1999

Young WD [Judge]. Tennessee Circuit Court, 1989. Quoted by Msgr James J Mulligan q v supra. In the matter of Junior L. Davis vs Mary Sue Davis

Zakowski P. Psychosurgery. Jour Legal Med, Pgs 26-28, April 1976

Zalewski D. Ties that bind: Do Corporate Dollars Strangle Scientific Research? *Lingua Franca*, June-July 1997

Zimmerly JG. Legal aspects of loss of chance. In Health Care Law And Ethics by Richard McK F Southby, Ph.D. and Harold L. Hirsh, MD q v supra

Zimmermann M. McGivney lecturer derides cloning experiments. Catholic Standard, P 7, Nov 4, 1993

Zoloth L [Assoc Prof, Social Ethics Chair Jewish Studies, San Francisco State Univ]. Religion and the public discourse of bioethics. Medical Ethics, Pgs 1-2, Fall 1999, Publication of Lahey Clinic, Mass

Zukerman H. *Scientific Elite: Nobel Laureates*. New York: Free Press, 1977